Speech Correction in the Schools

SPEECH CORRECTION

Jon Eisenson

SAN FRANCISCO STATE UNIVERSITY

IN THE SCHOOLS 4_{Ed}

Mardel Ogilvie

HERBERT H. LEHMAN COLLEGE OF THE CITY UNIVERSITY OF NEW YORK

Macmillan Publishing Co., Inc.

NEW YORK

Collier Macmillan Publishers

LONDON

Macmillan Publishing Co., Inc.
866 Third Avenue, New York, New York 10022

Collier Macmillan Canada, Ltd.

Library of Congress Cataloging in Publication Data

Eisenson, Jon, (date)
    Speech correction in the schools.

    Includes bibliographies and index.
    1. Children—Language. 2. Speech therapy.
I. Ogilvie, Mardel, (date)   joint author. II. Title.
LB1139.L3E4   1977   371.9'14   76-15357
ISBN 0-02-332070-2

Printing: 1 2 3 4 5 6 7 8   Year: 7 8 9 0 1 2 3

Preface

Speech Correction in the Schools is intended for readers who will work with speech, language, and/or hearing handicapped school children either as classroom teachers or as speech clinicians. In preparing the fourth edition of the book, we have taken into account the reactions of faculty and students who have used the third edition and have revised portions of the book accordingly. We are grateful for the help received from these comments and suggestions. We have also revised portions of the book by taking cognizance of new developments in the field and the impact of recent research on normal and deviant language and speech development.

Because of the current emphasis on language learning for the learning disabled and for the normal child, the classroom teacher is aware of the need to stimulate the development of language. The clinician is equally concerned with this area of development. Consequently, the teacher and clinician must understand their own and each other's functions as members of a language team for school-age children. In addition, both the teacher and clinician must be concerned with the communicative act in teaching as well as in clinical roles.

Cooperation between the classroom teacher and the clinician must be continuously maintained. The teacher should understand the nature of speech therapy and the work of the clinician. On the other hand, the clinician must be able to advise the teacher on ways of reinforcing clinical work and discovering measures for preventing speech and language impairments. The speech and language handicapped child will develop useful and effective oral communication when both the teacher and clinician mutually respect each other's contributions and work together for the good of the child.

We have retained the original title of the book: *Speech Correction in the Schools.* Other titles such as *Teaching the Speech and Hearing Handicapped, Communicative Disorders in the Schools, Therapeutic Approaches to the Public School Speech, Language, and Hearing Handicapped* are appropriate. Similarly the speech and language clinician may have one of several titles which may include: speech therapist; speech and language consultant; language clinician; teacher of the speech, language, and hearing handicapped; and speech, language, and hearing therapist. But the individual, regardless of title, is trained in diagnosing and treating children with communicative disabilities or impairments. In addition, some school systems employ an audiologist, a specialist competent in the assessment and treatment of the hearing handicapped child.

The first half of the book deals with general considerations and background knowledge basic for the teacher's and clinician's understanding and appreciation of the child with a communicative impairment. We begin with a chapter on the classification and incidence of speech defects and follow with a chapter on speech and language clinical services. The ensuing chapters are based on the assumption that fundamentals of information about normal speech and language precede a discussion of defective speech and language. Accordingly, we have included material about speech standards, the mechanism for speech, the production of speech sounds, the development of language in children, and stimulation of language development.

The second half of the book contains a discussion of the specific speech, language, and hearing handicaps found in public school children. We have explained the nature and cause of the speech disorder and the types of therapy involved. Here again we have indicated how teachers can supplement and reinforce the work of the clinician.

J. E.
M. O.

Contents

1. Classification and Incidence of Speech Defects

Approximately 5 per cent of school-age children have difficulties in communication related to defects in the manner or control of their oral productions. Such defects may be expressed in deviant speech sounds, in voice (vocal quality, rate, or loudness), in rhythm, in the number or choice of words, or in the way the words are "strung" to make utterances. Whereas some of the children seem to be aware of their defects and may be apprehensive about speaking, others show a benign indifference to their speech or to the reactions of listeners to them. Classroom teachers and professional workers[1] are likely to make similar judgments about these children. For example, the teacher and clinician are likely to agree that the five-year old who continues the infantile *wawa* for *water*, or *gogo* for *doggy*, has defective speech sound production. The child may, of course, have other indications of infantile language proficiency which, as we learn later, may be expressed in vocabulary or in syntax. The eight-year-old whose utterances are characterized by frequent starts, stops, sound, syllable, and word repetitions; and of whom his classmates say, "Jackie doesn't get his words out right" has, superficially, at least, a production speech problem. The child's difficulty may be based on poor formulation of the utterance accompanied

---

[1] The professional workers directly concerned with remediation of language and its oral expression have a variety of titles that include speech correctionist, speech therapist, speech and language clinician, speech clinician, language clinician, and speech pathologist.

1

by pressure to talk despite a lack of readiness relative to the formulation. Unconsciously, both adults and the child's peers are comparing Jackie with other children of his age who, in similar speech situations, speak with relatively greater ease and fluency.

When Helen, a five-year-old kindergartner, says *thay* for *say*, or *thoap* for *soap*, no one is likely to take particular notice. Such substitutions are not at all unusual for a child of this age. However, when Nancy, an eighth grader, uses a *th* for an *s*, even though an indulgent classmate may consider Nancy "cute" and observe, "I love to listen to Nancy. I wait for her *th*'s," we may conclude that, however cute, Nancy does have a speech defect. Her classmate's observation suggests that Nancy's lisp directs attention to how she is talking rather than to what she is saying, and thus gets in the way of what she is presumably trying to communicate.

Some barriers to communication that are often confused with speech and language defects may not fall within the province of the speech clinician. These barriers include (1) nonstandard pronunciations and language usage, (2) regional dialects, (3) poor oral reading, (4) articulation and fluency patterns that are not adult but are normal for the developmental stage of the child, and (5) a psychological disturbance that manifests itself as a speech symptom. The classroom teacher, usually with the help of other specialists, is responsible for handling these particular problems. The cooperating specialist frequently is the speech clinician who helps the teacher plan a program of speech and language improvement.

An eight-year-old girl says, "I din't recognize dat neighbor wid de fedders in her hair—de one who's awiz pretendin'. She's actin' in de Cender play." This girl is not in need of help from the speech clinician. Half of her classmates and even her parents say *dat* for *that* and *de* for *the*. Her observation gives evidence of a fairly sophisticated use of language for her age. Her classroom teacher, however, plans a program to improve the level of speech and language of all the students in the class. Undoubtedly, this child communicates effectively at home and with most if not all of her classmates. But time and occasion will arrive when such non-Standard pronunciations may handicap her. We discuss this problem in Chapter 3.

Children may transfer from sections of the country where people speak differently from most people in the area where the children now live. The teacher and classmates of these children may be very conscious of the differences in pronunciations and melody patterns in the speech of these children. In fact, at times the teachers and classmates may be unable to understand what these transferred children are saying. But as the children live in their new community for some time, the differences in their speech patterns will tend to disappear, and they will acquire the speech patterns of their playmates. The teacher can help the adjustment of the transferred children by accepting their speech and by explaining the differences in their speech to the other members of the class. Regional differences in speech are discussed in Chapter 3.

Oral reading presents problems for some children because of their difficulty in understanding the meaning of the printed page. As a result, their oral reading is uncommunicative; it is hesitant and hard to understand. The conversation of the same children, however, may be quite adequate. Their main problem in communication is one of oral reading although, as mentioned in the chapter on articulatory defects, reading, speech and language problems are often related. It has been our experience that as children improve in one ability, they frequently improve in another.

Kindergarten and first-grade teachers find that many of their children articulate inaccurately. Pendergast (1966), in a study of 15,000 first-grade children, found that slightly more than one fourth of first-grade children misarticulated one or more sounds. Similarly, in a study rating the articulatory performance of children in grades 1–12 (Hull and Mielke 1971), the percentage of acceptable articulation increased from 37.4 per cent in the first grade to 66.4 per cent in the twelfth grade, and extreme deviation of articulation decreased from 9.7 per cent in the first grade to 0.5 per cent in the twelfth grade. Some of these changes result from speech therapy, but others result from the children's own phonological development. In many instances, a child's "inaccurate" articulation is the result of the stage in development rather than of a deficit in development. Speech clinicians, therefore, prognosticate which children must have clinical help. Ways of successful prognostication for correcting deficient articulation are discussed in Chapter 10.

Similarly, children in kindergarten sometimes exhibit disfluencies that are part of the normal development of children. The aspects of language development are discussed in Chapter 7.

In some instances, the major problem is not one of speech but of social adjustment. One little girl whose voice is consistently thin and weak and who speaks with little or no inflection surely exhibits a problem of voice. This problem, however, may be closely related to the child's concept of herself—she feels she cannot do anything very well. She says, "I feel like a big stupid lug most of the time." Her stooped posture, her halting walk, her untidy dress, her sloppy compositions, her lack of enthusiasm, and her dull, thin, weak voice are all part of a syndrome. In such an instance, the voice is merely the symptom of a personality difficulty. The speech clinician can help only in cooperation with other members of the school personnel.

Communication, Speech, and Language

Rees (1974) examines the relationships among language, communication, speech, and reading:

> *Language* is a code with structural properties characterized by sets of rules for producing and comprehending sentences. *Communication* is the process of sharing or giving information, feelings, and attitudes. Language may serve as a tool in the process of communication, and also as an instrument for learning. *Speech* occurs when the rules of the language are applied in oral production; more specifically, speech is the articulatory-acoustic output of the linguistic code. *Reading* is the process of retrieving meaning from visual symbols that represent the phonological units of the spoken language.

Speech, the physical output of the linguistic code, is then the manner of communication with its many functions as distinguished from the means—language. The manner, the means, and the functions of communication cannot be separated—they are inexorably interwoven. At this point we discuss some of the necessary language abilities. In later chapters we describe the development of language and how to stimulate its development.

Language Abilities of the Child

Classroom teachers who teach in language arts programs make judgments about children's language. They categorize their groups into those with superior language, those with poor language, and those with adequate language. The members of the superior group speak clearly and intelligibly, listen critically and with discrimination, comprehend readily, and communicate even fine distinctions of meanings. Members of the inferior group speak unintelligibly and listen inadequately, in that their brains have only limited capacity to process in time, to form patterns, and to retain what is heard; consequently, they do not comprehend readily. When they express themselves, their speech is often characterized by concreteness, lack of generalizations, overly simple syntactic structure, syntactic and morphological errors, and an excessive use of nonverbal clues. In between these two extremes, teachers label speech and language adequate.

What, then, is involved in learning to use language? These abilities include the capacity to listen, to process various types of incoming information, to remember and relate ongoing experiences with previous experiences, to recall these experiences in meaningful terms, and to express ideas and concepts in an appropriately mature manner for the child's age.

Classroom teachers usually assess language ability through a descriptive approach of what they hear in the class in the children's communication of ideas in a variety of curricular areas such as science, mathematics, social studies, children's literature, music, or art. Today much of this classroom study is experientially based and is designed to further communication between the teacher and the students. For example, kindergartners visit the supermarket and upon returning to the classroom talk about the manager, the customers, the checkout girl or boy, and the arrangements of the products. Or in their housekeeping corner, they play "Mother," "Daddy," "Doctor," and "Sister." After the second graders have planted corn seeds, pumpkin seeds, avocado seeds, and cuttings from such plants as coleus or wandering jew, they read about and talk about various ways of propagation and the need for light and water for growth; that is, they set up criteria for growing living plants.

If a teacher had a child such as six-year-old Eloise in class and heard her explain that Sabine, a rag doll, "has absolutely no face at all partially because she came from Jamaica by Air Express" and that her very large doll Saylor is armless because "she was in the most terriblest accident and she bleeded so hard she almost choked in the night and this ambulance came and took her to this hospital and it was an emergency,"[2] she would describe the language as imaginative and giving evidence of considerable vocabulary and syntactic development. She would be pleased that Eloise had provided a reason for the armless state of Saylor and for her choking in the night. She would not be concerned with *bleeded* or *most terriblest*, for these show some understanding of the rules.

A variety of factors further the stimulation of language development in the classroom. Some of these factors are related to the teacher such as positive and sympathetic attitudes, ability to comment on and to expand children's expression of their ideas, and language patterns adapted to the children; other factors are related to the message of the teacher, such as relevancy of the materials or the experiential base of the message; other factors are related to the children, such as their positive self-concepts; and still other factors are related to adequate and effective feedback (see Chapter 4). The important need is for the

---

[2] From the child's book *Eloise* by K. Thompson New York: (Simon & Schuster, Inc., 1955).

children to interact. In other words, it is less important that Eloise say *bled* rather than *bleeded* than that the teacher encourage her to communicate by listening, appreciating what she is saying, and responding to her ideas. Similarly Eloise is listening, responding, and hopefully developing language competence.

Speech and language clinicians, who assess language from a descriptive approach, assess language from a quantitative one, as well. They are interested in finding out how the child deviates from normalcy. They may administer an inventory such as the Illinois Test of Psycholinguistic Abilities (ITPA) (Kirk, McCarthy, and Kirk 1969), which has the following 12 subtests:

1. Auditory reception (auditory decoding)—understanding what is heard.
2. Visual reception (visual decoding)—understanding what is seen.
3. Auditory vocal association—drawing meaningful relationships from what is heard.
4. Visual motor association—drawing meaningful relationships from what is seen.
5. Vocal expression (vocal encoding)—expressing ideas verbally.
6. Manual expression (motor encoding)—expressing ideas through gesture.
7. Grammatic closure—using grammatical structures automatically.
8. Auditory closure—filling in missing parts that were deleted in the auditory presentation. Example: Tele/one? Bo/le?
9. Visual closure—identifying a common object from an incomplete visual presentation.
10. Sound blending—synthesizing sounds of a word into a word.
11. Auditory sequential memory—recalling a series of digits auditorily.
12. Visual sequential memory—recalling a series of geometric forms visually.

These subtests are intended to assess the following areas of language functioning: (1) decoding (receptive functions), (2) encoding (expressive functions), (3) associations between encoding and decoding, (4) ability to integrate discrete units into a whole, and (5) memory processes.

Although the ITPA is one of the most frequently used tests, it has come under criticism on two counts: (1) cultural bias in favor of middle-class children and (2) lack of discreteness of the subtests (the result of research based on factor analyses of the subtests).[3] It is still regarded, however, as a very useful tool in assessing language development.

Types of Speech Defects

Accordingly, speech and language clinicians view speech and language as more than an ability to articulate sounds. They must be prepared to evaluate not only the child's phonological ability but also the channels of communication; the psycholinguistic processes involved in recognizing and understanding what is heard and in expressing ideas and responding either vocally or through gesture; the organizing process involving the internal manipulation of precepts, concepts, and linguistic symbols; and the degree to which habits of communication are organized within the child.

When clinicians discover the child who substitutes one sound for another or who omits sounds, they must decide whether the articulatory problem coexists with other problems of language. The test just described is one means of measuring the child's competence and performance with certain aspects of language. Ferrier's research (1966) points to the concept that articulatory problems coexist with language deficiencies. He studied 40 children of ages 6 through 8.7 with normal intelligence and normal hearing, but who had articulatory difficulties. The means on the ITPA scores of the group were all below the norms with auditory vocal automatic, auditory vocal sequential, visual vocal sequential, and vocal encoding being the lowest. Ferrier also observed that defective articulation appears to affect vocal encoding performance by reducing the total amount of verbalization. He further notes that these children also performed inadequately on the visual motor channels, although to a lesser extent than on the auditory channels. Ferrier gives as possible reasons an effect of verbal ability on the visual motor channels and the degree of availability of names for objects. The

---

[3] See V. G. Cicirelli, B. Graner, et al., "Performance of Disadvantaged Children on Revised ITPA," *Psychology in Schools*, **8** (July 1971), 240–246. G. W. Burns, and B. L. Watson, "Factor Analysis of the Revised ITPA with Underachieving Children," *Journal of Learning Disabilities*, **6** (July 1973), 371–376. B. A. Hare, D. D. Hammill, and N. R. Bartel, "Construct Validity of Selected Subtests of the ITPA," *Exceptional Children*, **40** (September 1973), 13–20. G. Cronkhite, and K. Penner, "A Reconceptualization and Revised Scoring Procedures for the ITPA Based on Multivariate Analysis of the Original Normative Data," *Journal of Speech and Hearing Research*, **18** (September 1975), 506–520.

clinician does well to investigate performance on other language abilities: morphological and syntactic accuracy, syntactic complexity, vocabulary, and sound discrimination.

Speech and language problems include (1) retarded language development, (2) articulatory defects, (3) stuttering, (4) vocal defects, (5) cleft-palate speech, (6) cerebral-palsy speech, (7) language impairment, associated with brain damage, and (8) speech defect caused by impaired hearing.

RETARDED LANGUAGE DEVELOPMENT

The child who is retarded in language development may initially also be somewhat delayed in language onset. Although one aspect of oral language proficiency may be conspicuously deviant, the likelihood is, as we learn later, that there is some degree of retardation—of lack of proficiency—in most of the components of speech. Thus, the child may be obviously retarded in speech sound production and appear infantile because of sound omissions and/or the persistence of infantile pronunciations. However, the child is also likely to have a smaller productive vocabulary and use shorter phrases and "simpler" sentences than most children of the same age.

To draw the line between retarded language development and an articulatory defect is sometimes difficult. The sound omission or substitution may well be but a symptom of retarded language development. Other aspects of the child's language must be examined before the label "articulatory defect" is applied. The Ferrier study mentioned previously points to the coexistence of articulatory and language problems. That the term *baby talk* is often used to label an articulatory defect is an indication that more than articulation is defective. Therefore, an assessment of the various language abilities is important.

ARTICULATORY DEFECTS

Among articulatory defects are (1) the omission of sounds. The nine-year-old boy who says *pay* for *play* and *banket* for *blanket* exemplifies the omission of sounds. (2) The substitution of one sound for another. The ten-year-old who says *wabbit* for *rabbit* and *wun* for *run* illustrates the substituting of one sound for another. (3) The distortion of sounds (substitution of a sound foreign to our language). An example of a distortion of a sound is the 12-year-old whose *s* has some of the characteristics of *sh*. A child with an articulatory defect may make any or all of these three errors. When the consonants that occur frequently, such as *s*, are involved and when some sounds are missing entirely, the child's speech may be unintelligible. Children on occasion either may include a sound they usually omit or make the sound acceptably. Frequently they make a sound accurately in its initial position but not in the final position or in a cluster such as *bl*. They may substitute an *f* for *th* but at the same time substitute a *p* for *f*. In other words, they are seemingly inconsistent in their articulatory errors. Ordinarily, however, a pattern exists even though the same individual uses several different substitutions for one sound. The substitution depends on the position of the sound in the word and its proximity to other sounds. A careful analysis of the child's articulatory errors will often point to a particular pattern.

Articulatory defects present an important problem of the speech program. Over half of the speech defects in a school population are articulatory defects and of this group, one half have difficulty with *s* and *z*. Many parents are unconcerned about these difficulties because they have become so accustomed to their children's articulatory errors that they do not even hear them. To older children particularly, however, these difficulties in their speech often bring anxiety. Their classmates think they sound like babies and at times may treat them as babies.

Other terms included in this category are lisping and lalling. Lisping refers to a defect of any of the sibilant sounds: *s*, *sh*, *z*, and *zh*. For example, *s* may be whistled, sound somewhat like an *sh*, or have a *th* quality about it. Lalling points to a speaker's difficulties with the *l* and *r* sounds. The child may substitute a *w* for these sounds or may make them in such a weak manner that they are not readily distinguishable. We suggest tests for assessing articulatory difficulties in Chapter 10.

STUTTERING

The stutterer's speech interferes with the reception of ideas by listeners. No stutterer's speech is exactly like another's although a disturbance of rhythm is obvious in each case. Symptoms of stuttering frequently include blocking on sounds, repetition or prolongation of sounds, repetition of syllables or words, and spasms of the speaking mechanism. One stutterer may speak abnormally slowly, another too quickly. The severity of stuttering varies for the individual stutterer. Almost always some situations exist where stutterers speak with comparative or complete fluency. There may be moments, however, when the fluency is so badly interrupted that both the speaker and the listener are unduly aware of the interruptions.

Although many parents remain quite unconcerned about their child's articulatory difficulties, most parents may be too aware of disfluencies. Some parents diagnose the very young child's normal disfluent speech as stuttering long before the child is aware of any difficulty. In the chapter on the development of language, we call attention to the number of times disfluencies occur in the young child's speech. Adults' concern and anxiety about disfluencies may be communicated to children, who in turn may become concerned and anxious. All of us should think long and carefully before diagnosing disfluent speech as stuttering. This idea is discussed at greater length in Chapter 13 on stuttering.

A type of rhythmic disorder sometimes confused with stuttering is cluttering. The child who clutters speaks at a rapid rate, omits and slurs syllables, and pauses in the wrong places. The clutterer always seems to be in a hurry.

Stuttering is not always easily discernible, because it is intermittent. If the children in the class are asked to read aloud, a stutterer may read aloud well. Furthermore the stuttering child may be able to speak easily to strangers but not to friends. The teacher who knows the child well frequently is the person who first notices evidences of incipient stuttering.

VOCAL DEFECTS

Vocal defects have to do with faults of pitch, quality, or intensity. A 16-year-old boy speaks at a pitch that is so inappropriate to his age and sex that it draws attention to itself. A 16-year-old girl speaks in a pitch so low that when she answers the telephone she is mistaken for her older brother. Both 16-year-olds have defects of pitch. A junior high school girl speaks with nasality and a strident quality. Her voice quality needs improvement. A 14-year-old girl speaks so softly that she is almost inaudible to her listeners. She needs to be helped so that she will have enough intensity of voice to make herself heard. Sometimes rate of speaking is also included in this category. In this instance, children speak so quickly or slowly that they are difficult to understand.

These terms are not quite as completely whole in themselves as they may seem. For example, Mary's voice sounds high, light, and barely audible. In her case, attributes of pitch, quality, and intensity are interwoven. Joan's voice sounds too low and husky. In Joan's case, the attributes of pitch and quality are interwoven. Separation of the entities of pitch, intensity, and quality in the diagnosis of voices is often impossible. In Chapter 12 on voice disturbances we discuss pitch of voice in detail.

Defects of intensity are easily recognizable, for voices are so soft that they do not carry or so loud that they irritate the listener. Here again, however, the lack of intensity and pitch may be interwoven.

Terms describing quality of voice tend to be more nebulous. Some persons will call a particular voice husky; others will call it hoarse; others will call it guttural; still others may call the voice a pleasant one though a bit throaty. But some of the adjectives describing vocal qualities are quite clear and well defined. Laymen may say that a person with a nasal voice talks through his nose. This term indicates excessive nasal resonance. Laymen portray a person with a denasal voice as always sounding as if he had a cold because his *m, n,* and *ng* lack sufficient nasal resonance. Some, however, label this an articulatory defect because it involves consonantal sounds. Furthermore, all of us easily recognize the breathy voice and the falsetto voice.

CLEFT-PALATE SPEECH

In cleft-palate speech, the cleft, either slight or extensive, may go through the teeth ridge and the hard and soft palates. It may extend through any one of these, or through the teeth ridge and hard palate, or through both palates. Consequently, the air passes freely between the mouth and the nose. This gives the speech a very nasal quality in unrepaired cleft palates. Even in repaired cleft palates the listener often perceives the voice as nasal. Many of the consonant sounds are distorted. The child with a cleft palate often has difficulty with the plosive sounds *p, b, t, d, k,* and *g,* for the child cannot build up enough air to explode these sounds. In addition, the fricative sounds *f, v, s, z, th, th, sh* and *zh* are often defective. The child may use a glottal stop or a nasal snort as substitutions. In severe cases the speech is unintelligible. The combination of physical defect and the symptoms of speech defects make cleft-palate speech quite obvious.

CEREBRAL-PALSY SPEECH

Cerebral palsy is a disturbance of the motor function resulting from damage to the brain before, during, or shortly after the birth of the child. The speech of the cerebral-palsied child may be normal when the muscles of the articulatory and respiratory organs are not affected. But, in about 75 per cent of the cases, the speech is slow, jerky, and labored, and the rhythm is faulty with unnatural breaks. The consonants, particularly those that require precise articulation, are likely to be inaccurate. Language development may be retarded.

LANGUAGE IMPAIRMENT

Language impairment associated with brain damage falls into two large categories. The first category includes the developmental failures and the unevenness of development in the child's ability to understand speech, to speak, and later to learn to read and write. The second category includes the involvements in oral and written functions resulting from brain damage incurred after the individual had learned to use language. These are generally referred to as aphasic language disorders. Some persons would include the first of our categories under retarded language development. The second category is primarily a problem for those beyond school age. We, therefore, do not consider this category in our text.

SPEECH DEFECT CAUSED BY IMPAIRED HEARING

A speech defect that is a result of impaired hearing shows itself largely in articulatory errors, voice aberrations, and language problems. Children with impaired hearing cannot pattern their speech on that of others because they cannot hear well enough. Consequently, their sounds are not articulated accurately and their voice reflects their lack of hearing by being too loud, too soft, or devoid of inflection. Because they cannot hear others, their vocabulary and morphological and syntactic development are impaired. How their hearing is impaired influences their articulation and voice. This is discussed in Chapter 14.

To help the classroom teacher decide whether students have speech difficulties, we have prepared the following questionnaire. When a preponderance of *yes* answers appears for any child, the teacher should consult a speech clinician.

Analysis of Speech Defects

RETARDED LANGUAGE DEVELOPMENT

1. Is the child's speech generally retarded when compared with that of his/her classmates?
2. Does the child
   a. Have a vocabulary limited for his/her age?
   b. Omit and substitute sounds substantially more frequently than his/her classmates?
   c. Use shorter and simpler sentences than his/her classmates?
   d. Use fewer phrases and prepositions than his/her classmates?
   e. Make errors in word order?
   f. Use many pronouns inaccurately?
   g. Use many tenses inaccurately?

   h. Use many comparisons and superlatives of adjectives inaccurately?

   i. Make many plurals inaccurately?

   j. Simplify words by deleting syllables as *fortable* for *comfortable*?

   k. Simplify words by repeating syllables as *Baba* for *Barbara*?

   l. Simplify clusters of sounds as *sap* for *slap* and *bue* for *blue*?

ARTICULATORY DEFECTS

1. Does the child
   a. Substitute one sound for another?
   b. Omit sounds?
   c. Change the utterance of a sound conspicuously?
2. Is the child very hard to understand?

STUTTERING

1. Is the child disturbed by his/her disfluency?
2. Does the child
   a. Repeat sounds or syllables or words more than his/her classmates?
   b. Have decidedly arhythmical speech?
   c. Block frequently?
   d. Have difficulty getting his/her words out?

VOCAL DIFFICULTIES

1. Is the child's voice
   a. Noticeably unpleasant in quality?
   b. Pitched higher or lower than that of other members of the class?
   c. Monotonous?
   d. Light and thin?
   e. Husky?
   f. Too loud?
   g. Too weak?
   h. Difficult to hear in class?

CLEFT-PALATE SPEECH

1. Is there an obvious cleft of the teeth ridge and/or palate?
2. Does the child's voice sound excessively nasal?

3. Are the sounds *p*, *b*, *t*, *d*, *k*, and *g* inaccurate?
4. Are some of the other consonants distorted?

CEREBRAL-PALSY SPEECH

1. Does the child have obvious tremors of the phonation and breathing musculature?
2. Is the child's speech slow, jerky, and labored?
3. Is the child's rhythm of speech abnormal?

LANGUAGE IMPAIRMENT

1. Is the child's comprehension of language markedly retarded?
2. Does there seem to be inconsistency in the child's ability to understand as well as to use language?
3. Is there a marked disparity between the child's ability to understand and to use language?
4. Is the child's profile of linguistic abilities uneven? (For example, can the child read much better than he can spell? Is the child surprisingly good in arithmetic and yet quite poor in either reading or writing?)

SPEECH DEFECT CAUSED BY IMPAIRED HEARING

1. Does the child
   a. Have frequent earaches and colds?
   b. Omit sounds or substitute one sound for another?
   c. Speak too loudly?
   d. Speak too softly?
   e. Frequently ask you to repeat what you have said?
   f. Move his/her head to one side as you speak?
   g. Watch you closely as you speak?
   h. Misinterpret your questions or instructions frequently?
   i. Do better when given written instructions than when given oral instructions?
   j. Seem more intelligent than indications from his/her work or tests?

Incidence and Types of Speech Defects

The teacher may have three children with speech defects in class one year and none the next. But on the average he/she can expect at least one child with a speech defect almost every semester. A 1969 report of the

National Institute of Neurological Diseases and Stroke gives the following estimated prevalence of speech defects in the United States. This report is an updated revision of the 1952 ASHA Committee on the White House Midcentury Conference report. *Journal of Speech and Hearing Disorders, 17* (1952), 129 137.

Estimated Prevalence of Speech Defects in the United States *

Type of Speech Problem	Ages 5–21		All Ages	
	Per cent	Years Number	Per cent	Number
Functional articulatory	3.0	1,500,000	3.0	6,000,000
Stuttering	.7	350,000	.7	1,400,000
Voice	.2	100,000	.2	400,000
Cleft-palate speech	.1	50,000	.1	200,000
Cerebral-palsy speech	.2	100,000	.2	400,000
Retarded speech development	.3	150,000	.3	600,000
Impaired hearing (with speech defect)	.5	250,000	.5	1,000,000
Total	5.0	2.500,000	5.0	10,000,000

* From National Institute of Neurological Diseases and Stroke, *Human Communication Its Disorders, An Overview*, Bethesda, Md.: United States Department of Health, Education and Welfare, 1969.

A survey by Gillespie and Cooper (1973) gives the number of speech defects of 5,054 junior and senior high school students of Tuscaloosa, Alabama; of this population, about 5 per cent possessed speech problems. The investigators listed stuttering and articulatory disorders as occurring most frequently (both 2.1 per cent). The prevalence of voice disorders was 1.2 per cent and of rate disorder 0.1 per cent. The table that follows illustrates the prevalence of speech disorders as indicated in this study.

Neal (1972) indicated that in his study of public school clinics, the case load distribution was as follows:

Articulation disorders	65.6%
Language disorders	21.4
Stuttering	3.2
Hard-of-hearing cases	3.0
Voice cases	2.6
Cleft palate	1.2
Cerebral palsy	.9
Others	2.1

The Prevalence of Various Types of Speech Problems Among 5,054 Junior and Senior High School Students in the Tuscaloosa, Alabama, City Schools, According to Grade*

Speech Problem	Grade Level												
	7		8		9		10		11		12		Combined	
	N	%	N	%	N	%	N	%	N	%	N	%	N	%
Articulation	32	3.4	20	2.4	10	1.0	15	2.0	16	2.3	11	1.4	104	2.1
Stuttering	29	3.1	25	3.0	17	1.7	20	2.7	12	1.7	4	0.5	107	2.1
Voice	14	1.4	11	1.0	10	1.0	10	1.3	8	1.2	8	1.1	61	1.2
Rate	0	0.0	0	0.0	2	0.2	0	0.0	2	0.3	0	0.0	4	0.1
Total	75	7.9	56	6.4	39	3.9	45	6.1	38	4.5	23	3.0	276	5.5

* S. K. Gillespie and E. B. Cooper, "Prevalence of Speech Problems in Junior and Senior High Schools," *Journal of Speech and Hearing Research*, **16** (December 1973), p. 740.

An examination of surveys of speech defects in school systems reveals that up to 10 per cent of our school population is defective in speech. In most surveys, the writers are counting those children with speech that is sufficiently different from normal speech to call undesirable attention to itself in conversation. We may arrive at various reasons for the differences in the incidence of speech defects found in publications as well as for estimates in excess of 5 per cent. (1) Clinicians may have to examine too many children too rapidly, so that they are not thorough enough in their analysis. (2) Classroom teachers with little training in speech may be reporting. They may be inaccurate in their diagnosis. (3) The basis of judgment varies. What may be a decidedly unpleasant voice to one teacher or clinician may be less offensive to another. One person may include a child with an articulatory defect, another may decide not to include such a child, feeling that the difficulty is the result of the child's immaturity, whereas the other person may consider it a serious defect.

The last two reasons are partially supported by a study that raises questions concerning intragroup agreement of ratings of the severity of speech problems, that is agreement among (1) the clinicians themselves and (2) the teachers themselves, and concerning intergroup agreement of rating, that is between the teachers as a group and the clinicians as a group (Wertz and Mead 1975). Classroom teachers of kindergarten, first grade, second grade, and third grade, and public school speech clinicians ranked four speech disorders: voice, cleft palate, articulation, and stuttering. Results showed that in this study the classroom teachers and speech clinicians rate stuttering as a more severe speech disorder than voice, cleft palate, or articulation. Only the third-grade teachers rated articulation as most severe, differing from the other teachers and the speech clinicians. All teacher groups and speech clinicians rated the voice disorder as the least severe disorder. No consistent agreement among groups was observed in rating cleft palate and articulation. Intragroup agreement was much better among teachers than among speech clinicians. The authors, in pointing to the difference in judgment among the clinicians, give these possible reasons: Clinicians may have been influenced by the extent of their clinical experience with the disorders, previous success or failure, or the influence of different academic and clinical training.

Teacher's Role in Locating Speech Defects

Classroom teachers frequently refer the speech-defective child to the speech clinician—often carrying the major responsibility for locating the speech-defective child. When the speech clinician does not screen the school population, the teacher should be trained to hear and identify symptoms of the various speech defects. The training may be accomplished by college courses, in-service courses, or a series of lectures by the speech clinician.

In the light of a study by James and Cooper (1966), this training seems essential. James and Cooper investigated how successfully classroom teachers who were given the aid of a written statement defining and describing speech handicaps could identify speech-handicapped children, and determined the relationship of the teachers' ability to identify speech-handicapped children with the type and severity of the speech disorder. The experiment involved 30 third-grade teachers who had no training in speech correction, and 718 children were screened. The speech clinician found 242 children with speech difficulties; the teachers referred only 98 of them. The teachers were least accurate in their referral of children with voice disorders and most accurate in their referral of stutterers. They referred 87.5 per cent of the severely disordered, 51.9 per cent of the moderate, and 28.7 per cent of the mild. Their percentage of accuracy of referral varied from 10.1 for voice, 41.4 for articulatory defects, and 80.0 for stutterers.

The findings of this study are supported by Prahl and Cooper (1964). They compared teacher referrals with the results of screening by a speech clinician and reported that the percentage of accurate referrals rose as the severity of the disorder increased. Prahl and Cooper suggest two alternative interpretations for these findings. The first is that teachers fail to identify a large percentage of speech handicapped children. Obviously teachers need to be trained to identify speech defects, particularly in school systems where the classroom teacher is responsible for referring those children who need speech therapy to the speech clinician. From the evidence of the studies just cited, the detection of voice disorders needs special attention with clear explanations and with illustrations.

The need for training teachers to recognize speech handicaps is also emphasized in a survey of teachers conducted by Clauson and Kopatic (1975). They report that teachers are uncertain about the particular speech handicaps that the school speech and language clinician handles; in fact, only one teacher out of 50 answered the question pertaining to this subject correctly. Only 58 per cent of the teachers felt certain they could recognize a speech-defective child in their class. A majority of the teachers believes that children will outgrow their speech problems even when the children are past the third grade.

The second interpretation of Prahl and Cooper (1964), that clinicians are unnecessarily severe in their judgments of defective speech and have consequently lost perspective of what constitutes a "speech problem," needs to be examined. If the s deviation is such that no teacher, parent, or classmate detects it, is it a problem? Certainly, it does not seriously interfere with communication and in most instances the speaker is unaware of the "handicap." If the r is weak but its weakness is not discernible to anyone but the clinician, does a speech problem exist? The answer must be, "Only in the ears of the clinician."

The classroom teacher does not ordinarily do audiological testing.[4] Audiological testing is accomplished by a variety of specialists in the public school system, including speech and hearing clinicians, nurses, physicians, school audiologists, and health department personnel. Almost all schools, however provide for regular audiological screening.

The Classroom Teacher and Speech and Language Problems

It is very important for classroom teachers to have training recognizing speech and language difficulties, in planning strategies for the reinforcement of clinical work, and in being able to differentiate between what language and speech work falls into the realm of speech and language therapy and what falls into the realm of speech and language improvement and stimulation. The evidence for teachers' need for training in the identification of speech defects has already

---

[4] See Chapter 14 for a more detailed discussion.

been given. As stressed earlier, the need for this training is particularly important because the teacher frequently carries the responsibility for referral of speech- and language-handicapped children to the school speech clinician.

Teachers should also know what is going on in the speech clinic, for when this work is reinforced in the classroom, the improvement in communication is more rapid. If the child uses one set of rules for speech and language in the clinical setting and another set in the classroom, the improvement in the child's speech can be hindered. Furthermore, the teacher and clinician should approach the problem from the same basic philosophy; otherwise the reinforcement may be negative rather than positive. For example, while the clinician may be helping children to accept their stuttering, the teacher may be asking them to stop, to think before they speak. The combination of these two behaviors is counterproductive. We suggest close cooperation between the teacher and the specialist. The members and the roles of the speech and language team are discussed in the next chapter.

Teachers must also be able to recognize which language and speech problems are in their province and which are in the province of the speech clinicians. For instance, teachers show good judgment in re- fusing to accept primary responsibility for the rehabilitation of the speech of the stutterer, of the speech and voice of the child with a cleft palate or with a hearing defect, or of the voice of the child with a serious vocal handicap. However, teachers often have had the training and have the competence to handle the child with a minor functional articulatory difficulty, such as the child who says *tree* for *three*. And teachers should be able to distinguish whether this substitution is a dialectal difference or a functional articulatory error. In some in- stances, most of the children in the class may say *tree* for *three*, for this substitution is a product of their environment. The classroom teacher, however, is almost always responsible for the program that stimulates speech and language development of the entire class. Frequently, the speech clinician or another educational specialist, such as the learning disabilities resource teacher, aids in planning this work. Kindergarten teachers stimulate language development in many ways: They teach listening skills (or auditory decoding) by asking children to follow simple directions such as to touch his/her ear, eye, nose, or arm, with these actions being accompanied by song. Or they ask children to follow somewhat more complicated directions:

Stand in front of your chair. Now behind your chair.

Jump twice and then put your hands over your head.

Or kindergarten teachers may teach verbal expressive skills (verbal encoding) by asking the child to pick an article, such as an apple, out of a grab bag. The child does not let the other children know what was picked, but tells them enough about the apple so that the other children can guess what it is. Or teachers may teach verbal associations by filling a glass with water and then emptying it, thus establishing the difference between *full* and *empty*. Most teachers are imaginative in such activities and, as a result, the children's behavior is imaginative. Activities, such as these, which help stimulate language development, are dealt with in Chapter 8.

Problems

1. Visit a lower-grade classroom and try to screen the children into the following categories: (a) those who have speech and language that will probably meet their social and educational needs; (b) those whose speech and language may be faulty but likely to improve with maturation; (c) those who need language stimulation; (d) those who have more serious difficulties that will require the attention of a speech clinician.
2. Visit one of the sessions held by a speech clinician. Indicate the problem of one of the children and the kind of help he/she received.
3. Visit a kindergarten and a fifth-grade class. Indicate whether the number of articulatory errors decreases or increases and whether the disfluencies decrease or increase in the two grades. Lastly, indicate some differences in vocabulary and syntactical development between the groups. Be as specific as you can.
4. Answer the questions on pages 12–14 in reference to five particular children. Try to choose one child whom you suspect of having a speech difficulty.
5. Visit a session held by a speech clinician. Indicate in two specific ways how you as a classroom teacher could reinforce the teaching done in this session in your classroom.

or

Visit a first- or second-grade class. Indicate suggestions you might make as a clinician to the teacher to help a particular child with a specific language disability.

References and Suggested Readings

American Speech and Hearing Association Research Committee, "Public School Speech and Hearing Services," *Journal of Speech and Hearing Disorders*, Monograph Supplement **8** (July 1961).

Clauson, G. M., and N. J. Kopatic, "Teacher Attitudes and Knowledge of Remedial Speech Programs," *Language, Speech, and Hearing Services in Schools*, **6** (October 1975), 206–210.

Ferrier, E. E., "Investigation of ITPA Performances of Children with Functional Defects of Articulation," *Exceptional Child*, **32** (May 1966), 625–629.

Frostig, M., and P. Maslow, "Language Training: A Form of Ability Training," *Journal of Learning Disabilities*, **1** (February 1968), 105–115. (Describes developmental functions, language deficits, influence of education. Talks about a program for training language abilities.)

Gillespie, S. K., and E. B. Cooper, "Prevalence of Speech Problems in Junior and Senior High Schools," *Journal of Speech and Hearing Research*, **16** (December 1973), 739–743. (Indicates that in Tuscaloosa, Alabama, 5.5 per cent of junior and senior high school students have speech problems.)

Hull, F. M., P. W. Mielke, Jr., R. J. Timmons, and J. A. Willeford, "The National Speech and Hearing Survey: Preliminary Results," *ASHA*, **13** (September 1971), 501–510. (Describes the procedures in the survey and gives statistics on articulatory difficulties and on hearing disabled.)

James, H. P., and E. B. Cooper, "Accuracy of Teacher Referral of Speech-Handicapped Children," *Exceptional Child*, **30** (September 1966), 29–33.

Kirk, S. S., J. J. McCarthy, and K. A. Kirk, *Illinois Test of Psycholinguistic Abilities*, rev. ed., Urbana, Ill.: Institute for Research on Exceptional Children, 1969.

Neal, W. R., "Speech Pathology Services in the Secondary Schools," *Language, Speech, and Hearing Services in Schools*, **7** (January 1976), 6–16.

Pendergast, K., "Articulation Study of 15,255 Seattle First-Grade Children with and Without Kindergarten," *Exceptional Child*, **32** (April 1966), 541–547.

Prahl, H. M., and E. B. Cooper, "Accuracy of Teacher Referrals of Speech-Handicapped School Children," *ASHA*, **6** (October 1964), 392.

Rees, N. S., "The Speech Clinician cum Language Clinician," *Language, Speech, and Hearing Services in Schools*, **4** (October 1974), 185–186. (Gives knowledge and therapeutic strategies that the speech clinician needs. Contains definitions of *language*, *communication*, and *speech*.)

Van Riper, C., *Speech Correction: Principles and Methods*, 5th ed., Englewood Cliffs, N.J.: Prentice-Hall, Inc., 1972, chap. 2. (Describes the types of disorders of speech.)

Wertz, R. T., and M. D. Mead, "Classroom Teacher and Speech Clinician Severity Ratings of Different Speech Disorders," *Language, Speech, and Hearing Services in Schools*, **6** (July 1975), 119–124.

2. Speech and Language Clinical Services

The number of school personnel dealing with speech and language disorders is increasing. Before 1940 only nine states had legislation recognizing the need for providing financial support for the speech-handicapped child (Irwin 1959, p. 127). Today, in contrast, most states recognize the needs of the speech-, hearing-, and language-handicapped children through enabling legislation and through upward trends in certification requirements for school clinicians (Causey, Johnson, and Healey 1971). The growth is also evident in the increase in the American Speech and Hearing Association membership, a 15.8 per cent increase in 1974 alone. Of the total ASHA membership, 40.8 per cent are employed in an elementary or secondary school (*ASHA* 1975, p. 413).

Organization of Speech Therapy Services

Speech and language programs within schools differ in their administration and organization in many ways. Sometimes the teacher, the principal, parents, school nurse, reading specialist, learning disabilities specialist, psychologist, or guidance director refers the speech- and language-handicapped child to the speech clinician; at other times, the clinician makes a clinical survey. The clinician's case load varies from

25 children in some places to 300 in others. A clinician may help a child for as short a period as ten minutes or as long a period as 50 minutes either individually or in groups varying in size from three to 18. The groups are homogeneous or heterogeneous in terms of the speech difficulty and age. Each of these facets of organization is discussed.

IDENTIFICATION OF THE SPEECH, HEARING, AND LANGUAGE HANDICAPPED

Clinicians locate children with speech and language problems primarily through teacher referrals and survey. The identification process, however it is handled, is time-consuming, because speech screening usually takes from one to three weeks of the clinician's time each year. In some cases the testing begins before the children's entrance to kindergarten (Glick, Ueberle, and George 1973); in others, it begins either in kindergarten or in the first grade. In the upper grades, frequently only newly entering students are screened. Audiological screening, provided in almost all schools, is usually under the supervision of either a nurse or a speech and hearing clinician.

The Task Force Report on School Speech, Hearing, and Language Screening Procedures (Task Force 1973) gives in detail the basic principles of screening, methods of screening, use of team screening, hearing screening, and factors in choosing the population to be screened. A quick screening procedure (five minutes) is suggested:

1. Tell full name, age, and address.
2. Describe an action picture involving children of the same age for sentence use and fluency.
3. Follow a one-step and then a two-step command for memory span and knowledge of prepositions and verbs.
4. Points to parts of the body; describe clothing.
5. Name objects as shown in the Templin-Darley Screening Test, the Hejna Developmental Test, or Ferwill Object Kit Test of Articulation.

The children are then rated on a five-point scale with those with the lowest rating needing instant referral, those with the next lowest needing further diagnosis, and those in the middle needing follow-up.

CASE LOAD

Case loads vary from 25 to 250 or 300. The tendency of recent years is for the speech clinician's case load to decrease. Neal (1976) reports that his survey found a 72.68 student average case load. Various factors are involved in establishing the size of the case load: (1) limitation by state law, (2) the total number of children with speech and language problems, (3) the rationale for selection of children on the part of the director of the program.

Brown (1971, p. 540) suggests that the speech clinician ask the following questions when selecting a case load:

1. Does the child have an emotional reaction to communicative effort?
2. Does the child's speech and language interfere with communication?
3. Does the child's communication problem interfere with classroom achievement?

INDIVIDUAL AND GROUP THERAPY

Whether to handle speech- and hearing-handicapped children individually or in groups is usually left to the discretion of the therapist. In public schools most of the children who require help receive group therapy. But the individualized needs of the child are taken into account —and where necessary, a child is given individual therapy. In schools today with emphasis on productivity, it is apparent that much of the therapy will occur in groups. For some kinds of cases group therapy is beneficial. In his study, Sommers (1966) found that in the correction of articulatory defects group therapy was as effective as individual therapy, regardless of the severity of speech defectiveness or the grade levels of the children involved. In this study, Sommers used 12 experimental groups of 40 children who were given the McDonald Deep Test of Articulation before and after a period of eight and one-half months of speech correction. These 12 groups provided for the investigation the following sources of variation: (a) therapy—half of each group of 40 received group therapy; the other half received individual therapy; (b) severity—half of each group had "mild" articulation problems; and half had "moderate" articulation problems; (c) grade—four of the groups were from grade 2, four from grade 4, and four from grade 6. The average size of the groups was 4.5 with the largest group containing six and the smallest three.

WORK OF THE CLINICIAN

Speech and language clinicians identify those children who are language, speech- and/or hearing handicapped; diagnose and evaluate their problems; and then plan, schedule, and conduct a program to handle these problems. They confer with parents concerning their children's difficulties. In addition, they may offer in-service courses to teachers and may serve as consultants for those classroom teachers who carry on a program of language stimulation for children who show inadequacies in pronunciation, vocabulary, syntax, decoding, encoding, and associative and sequencing language functions. Because schools revolve around verbal skills, such programs help children to be more successful in their school environment. Chapter 8 deals with these aspects in some detail.

To summarize, the teaching of the broad language-arts skills is the responsibility of the professionally trained classroom teacher. The area of language stimulation and development for all students involves both the classroom teacher and the clinician who serves as a consultant for the teacher. Finally, the special services to be rendered to the speech-, language-, and hearing-impaired child are the responsibility of the speech and language clinician.

LIMITING THE CASE LOAD

A frequent problem in schools is a case load that is too large for the clinician to handle efficiently. With a therapy schedule that cannot effectively accommodate more than 75 to 100 cases, 150 to 200 cases often need to be scheduled. Such a situation allows a variety of options:

1. To give a little help in large groups to all the handicapped children.
2. To train the classroom teachers to take care of the less severely handicapped children.
3. To limit the case load to 75 or 100 cases.

The first alternative, to give some therapy to all the handicapped, does not seem feasible, because a small amount of training usually results in a small amount of improvement, and marked success requires effectively treated students. Feasibility of the second alternative depends on many factors: the speech background of the classroom teachers; the availability and ability of the clinician to train the teachers; the size of the various teachers' classes; their schedule and that of the clinician; and the attitudes of the administration and the teachers to the problems of the speech-handicapped. In a few instances, the clinician may be able to give the necessary training to some of the teachers

Usually, however, the clinician will choose the third alternative of giving training to approximately 75 to 100 students, selecting the students on the basis of valid principles. Disgruntled parents whose children have been deprived of speech therapy may demand an explanation. So may those parents whose children have been asked to take it. The reasons for selection should be arrived at thoughtfully and carefully and in consultation with the administrative officers of the school.

Such factors as the severity of the handicap, ability to benefit from training, and placement in grade and school are all important. In discussing case selection most authorities agree that children with voice problems, those with speech difficulties that are related to organic involvements, and those who stutter should be enrolled in the speech therapy program. Many authorities believe that children with speech defects that are a cause of concern to them, their parents, or their teachers, or that seriously interfere with communication, with inter-personal relationships, or with school progress ought to be included in the program. That the words "seriously interfere with communication" means something different to speech clinicians and classroom teachers is obvious from the research reported in Chapter 1.

Most writers cite ability to benefit from training as an important factor in selection. They suggest that measures be used to prognosticate articulatory improvement, such as the child's ability to produce a sound in a nonsense syllable, or to discriminate the correct production of misarticulations from acoustically similar sounds. They also suggest other measures dependent on standardized tests: intelligence tests, language tests, sound discrimination tests.

Some clinicians emphasize therapy in the upper grades rather than the lower grades; others emphasize helping children in kindergarten, first, and second grades. A rationale can be made for both positions.

It is important that speech clinicians base their selection of cases on a logical, appropriate rationale and that they use this rationale in defending the inclusion or omission of a child from the case load. When teachers and administrators have been involved in working out this rationale, a parent, concerned about the omission of a particular child, is more likely to accept the decision gracefully.

When classroom teachers have not participated in the discussion of the rationale for placing children in speech therapy, the principles should be carefully explained to them. They will be better equipped to explain the principles to disgruntled parents, however, when they have been included in the discussion that led to the formulation of the principles.

The Team Approach

Although the administration and organization of speech therapy programs may differ, the clinician always keeps the classroom teacher informed of what he/she is doing. The teacher, in turn, reinforces the learning acquired in speech sessions. Almost always both the clinician and the teacher confer with the parents. Both teacher and clinician often consult with the school health authorities. In other words, a team approach is appropriate. The composition of the team may vary somewhat, but typically the classroom teacher, the clinician, the school health personnel, the learning disabilities teacher, and the school psychologist make up the team. Its members meet to discuss the problems of the handicapped children and to work out programs for particular children. At times they invite other specialists such as an otologist, an orthodontist, a neurologist, or a psychiatrist to join the group.

For example, Shearer (1972) reports on a team approach to the diagnosis and treatment of voice disorders in schoolchildren established at Northern Illinois University at the request of local school speech clinicians. The diagnostic team, meeting four times a year, consisted of a speech pathologist, a laryngologist, and a school psychologist, with the college clinic providing audiological services. The school clinicians referred the children, mostly because of hoarseness, and followed through with the team. The diagnosis revealed vocal nodules in 57 per cent of the children. The team approach in this instance became a learning situation for the clinicians both in the diagnosis and treatment of vocal disorders.

ROLES OF THE MEMBERS OF THE TEAM

THE CLASSROOM TEACHER

Surely classroom teachers know the children better than other members of the team, for they are with the children all day. Because they are interested in all of the child's development, they see the child's speech and language as part of a total development. Of the members of the team, teachers in all likelihood have the most opportunity to observe and understand the child. They know how the child acts in the playground and in class. They recognize the child's ability to lead, to be a good student, to build birdhouses, or to throw a baseball. Furthermore, they usually have more contact with the parents than any of the other members of the team. Consequently, they are the ones most intimately acquainted with the child. ·

Ideal classroom teachers for the language- and speech-handicapped children are good teachers for both the children with normal speech and those with defective speech. First, and most important, they accept children with handicaps, whether the handicaps be speech, physical, or emotional, and help the classmates of these children to be accepting. When teachers control their feelings of sympathy and accept handicapped children with their difficulties in a matter-of-fact way, the handicapped children and their classmates are likely to adopt a similar attitude. Second, teachers make sure that their classrooms invite oral communication. When the children plan their work together, when they like to play with each other, they talk and listen. As they go on purposeful trips, as they act in a play, or as they build a bookcase, they have worthwhile discussions. Their classroom, with its interesting bulletin board, with its work corner, invites conversation. Chapter 8 contains suggestions on how to stimulate speech activities. Third, the teacher fosters good human relationships among the children. When a warm friendly feeling exists in the classroom, when youngsters like each other and their teacher, when the teacher helps to build a positive concept of self in the child, when activity is stimulating, speaking is both necessary and enjoyable. As children participate in decisions, as they realize that they are the most important part of the school program, they have a feeling of belonging to their school group. Last, the good teacher is a cooperative person who reinforces the learning taught by other teachers and who contributes factual information about the child to other colleagues when it will prove useful.

In addition, classroom teachers who are to be successful in helping children with handicapped speech and language must have certain other qualifications that more directly relate to speech: (1) Their own speech and voice must be worthy of imitation. This is discussed in Chapter 4. (2) They must have a discerning ear so that they hear the errors their children make. (3) They must have an accurate knowledge of how the American-English vowels and consonants are made. The chapter on the production of speech sounds covers this area. (4) They must be able to plan a program of language stimulation for all their children. Whereas only a small number of children needs speech and language therapy, almost all students have a need for language stimulation. This need is explained in Chapter 8. (5) They should have enough knowledge of communicative disorders to reinforce the teaching of the clinician. They must, therefore, be able to understand the clinician's goals, objectives, and strategies. In this book the chapters on the various speech defects contain this material. (6) They should be able to pick out those students in their class who need clinical help. The chapter on the definition of speech defects includes some of this information.

Teachers can cooperate in other ways too. For example, classroom teachers can help students above the first grade to carry the responsibility of watching the clock for the time when they are to go for speech help. Frequently, the teachers write the time on the blackboard on the day the child is to go for help. Through some means, the teacher should help the child to get to the clinician at the scheduled time.

THE CLINICIAN

Clinicians must appreciate that they are working members of an educational team. As such, they must have a professional awareness and attitude, and must get along with students, parents, and school personnel. In addition, they must be able to gain the help of other school personnel, set up their programs effectively and cooperatively, and report on their progress capably and efficiently.

Cooperation with the Classroom Teacher. Since the teacher reinforces the therapy provided by the clinician, the clinician must make sure that the teacher has the necessary information about the child's problem and the knowledge and skill for the reinforcement. When the clinicians seek reinforcement in terms of behavioral objectives, they are more likely to succeed in achieving the desired goals. For example, the objective may be that the child correctly articulate the *r* sound in conversation in 25 words. A scorecard may be provided for the teacher to record the child's behavior. Or the objective may be that the child differentiate between *same* and *different* in ten pictures with same and different articles. Or the objective may be that the child communicate accurately his/her name and address. When the reinforcement can take place in the classroom with other children, as could be done in these examples, the teacher is likely to be more willing to cooperate and the interaction motivates successful communication.

Cooperation also is essential in the area of language disabilities. Many severely language-disabled children are mainstreamed, placed in a regular class rather than a special class. For these children, speech clinicians are often the resource teachers, since they have a background in the theory of language development, in phonology, morphology, syntax, and semantics and in learning theory. Clinicians, therefore, serve as diagnosticians and as programmers. For instance, they suggest strategies to the teacher for developing such concepts as categorization or the use of prepositions as *in* and *under* or *above* and *below*.

Indeed, because of the growth in the field of learning disabilities and because of advances in linguistic research, the interdisciplinary approach to the child with language-learning problems has become an integral part in planning for intervention of language difficulties. The speech clinician plays an important role on this team because of his/her knowledge of the language processes. Robertson and Freeman (1974, p. 188) list the following facets of this role:

1. Providing a comprehensive summary of the child's linguistic competencies.

2. Identifying and interpreting relationships between the child's linguistic competency and performance on psychological and educational assessments.
3. Establishing correlations between the child's observable motor, adaptive, and personal-social development and his/her language behavior.
4. Formulating generalizations regarding the child's learning patterns for language as they relate to the academic environment of the classroom.

Professional Status and Attitudes. Now that the study of speech disorders has reached maturity, clinicians should be aware of the need for maintaining professional status and attitudes. The first factor in awareness is gaining the necessary training. The American Speech and Hearing Association lists the requirements for the certificate of clinical competence. Speech clinicians who work in the schools should preferably meet these requirements upon beginning their employment. If they do not, they should take summer work to meet these requirements as quickly as possible. In a recent study, Neal (1976) notes that of the clinicians in public schools that he surveyed, 81 per cent held the American Speech and Hearing Association's Certificate of Clinical Competence in Speech Pathology, 89 per cent held a Master's degree, and 2 per cent held a doctorate degree. A second factor is the clinicians' relationships with other professions. They must recognize the delimitations of their field from those of the doctor, psychologist, psychiatrist, dentist, and physical therapist. Clinicians should neither criticize these workers nor make even a hint of a diagnosis in a field other than their own. The third factor is the knowledge of their own limitations. When clinicians do not understand a voice case or when they have difficulty with parents, they must seek help from someone who knows more than they do. Professors in universities, experienced workers in the field, and administrative officials of a school are all glad to help young clinicians.

Because the clinicians are working with individuals and with small groups, they must be particularly careful to maintain a professional and workmanlike attitude and to allow no undue familiarity between them and their students. They should be friendly but at the same time keep the necessary professional distance. They should not respond emotionally to a child's problem, for their attitude must remain objective. Although they undoubtedly desire a permissive atmosphere for their speech therapy, clinicians should set their limits and hold strictly to them. A permissive attitude should not mean a laissez-faire attitude. Some behavior should be discouraged.

Human Relationships. Another part of being an effective clinician is getting along well with others—having good personal relationships with the members of the community, with the school personnel, and with the parents of their children. Clinicians must be able to work and interact with people effectively. The success of their programs depends to some extent on how well the members of the community receive the programs. Clinicians must be able to explain their programs to the Rotary Club or the Lions Club, and to others who are already sympathetic to the handicapped child. Clinicians must, however, be able to make them understand that the language-, speech-, or hearing-handicapped child can receive help and that their community is responsible for offering this help. One clinician, talking to a club in the town about the kind of help being given to three children with quite different difficulties, persuaded its members of the advantages of the program; in turn, these men and women were supportive of the program when the need arose.

Clinicians need the cooperation and help of the classroom teachers. In turn, they must appreciate the teachers' work. One clinician made it his duty to visit a classroom when he had some free time because of the absence of a child in his case load. His few warm words of appreciation to the teacher at the end of the visit aided in building a good relationship between the two.

The support of the parents of the handicapped children is as important as that of the classroom teacher. One father remarked recently, "I'll only live in this town three years, but I'll always be thankful for Davy's speech help. Suppose I'd happened to be in a place where there was no help." Sincere appreciation by parents is an asset in firmly establishing and maintaining a speech therapy program. The conferences with parents and the home visits are most important. The clinician must be able to gain the confidence of the parents so that they will cooperate for the good of the child and the success of the program.

Parent Counseling. Many speech clinicians meet regularly with the parents of the children they service. In one area of an inner city, the clinician meets frequently with the parents of her children in groups of about 25. Their discussions have ranged from helping the child to build a strong self-image to the verbalizing of feelings of guilt and anger by the parents. Members of this group talked frankly about their relationships with their youngsters and about their own needs and feelings, which were often reflected in their children's attitudes and behavior. As they discussed these problems with each other and with the clinician, they were better able to understand their own feelings and the feelings their children had about themselves and about their parents.

One parent lived in fear that his son, a stutterer, would become a dope addict. He kept repeating, "I try to set him straight." When questioned, he acknowledged that the reason for his fear was the boy's anger, which was often expressed in "beating up" his younger brother and other kids on the block. He began to understand why the boy felt angry and to be able to communicate this understanding to him. Even though the boy's behavior was unacceptable, the father *did* accept the fact of his anger, even when it was unprovoked. As the boy perceived his father's understanding and acceptance of his feelings, he began to communicate. The father, who had communicated mostly nonverbally, to reprimand, began to communicate verbally, and particularly at times such as when the boy was elated at his success in writing poetry. The father previously had looked on this activity as a foolish waste of time. Admittedly, the severity of the boy's stuttering did not diminish, but he became a happier and much more communicative member of his family and of his school community. The other parents in the group, mostly mothers, were instrumental in helping the father to look at himself and his son realistically and honestly.

Webster (1966) says that parent conferences provide parents with three vital aids:

1. Important information about the child's specific disorder.
2. Opportunities for parents to experiment with tools for promoting better communication: (a) trying to understand the child's feelings and verbalizing this understanding, (b) trying to accept the child's feelings, even when the behavior is unacceptable, (c) allowing the child time with his parents when they can concentrate on communicating, (d) giving the child a chance to communicate at times when he feels success and satisfaction, and (e) attempting to communicate with the child on his own level.
3. A chance to verbalize frankly about vital issues in their relationships and the forces that motivate them.

In-Service Courses. In some schools, clinicians not only treat the children but also lead discussions and give lectures or in-service courses so that teachers can reinforce the clinician's work given in therapy sessions. Clinicians give the teachers the necessary training to locate the children with speech difficulties and send out mimeographed bulletins to help the teachers understand the various speech and language handicaps of the children. Clinicians explain to teachers the relationship of speech and language difficulties to academic achievement, such as reading, and to behavior problems. They report to teachers on research that relates the study of language and speech disorders to classroom teaching.

As clinicians talk to teachers and parents, they will keep their use of technical terms to a minimum. They will not say that Mary has dysphonia and that Johnny has a lall; rather they will explain that Mary's voice is hoarse and that Johnny substitutes *w* for *r* and *l*. Parents particularly are wary of specialists' terms; therefore, both the classroom teacher and the clinician should not talk about "cases," "clinicians," or "clinics" unless absolutely necessary.

Preparing Schedules. Last, the clinician must serve as a team member in preparing a schedule of classes and in making reports. Many variables make the preparation of a therapy schedule difficult. The clinician may want to place students homogeneously in terms of defect and age, to work with certain cases in the morning, or to cut across several classes and age levels for stuttering groups. In addition, the clinician usually has to work around the schedules of the classroom teachers and other specialists; for example, the classroom teacher may not wish a child to lose certain fundamental work that is usually given at a particular time. Because so many of the school personnel are involved, their cooperation and that of the administration is essential in working out a schedule. Consultation with the teachers and the administration helps to ensure the prompt and regular attendance of the speech-handicapped children.

Clinicians generally use one of the following two types of scheduling or a combination of both: (1) Block scheduling that involves a concentrated program with as many weekly therapy sessions as five in a block of three to six weeks. Some research studies indicate higher dismissal rates for such difficulties as stuttering in this type of scheduling. (2) The traditional scheduling of once or twice a week for a full term. Recent research on articulation progress favors this system (Weston and Harber 1975). (3) A combination of these two methods. Some clinicians believe that the block scheduling is superior because they can provide intensive treatment for those who need it. Less traveling and transporting of materials is required, and while they are there, they are a more integral part of the school.

The resulting schedule should be placed in the hands of the administrator and the teachers involved. All the members of the team should adhere to the schedule except for necessary absences.

When assigning students to the speech-correction classes, the clinician should also notify the parents. In this activity, the advice of classroom teachers is important, for most teachers meet with the parents at least once a semester. With the advice and consent of the supervisor or principal, the clinician or director of language, speech, and hearing services sends a letter such as the following to the parents of children to be enrolled in speech-correction classes:

> Dear Mrs.————————:
>
> A recent test shows that your son can profit from work in speech. I have, therefore, scheduled him to work with me twice a week during which time I shall try to teach him to speak more clearly.
>
> I shall be glad to have your help. You can, I am sure, give me information and advice that will make my work with your son more effective. Won't you come to see me next week when I have planned conferences with parents? Would Tuesday at 3:00 be a possible time? If it is not, please call me between 3:00 and 5:00 on Friday at Forest 6–7000, extension 7, and we can arrange another time.
>
> Sincerely yours,

Before enrolling a child in speech-therapy class, the clinician should make sure that the child is not receiving help from a speech and hearing center or from a private individual. Speech instruction from both a school and another source usually are not advantageous to the child, although overanxious parents often believe that the more help their child receives the better, and consequently enroll the child for private help without informing the school. Local centers and school personnel should cooperate to do what is best for the youngster. In some instances, the child is better treated at a center; in other instances, at school. A school administrator may coordinate the work by approving the child's taking therapy from an outside source and by excusing the child from school therapy. A signed slip is then sent to the outside source. The superintendent or another official should also request information on the amount and kind of therapy being given the child by outsiders. The work between the agency and the school should be related.

Records. Clinicians keep records for several reasons: (1) Clinicians want to know as much as they can about each child. From interviews with the child, teachers, and parents, they acquire information about the child's interests, personality, medical history, and academic attainments that can be helpful in handling the child. When such information is recorded, the next clinician has a basis for understanding the child. (2) The clinician needs to know what has been done with a child and how effective the therapy has been. (3) Teachers, administrators, and other school personnel need to find out what has taken place in the speech-therapy program. (4) Administrators frequently want reports o that they can justify the program to their governing bodies. (5) State Departments of Education often require reports to serve as a basis for financial aid to the local community. All clinicians keep some form of a case history.

A number of recent articles deal with case histories: Rees (1969) describes the development of a standard case record form by a group of clinicians and supervisors in the Los Angeles area who found the transfer of information among school speech clinicians inefficient. This form includes the usual obvious identification data such as name and address and material on spontaneous speech and language including dialect, length of responses, vocabulary, grammar; on articulation; on fluency; on voice; on intelligibility; on the speech mechanism; on communicative responsiveness; on general health history; on observed physical behavior; more detailed identification data including case identification, years of therapy, type of class, grade level, test result from such tests as WISC, Binet, Peabody, and CIMM, reading scores, arithmetic scores, an articulation record, and a hearing test record. Such a detailed source of data accumulated over years can supply answers to many questions, including queries about case selection, prognosis, dismissal criteria, associated learning difficulties, and related family and health conditions.

Wing (1975) illustrates a data recording system that could easily be placed on a 5 inch by 7 inch card. The data includes the name of the child, referral date and source, evaluation dates, outside referral, classification, etiology, severity, therapy dates, prescriptive program dates, resource room, ongoing assessment dates, no program, waiting list, parent conferences, teacher conferences, and recommendations.

Other reports frequently made by clinicians include results of hearing-, speech-, and language testing; schedules of schools and classes; therapy progress reports; and final reports (*ASHA* 1961, p. 42). Final reports frequently are sent to superintendents and could well include the number of students receiving clinical help during the year broken down into type of disorder, number of students dismissed and reasons for their dismissal, number of students added during the term, number of conferences with parents, number of home calls, number of referrals indicating to whom referred, and number of meetings with parent groups. The Task Force Report on Data Collection and Information Systems (1973) includes an outline for data collection systems. This form includes data concerning the program such as current case load, waiting list, and child-clinician ratio. Keeping such records is particularly important in these days of accountability, and they should be kept in a systematized, organized fashion so that outsiders can interpret them readily.

Facilities. Space in schools is increasingly hard to find. Because of the demand for space, clinicians may find themselves in nurses' outer offices, under stairwells, in locker rooms, and, more fortunately, in well-equipped, especially planned "speech rooms." When clinicians are asked to plan such a room for a new building, they may wish to put in writing their needed facilities. A committee of ASHA has listed room requirements, including lighting, heating, ventilation, necessary furniture, storage facilities, and equipment in the April, 1969, issue of *ASHA* (*ASHA* 1969).

Competencies of Speech Clinicians. All of the duties mentioned previously point to the need of general effectiveness of the speech clinician. We assume that all clinicians will have solid academic backgrounds in human development, including knowledge about language acquisition and its relationship to the normal development of children, in the areas of language and language behavior—an understanding of the ana-tomical, physiological, acoustic, psychological, and linguistic para-meters underlying linguistic competence and performance; in the theory of the causes, diagnosis, and treatment of the various types of speech, hearing, and language disorders; and in the current philosophies, curricula, and organizations of the public schools. With this assumption, we present the following list of competencies for the public school clinician.

1. To identify accurately and efficiently those individuals who exhibit disorders of speech, language, and/or hearing.
2. To plan a program of remediation for each individual.
3. To carry through this program effectively, modifying the speech and language behavior of these children.
4. To evaluate in an organized fashion the effectiveness of the program.
5. To plan and supervise the activities of the aide or aides that the school assigns.
6. To serve as a resource teacher for the classroom teacher for stimulating language development and for the learning dis-abilities specialist in the prevention and intervention of language disorders.
7. To interpret a child's speech problem for his parents.
8. To function usefully as a member of the learning disabilities team and to determine the nature, etiology, and severity of the specific handicaps of those children with language handicaps.
9. To program one's own continual professional growth through

association activities, attendance at summer schools, and reading.

10. To distinguish between language differences such as dialectal speech and language disorders.
11. To measure results of one's own speech, language, and/or hearing strategies in the treatment of these disorders.
12. To measure data collected from the program against other published data.

PSYCHOLOGIST

The psychologist helps the teacher, the clinician, and the parents to understand the child. The results of the testing program may help all three in handling the child. For example, in one case a psychometric test showed a child to be far brighter than the teacher, clinician, or parents had thought. In another case, the administration of the Children's Thematic Apperception Test revealed a definite adjustment difficulty for the child. Because of the information and advice given by the psychologist, both the teacher and the clinician were able to treat these children more wisely.

In still another case, the counseling services of the psychologist were of inestimable value. A stutterer was determined to become a lawyer. The choice definitely appeared to be his own. But the psychologist discovered in talking with him that the choice was really his grandfather's. The boy was deeply interested in science and mathematics. As a result of conferences with the psychologist and the boy's parents, the boy changed his high school major from social science to science and mathematics. The pressure to major and to do well in social studies, about which he was not enthusiastic, was removed.

A mother and father, both college graduates, set high academic standards for their boy—who was struggling through an academic high school course. The psychologist helped the parents to understand their son and his academic problems—and in the process to better understand themselves. The boy is now doing very well in a general course. He spent some of his free time selling Christmas cards, which until recently was a forbidden activity. The suggestions and advice of the psychologist are particularly helpful in the adjustment of children such as these.

The psychologist's services may be of a more general nature. The problem may be one of social adjustment. Some children with speech difficulties need help in becoming a vital part of a group. According to a study by Marge (1966), sociometric results have indicated that there is a trend for the speech-handicapped child to hold a lower social position than that of the normal-speaking child in certain social interpersonal relationships. In the areas of study and work activity and of desirability as a dinner guest, the speech-handicapped child has a significantly lower social position than his normal-speaking peers.

MEDICAL PERSONNEL

When a speech defect is the result of an organic or psychological difficulty, the health authorities contribute to solving the speech problem by arranging for appropriate medical treatment. They talk the health problem over with the parents and frequently refer the child to medical specialists. For instance, the nurse's home visits may be the beginning of a sound health program for the child. At times the need for the help of other specialists is obvious. For example, when the results of the audiometric examination reveal a hearing loss, the child is referred to an otologist. The child with a cleft palate will be under the care of an oral or a plastic surgeon and an orthodontist. A stutterer with a serious adjustment difficulty may require psychiatric help. The situation where many specialists work together for the benefit of the child is ideal.

As the specialists work together, an appreciation for and an understanding of the work of the others comes about. Inevitably, some overlapping takes place. The speech clinician, for example, surmises that certain problems of the speech-handicapped child need investigation by the psychiatrist, psychologist, or doctor. The pediatrician, on the other hand, is concerned that a child has developed a stutter and recognizes that the child's speech difficulty needs treatment. The psychologist, in examining the speech-handicapped child, may uncover a deep-seated personality problem that the psychiatrist must handle. Each specialist is learning from those in other fields, and each is primarily interested in helping the child to develop into an effective and well-functioning human being.

AIDES

Aides or paraprofessionals contribute to most school systems. Speech clinicians usually find that aides have added support to speech and hearing programs in that they have done work that frees clinicians for language, speech, and hearing problems that require their special expertise. In almost every instance, aides begin with a training program that varies in length but normally is around two to three weeks. During this time, the aides observe the work in the speech and hearing clinic and are introduced to such areas as public school organization and administration of speech, language, and hearing therapy; the speech and hearing mechanism; disorders of speech, language, and hearing; the evaluation and rehabilitation of these disorders; and the system for recording data. Alpiner, Ogden, and Wiggins (1970, p. 600) report that in one Colorado program, the activities in which aides engaged in order from the greatest percentage of time to the least percentage were

1. Assisting with articulation therapy — 51%
2. Clerical work — 29%
3. Assisting with language therapy — 14%
4. Assisting with hearing therapy — 4%
5. Assisting with rate and rhythm therapy — 1%
6. Professional-family contacts — 1%
7. Assisting with phonation theory — 1%

The activities that an aide could carry on are described for the first three categories. Aides can be helpful in providing opportunities for carry-over of learned, corrected articulatory behavior. For example, while working with a group of three children on (1) initial *s*, (2) initial *l*, and (3) initial *r*, an aide might play a name game with a flannel board filled with cutout boys and girls wherein each child might give a name with his/her sound to one of the cutouts. In a language therapy group, a categorization drill might take place. One child serves as the supermarket departmental head who accepts or rejects products as children place them in the section for canned fruits, for dairy products, for fresh produce, for paper products, or for cleaning products. The aide produces the pictures of the products. There is a wealth of published materials such as the Peabody Language Kit, which can be used for the purposes of reinforcement. A list of houses that publish such materials is included in Chapter 11. Most of these houses will be glad to furnish catalogs with descriptions of such materials.

Accountability. Accountability is a concept that is recently being applied to most programs in a school system. In a program of speech, language, and hearing rehabilitation, this concept has two applications: (1) success of the rehabilitation aspects of the program and (2) the cost of the rehabilitation processes.

The first application is concerned mainly with the number and degree of changes in observable behavior in the speech and language of children enrolled in the program. Most clinicians give pretests and posttests that give them some general information in this area. More specific information is needed. Mager (1962) asks: (1) What is the desired behavior? (2) Under what conditions is it to be performed?

and (3) To what level of proficiency? The last two questions are particularly important in an objective analysis of the success of a program. A lisper is awarded a certificate of excellence because she has demonstrated that she can incorporate a perfect *s* in her conversation in the clinical situation. But at home the lateral lisp almost consistently appears in her conversation. She deserves the certificate for her behavior at the clinic under strict surveillance. But have other conditions been considered? Was there any attempt on the part of the clinician to check her speech behavior outside of the clinic situation? Another lisper no longer protrudes her tongue making a *th* for an *s*. But her *s* is still far from clear. At what level of proficiency is she operating? Clinicians need to determine under what conditions and at what level of proficiency they are performing. Perhaps levels of speech and language proficiency need to be established for each case. Perhaps the conditions for the desired behavior need to be defined.

Second, for clinicians to assess the cost of expenditure per pupils is important. Work et al. (1975) found after a cost accounting analysis that their program was less expensive than anticipated and less expensive than most clinic or private therapy programs. The authors of this article provide a model for establishing the program costs of services provided by an itinerant speech therapy staff. The population they worked with included 3,872 children with communication disorders and 35 staff clinicians. Their cost accounting model includes both direct costs such as salaries, fringe benefits, travel expenses, therapy equipment, office and storage equipment, office supplies, therapy materials, and indirect costs. The indirect costs include costs for regular school district administration, clerical and custodial services, and physical facilities needed for the support of the itinerant speech and language staff. To determine the total indirect costs for the itinerant program, the program costs for all supporting personnel services and physical facilities (including maintenance) were itemized, an estimate of the relevant time and usage was made, and the percentages of the total estimates were established for each category.

Problems

1. Outline the help your state provides for programs for language-, speech-, and hearing-handicapped children. How does this help compare with that of one of your neighboring states?

2. Indicate the general organization of the services for the language-, speech- and hearing-handicapped children in your town. What do you think can be done to improve them?

3. What are the certification requirements for a school language-, speech-, and hearing-clinician in your state? How do they compare with the requirements in one of your neighboring states?

4. Compare the competencies needed by the language and speech clinician with those you believe the classroom teacher requires.

5. Attend a section of an educational meeting having to do with children needing services from a speech, language, or reading specialist. Indicate how the concepts discussed in this meeting could further your education in the area.

6. Using as a base an article in *Elementary English*, *Reading Teacher*, or a language arts test, describe one strategy for reinforcing language remediation by a classroom teacher.

References and Suggested Readings

Ainsworth, S., "The Speech Clinician in Public Schools: 'Participant' or 'Separatist'?" *ASHA*, **7** (December 1965), 495–503. (Explains point of view of speech clinician, his responsibilities to the schools, professional responsibilities, and implications for training.)

Allen, E. Y., et al., "Case Selection in the Public Schools." *Journal of Speech and Hearing Disorders*, **31** (May 1966), 157–161. (A group of authorities answer two questions: "What guidelines do you use in determining which children to enroll?" and "What tests of articulation have you found appropriate and predictive for children in primary grades?")

Alpiner, J. G., J. A. Ogden, and J. E. Wiggins, "The Utilization of Supportive Personnel in Speech Correction in the Public Schools: A Pilot Project, *ASHA*, **12** (December 1970), 599–604. (Describes the utilization of aides in the public school speech therapy program.)

American Speech and Hearing Association, "ASHA Membership Reaches 20,000," *ASHA*, **17** (June 1975), 413–414.

———, "Meeting the Needs of Children and Adults with Disorders of Language: The Role of the Speech Pathologist and Audiologist, "*ASHA*, **17** (April 1975), 273–278.

———, "Public School Speech and Hearing Services," *Journal of Speech and Hearing Disorders*, Monograph Supplement **8** (July 1961.)

———, "The Speech Clinician's Role in the Public Schools," *ASHA*, **6** (June 1964), 189–191. (Details the functions and responsibilities of the speech clinician in the school setting.)

———, "Recommendations for Housing of Speech Services in the Schools, *ASHA*, **11** (April 1969), 181–182. (Describes room, equipment, furniture and storage space for the speech correction room.)

Anderson, J. L., "Status of Supervision of Speech, Hearing, and Language Programs in the Schools," *Language, Speech, and Hearing Services in Schools*, **3** (January 1972), 12–21.

———, "Supervision of School Speech, Hearing, and Language Programs— An Emerging Role," *ASHA*, **16** (January 1974), 7–10.

Andrews, J. R., "Applying Principles of Instructional Technology in Evaluating Speech and Language Services," *Language, Speech, and Hearing Services in Schools*, **4** (April 1973), 66–71. (Includes five questions that apply to the evaluation of speech and language therapy.)

Beckman, D. A., "Role of the Elementary-School Speech Therapist," *Today's Speech*, **14** (February 1966), 2–4.

Black, M. E., "The Origins and Status of Speech Therapy in the Schools," *ASHA*, **8** (November 1966), 419–425.

Bown, J. C., "The Communication Disorders Specialist as a Support Team Member of a Resource Program," *Language, Speech, and Hearing Services in Schools*, **4** (April 1973), 77–85.

———, "The Expanding Responsibilities of the Speech and Hearing Clinician in the Public Schools," *Journal of Speech and Hearing Disorders*, **36** (November 1971), 538–542. (Examines the boundaries separating the speech and hearing clinician from the resource teacher, the learning disabilities teacher, and the remedial reading teacher, and the duplication of services by this group.)

Caster, J. A., "Teacher: An Ally to the Clinician Serving Retarded Pupils," *Language, Speech, and Hearing Services in Schools*, **4** (January 1973), 41–44.

Causey, L. M., K. O. Johnson, and W. C. Healey, "A Survey of State Certification Requirements for Public School Speech Clinicians," *ASHA*, **13** (March 1971), 123–129.

Crabtree, M., and E. Peterson, "The Speech Pathologist As a Resource Teacher for Language Learning Disabilities," *Language, Speech, and Hearing Services in Schools*, **5** (October 1974), 194–197. (Gives a case study of a child whose language strategies were carried out by a speech pathologist serving as a resource teacher.)

Dopheide, W. R., and J. R. Dallinger, "Improving Remedial Speech and Language Service Through Clinician-Teacher In-Service Interaction," *Language, Speech, and Hearing Services in Schools*, **6** (October 1975), 196–205.

Galloway, H. F., and C. M. Blue, "Paraprofessional Personnel in Articulation Therapy," *Language, Speech, and Hearing Services in Schools*, **6** (July 1975), 125–130. (Describes a three-year project in which paraprofessionals were trained to administer programmed materials in first- through fifth-grade students with articulatory errors.)

Glick, M. J., J. K. Ueberle, and C. E. George, "ESEA Title III Project Design for Language-Handicapped Kindergarten and Preschool Children," *Language, Speech, and Hearing Services in Schools*, **4** (October 1973), 174–181. (Describes screening and evaluation practices for language handicapped.)

Healey, W. C., Coordinator, "Position Statement of the American Speech and Hearing Association on Learning Disabilities," *ASHA*, **18** (May 1976), 282–290. (Includes material on definition of a learning disability, the preparation of speech pathologists for servicing learning disabled children, the roles and responsibilities of speech pathologists engaged in the treatment of learning disabled children, and designs for services for learning disabled children.)

Irwin, R. B., "Speech Therapy in the Public Schools: State Legislation and Certification," *Journal of Speech and Hearing Disorders*, **24** (May 1959), 127–143. (Reviews state legislation and certification requirements for speech therapists in each state.)

Jones, S. A., "The Role of the Public School Speech Clinician with the Inner-City Child," *Language, Speech, and Hearing Services in Schools*, **3** (April 1972), 20–29. (Advocates that clinicians become involved in the total educational system.)

Knight, N. F., "Structuring Remediation in a Self-Contained Classroom," *Language, Speech, and Hearing Services in Schools*, **5** (October 1974), 198–203. (Indicates five basic language skills that need to be covered.)

Mager, R. E., *Preparing Instructional Objectives*, Palo Alto, Calif.: Fearon Publishers, Inc., 1962.

Mowrer, D. E., "Accountability and Speech Therapy in the Public Schools," *ASHA*, **14** (March 1972), 111–115.

———, "What the Speech Clinician Should Know About School Money," *Language, Speech, and Hearing Services in Schools*, **6** (October 1975), 217–222. (Gives the results of a survey of 70 clinicians' knowledge of school budgets.)

Neal, W. R., "Speech Pathology Services in the Secondary Schools," *Language, Speech, and Hearing Services in Schools*, **7** (January 1976), 6–16.

O'Neill, J. J., "The Possible Role and Position of Speech Pathology and Audiology in Regard to Language, Learning Disabilities, and the Hearing Impaired," *ASHA*, **13** (February 1971), 51–52.

O'Toole, T. J., and E. L. Zaslow, "Public School Speech and Hearing Programs: Things Are Changing," *ASHA*, **11** (November 1969), 499–501.

Pannbacker, M., "Diagnostic Report Writing," *Journal of Speech and Hearing Disorders*, **40** (August 1975), 367–379. (Reviews purposes and types of diagnostic reports and provides guidelines for report writing.)

Potter, R. E., "Perhaps We Have Been in This Business of Specific Learning Disabilities Longer Than We Know," *Language, Speech, and Hearing Services in Schools*, **4** (April 1973), 86–89. (Defines a learning disability and shows the overlap of the work of the specialist in this area with the work of the speech clinician.)

Prahl, H. M., and E. B. Cooper, "Accuracy of Teacher Referrals of Speech-Handicapped School Children," *ASHA*, **6** (October 1964), 392.

Pronovost, W., "Case Selection in the Schools: Articulatory Disorders," *ASHA*, **8** (May 1966), 179–181.

Rees, M., E. L. Herbert, and N. H. Coates, "Development of a Standard Case Form," *Journal of Speech and Hearing Disorders*, **34** (February 1969), 68–80. (Suggests the minimal information that would give a common body of information for all receiving school speech and hearing clinical help. Contains a simple form.)

Robertson, M. L., and G. C. Freeman, "Applying Diagnostic Information to Decisions About Placement and Treatment," *Language, Speech, and*

Hearing Services in Schools, **5** (October 1974), 187–193. (Discusses the role of the speech pathologist on the school team, his/her needed competencies in his/her role in language evaluation, and formulation of the language aspects of the child's educational program.)

Schubert, G. W., "Suggested Minimal Requirements for Clinical Supervisors," *ASHA*, **16** (June 1974), 305.

Shearer, W. M., "Diagnoses and Treatment of Voice Disorders in School Children," *Journal of Speech and Hearing Disorders*, **37** (May 1972), 215–221. (Gives results of a team approach by a speech pathologist, a laryngologist, and a school psychologist.)

Sommers, R. K., et al., "Effectiveness of Group and Individual Therapy," *Journal of Speech and Hearing Research*, **9** (June 1966), 219–225.

Task Force Report, "Task Force Report on Data Collection and Information Systems," *Language, Speech, and Hearing Services in Schools*, **4** (April 1973), 57–65.

———, "Task Force Report on School Speech, Hearing, and Language Screening Procedures," *Language, Speech, and Hearing Services in Schools*, **4** (July 1973), 109–117.

———, "Task Force Report on Traditional Scheduling Procedures in Schools," *Language, Speech, and Hearing Services in Schools*, **4** (July 1973), 101–109. (Discusses ways of scheduling cases in schools.)

———, "Task Force Report on Supervision in the Schools," *Language, Speech, and Hearing Services in Schools*, **3** (July 1972), 4–16.

Van Hattum, R. J., "The Defensive Speech Clinicians in the Schools," *Journal of Speech and Hearing Disorders*, **31** (August 1966), 234–240. (Talks about the basic issues in training the school speech clinician and suggests solutions.)

———, "Services of the Speech Clinician in Schools: Progress and Prospects," *ASHA*, **18** (February 1976), 59–63. (Discusses the changing role of the speech clinician in the schools with less emphasis on articulatory difficulties and more on language and with the clinician's contribution to the learning disabled professional team.)

Van Riper, C., "Success and Failure in Speech Therapy," *Journal of Speech and Hearing Disorders*, **31** (August 1966), 276–278. (Suggests that the therapist ask two questions, "What is it that this person needs?" and "What is it that he needs from me?")

Webster, E. J., "Parent Counseling by Speech Pathologists and Audiologists," *Journal of Speech and Hearing Disorders*, **31** (November 1966), 331–340. (Tells how to help parents modify the circle of poor communication with their children.)

———, W. H. Perkins, H. H. Bloomer, and W. Pronovost, "Case Selection in the Schools," *Journal of Speech and Hearing Disorders*, **31** (November 1966), 352–358. (Helps to develop criteria for choosing children who need speech correction services.)

Weiner, P. S., "The Emotionally Disturbed Child in the Speech Clinic: Some Considerations," *Journal of Speech and Hearing Disorders*, **33** (May

1968), 158–166. (Discusses the problem of whether the emotionally disturbed child should be accepted in a speech clinic.)

Weston, A. J., and S. K. Harber, "The Effects of Scheduling on Progress in Paired-Stimuli Articulation Therapy," *Language, Speech, and Hearing Services in Schools*, **6** (April 1975), 96–101. (Contrasts traditional and block systems of scheduling.)

Wing, D. M., "A Data Recording Form for Case Management and Accountability," *Language, Speech, and Hearing Services in Schools*, **6** (January 1975), 38–40. (Includes a data recording form for speech and hearing services.)

Wingo, J. W., "Student Speech and Hearing 'Teams' in the Public Schools," *ASHA*, **12** (December 1970), 605–606.

Work, R. S., et al., "Acountability in a School Speech and Language Program," *Language, Speech, and Hearing Services in Schools*, **6** (January 1975), 7–13. (Evaluates aspects of a school district's speech and language program: cost accounting, instructional materials analysis, and service effectiveness.)

3. Standards of Speech

The following scenes represent a variety of reactions to particular speech patterns:

Scene 1. Front porch of a large, white house.

YOUNG MAN, A PH.D., SON OF A COLLEGE PROFESSOR (*to a black cat*): Youz a beautiful kitty-cat.

FRIEND OF HIS FATHER'S: *Youz*! Ugh!

Scene 2. A reception room in a college dormitory.

HANDSOME SENIOR (*to his friend*): I say you're wrong again. (*again* rhyming with *rain*.)

FRESHMAN (*not so handsome*): Dumb guy—clothes, hair, walk, and *again*!

Scene 3. A train.

CONDUCTOR (*calling loudly*): Silver Creek. (Rhyming with *brick*.)

PASSENGER: Someone should tell him it's *Creek*. (Ryhming with *meek*.)

Scene 4. At the side of a large, comfortable house.

EIGHT-YEAR-OLD BLACK GIRL (*to her black friend*): I'll axe Mom for fifty cent.

MOTHER: Don't axe me for fifty cent; ask me for fifty cents!

In all four instances, the emotion of the tone and the inflection with which the comments are uttered are easy to identify but difficult to understand. If the young man feels good about saying *Youz* to the cat and if, in turn, the cat feels good about this salutation, why not?

46

Surely this young man would not say *Youz* to his research assistant. If the second young man has somewhere picked up his particular pronunciation of *again*, why not? If the conductor calls *Silver Crick*, fine. In the United States as a whole, his *crick* is used as commonly as the passenger's *creak*. The small black girl, communicating to a peer, could just as easily have said, "I'll ask Mom for fifty cents" but, like Martin Luther King, Jr., she uses one of two dialects depending upon the circumstances. Sometimes she combines the two dialects as she did here.

The amount of interest and even of emotion generated by the pronunciation and syntactic differences in such instances as these far outweigh their importance in communication. If we were teaching actors to read the lines in these four scenes, what motivations would they ascribe to the four speakers who did the commenting? Perhaps the first commentator would add these words to the script: *with some condescension*; the second, *with derision*; the third, *with ill-concealed superiority*; and the mother, *with annoyance*. This mother may not want her child ever to use any aspect of Black English dialect, regardless of the circumstances.

In the first place, such interest in pronunciation and in syntax arises partly because these aspects of spoken language are perceived as social skills. Educated, cultured speakers tend to sound alike, to communicate with many of the same speech patterns. Admittedly, their patterns do vary somewhat as they come from different regions, but the similarity of their speech patterns outweighs the differences. Dictionaries reflect this concept. For instance, *The Random House Dictionary of the English Language* (The Unabridged Edition 1966) contains these two definitions:

Standard English. The English language as written and spoken by literate people in both formal and informal usage, and that is universally current while incorporating regional differences (p. 1385).

Nonstandard English. Differing in usage from the speech or writing of those whose language is generally considered to be correct or preferred (p. 981).

In the second place, the emotional attitudes represented in the comments reflect one of the characteristics of language—that it is closely related to self. Our language is part of us and part of our family heritage. When a teacher criticizes children's language, they may feel rejected both for themselves and for their families. Many teachers believe that children who apply sets of "incorrect" pronunciation or grammatical rules must be brought into line. Their way of bringing the children into line may be humane and compassionate but negative feelings may still persist.

When teachers put the emphasis on clear communication of meaning and feeling to a particular audience, the situation is conducive to good feelings, to clear expression and reception of ideas, and frequently to the acquisition of Standard English. The understanding and feelings that are expressed and received must represent accurately the intentions of the speaker. Edwin Newman in *Strictly Speaking* (1974, p. 6) exemplifies this notion:

> Harry Truman used to say *irrevelant* and stress the third syllable in *comparable*. But Mr. Truman never had any trouble getting his points across.

Newman also observes:

> As a veteran, I was in an army hospital in 1947, and a fellow patient asked me what another patient did for a living. I said he was a teacher. "Oh," was the reply, "Them is my chief dread." A lifetime was summed up in those six syllables. There is no way to improve on that.

On the other hand, Newman pokes fun at such blocks to communication as *Y'know*. He says

> Some people collapse into *y'know* after giving up trying to say what they mean. Others scatter it broadside, these, I suspect being for some reason embarrassed by a silence of any duration during which they might be suspected of thinking what they are going to say next (p. 14).

Similarly, he ridicules with humor pompous, ponderous, lengthy, complex statements with many circumlocutions.

What Standards of Speech for the Classroom?

Every young child develops language to express ideas and feelings, using whatever language feels most comfortable. In a few instances, the young child's language necessarily may be almost entirely pantomimic. But it is better to communicate through gesture than not to communicate at all. Eventually the child can be weaned from pantomimic language to spoken language. In other instances, the child's language may possess many nonstandard features. In still others, it may represent the prestigious dialect of the community. Regardless of dialect, young children must first speak in sentences to develop their particular linguistic potential; furthermore, in their early years, they do better with their native tongue than with a superimposed one.

We believe, however, that at some point children must be able to read, speak, and write Standard English if they are eventually to succeed in school, in most jobs, and in almost all professions. They may, of course, later wish to pursue a life-style outside of the middle- and upper-class milieu. But the school should provide boys and girls with the tools to cope with the demands of education in elementary school, high school, and college, in certain vocations, and in most, if not all, professions. Thus, this concept conflicts with the one that children should communicate each as an individual in a dialect of choice that may well have a code and structure all its own and that fundamentally has as much right to attention as any other dialect.

Admittedly, some educators and some linguists, believing that teachers should not confuse the middle-class social stigma of a particular dialect with its linguistic capacities as a linguistic tool, are not concerned with presenting children with the option of learning the "prestigious" dialect. They consider the sum total of dialectal variations as self-contained, systematic, ordered systems that are different from but neither communicatively more or less effective than Standard English. They believe that a nonstandard dialectal system with its logical and consistent rules is an effective code for expressing ideas and concepts. Most educators today recognize that a Black English dialect is a viable tool for communication, that a speaker can use it to communicate abstractions on any level, and also that it is based on a variant of the linguistic system that is recognized as Standard American English. As communication is needed, language develops.

Whenever speakers of different languages are thrown together through business, war—or in earlier days at slave stations—they devise a language for the necessary communication, a contact language or pidgin. African pidgin was one language of this type. The Portuguese in their travels and conquests established pidgins around the world. A pidgin is a nonnative shared language resulting from intersocietal rather than intrasocietal contacts. Occasionally, when the need for communication disappears so does the need for the pidgin. In such cases, the pidgin may be learned as a native language and the process of creolization begins; consequently Creole then evolves like any other language (Bolinger 1975, p. 356).

Bailey advocates that teachers understand the creolization processes:

> Specialists in Creole linguistics believe that the verb system of the Negro speakers of non-Standard English is much more like that of the English-based Creoles than of Standard English, and that unless teachers understand that this is a valid system with its own grammatical rules, they cannot intelligently guide the children into an acquisition of the new system that is so much like their own that the possibility of linguistic

interferences increases at every turn. The Creole languages express the possessive relationship, the number distinction in nouns and verbs, the past tense in verbs, and the cases of pronouns by different means from the Indo-European languages, in which such relationships are indicated by suffixation of some kind. Grammatical relations in the Creoles are largely expressed by juxtaposition of words, by the aid of special function words, or by the stress and pitch patterns (Bailey 1968, p. 573).

We believe that language and culture are entwined. If in Hawaii, pidgin is part of an individual's culture and of his image of himself, it should not be ridiculed but accepted. However, it should be possible to learn Standard English as part of another culture. We believe that the child must learn first to communicate in his native born dialect. The kindergartner who omits the final *t* and *d* for the past tense in *I like her* for *I liked her* and *I lug the box* for *I lugged the box* is using a morphological system that is different from those of children speaking Standard American English. It is important for the teacher to accept this as one mode of communication but, at some point, the child must build a second mode of communication, for a nonprestigious social dialect in a local community can be a handicap. A candidate for district attorney who says "tooim" and "dis" and "dat" detracts from his "source image" or "ethical appeal" with some of his audience even though what he says may have real and significant import to the community.

When Do We Teach Classroom Standard Speech?

Having stated our position that at some point the teacher teach Standard English or the "prestigious dialect" as a second mode of communication, the question arises: When? Loban suggests that children start learning standard English during the third grade:

> The strategy is merely that the pre-school stage and kindergarten are much too early to press him to be concerned about using Standard dialect continuously. Such teaching only confuses small children, causing them to speak much less frequently in school. Usually from grade three and after, the children's daily recitation should adhere to standard English, but in the early years the teacher would accept "him a good dog." At this stage the teacher would be more interested in eliciting from the child, "him a good dog but with three fleas"; indeed, the teacher would be very much interested in such qualification and amplification (Loban 1968, p. 595).

Loban further talks about when to begin the discussion of social language discrimination:

> Eventually the time comes when the teacher must talk over with these pupils the facts of social language discrimination, and that time, to my way of thinking, usually is grade five, six, or seven. Teachers differ on the ideal age for introducing the concept, but I see no point in telling children this earlier. Before they can really see the value of learning standard English, pupils need to understand the social consequences the world will exact of them if they cannot handle the established dialect. Grade five, six, or seven, therefore, would be the point at which the concept would be discussed, although parts of the total concept might be sketched in earlier as answers to questions children ask. At this grade level I would select most carefully teachers who do not have snobbish attitudes about language, the scholar-linguist-humanists whom the school could most safely entrust with the important task of explaining sociological truth to these children, aged 11 and 12 (Loban 1968, p. 519).

How Do We Teach Standard Classroom Speech?

Having indicated *when* we would begin teaching Standard English, we now need to be concerned with *how*. The base of literacy is the child's existing language and the ability to use it proficiently and effectively. The first important principle in establishing the base combines two concepts: (1) Teachers speak in manners that are natural to them; they do not need to speak in the local dialect even when most of the children use it, and (2) Teachers understand and accept the children's particular dialects. The class may contain children with a variety of dialects: those coming from foreign countries and having a definite "foreign accent," those speaking Black English; those speaking little or no English; those speaking non-Standard English; those speaking Standard English. The second important principle is that the child be permitted, even encouraged, to respond to what he/she has read or experienced in his/her own language. The third principle is that as much of the curriculum as possible be experientially based. Our own preference would be that reading be taught through language experience. This strategy utilizes the child's own language patterns naturally reflecting the phonology, morphology, syntax, and grammar of native speech. The experiences in the class should be those that will expose the children to vocabularies they do not already possess, to more complicated sentence structure, to Standard English, and to experiences that will encourage talk.

RECEPTIVE LANGUAGE ABILITIES OF INNER-CITY CHILDREN

Current research seems to indicate that upon entrance to school, inner-city children are able to comprehend the Standard English of the teacher even though this dialect is different from their own. We have selected some recent reports of research that support this thesis: Quay (1971) tested 100 black four-year-olds with the Stanford-Binet Test using (1) Standard English and (2) Negro dialect and found no reliable difference in the two modes of expression. Levy and Cook (1973) studied the relationship between dialect proficiency in Standard and in Black non-Standard English and auditory comprehension of stories presented in Black non-Standard and Standard English. The subjects, 32 black second-grade boys and girls, did consistently better on performance based on stories that were told in Standard English. Similarly, Ramsey (1972) found no significant difference in the ability of first-grade Negro dialect speakers to answer literal comprehension questions about stories presented orally in Standard English and in Black non-Standard English. Again, Frentz (1971) found no relationship between the dialect of third-grade users and the comprehension of sentences presented orally in the two dialects.

This research has to do with the receptive aspects of language that precedes production aspects. In other words, young children understand many facets of the language before they are able to produce them. Teachers and clinicians need to understand the differences between the receptive and productive language processes and, in addition, be aware of what young children are listening to and understanding, to be supportive of the children's communicative efforts in their own dialects, and to de-emphasize the production of Standard English. They need to recognize that children may have more language proficiency than they exhibit in talking. Cohen and Kornfield (1970), investigating proficiency in vocabulary of inner-city children for learning to read, found that urban ghetto children possess an oral vocabulary that is similar to the vocabulary demanded by five major reading series.

Factors Involved in Adopting the Language of the School

In helping students to adopt the language of the school, teachers recognize a variety of factors: (1) that words are rarely spoken singly, but are almost always a part of a phrase or sentence and that in this process pronunciations of words change because of the influence of sounds in context; (2) that language is constantly changing; (3) that there are regional differences in speech; (4) that speech styles vary from one communicative situation to another and that the social group of the speaker influences the speaker's patterns; (5) that spelling is frequently not helpful in learning to pronounce words, and (6) that dictionaries, while useful guides, are not wholly dependable when a particular word is to be used in a conversational phrase. These factors are considered in more detail in the following pages.

CONTEXTUAL UTTERANCE

Words, almost never spoken singly, are usually part of a phrase or a sentence. As your friend asks, "Are you going to buy a red or blue dress?" you may respond, "Red." Even here, however, you are likely to respond with, "A red dress" or "I need a red one to match my shoes and purse." Speech moves or flows onward from word to word within a phrase. In onflowing speech contextual influence is always at work and the sounds of syllables of different words may be linked as "Aredress," [ərɛd:rɛs] for *a red dress*. *What is* usually becomes "Whats" or "Wats" [hwɑts] or [wɑts].

Children eat a *napple* [ənæpl] long before they become aware of *an apple*. Part of the change in pronunciation is the result of the influence of adjacent sounds. *Assimilation*, the modification of pronunciation, has usually occurred over the decades in the direction of simplicity and economy of effort. For instance, the past tense of *flip* is *flipped*. The final sound is not a [d] but a [t]. [p] is an unvoiced sound that influences the unvoicing of the sound [d] that follows. [t] is made like [d] except that it is unvoiced. In other verbs where the final sound of the verb in its present tense is voiced, the [d] of the past tense is preserved. For instance, the final sound in *begged* is [d] because [g] is a voiced sound; the same is true of plurals. The final sound in *taps* is [s] but in *tabs* is [z]. The [b], which is voiced, influences the [s] to become [z]. *Captain* sometimes becomes *Capm* [kæpm̩]. [p] is made with both lips and this position influences [n] to become [m]. But the nasal characteristic of the [n] is maintained. [t] is dropped entirely, however. In *horseshoe* [s], too, is completely lost; [ʃ] takes over [s].

Some assimilations are widely used; others are not. *Nature* and *picture* are commonly pronounced *nacher* [netʃɚ] and *pikcher* [pɪktʃɚ]. Almost all of us take these pronunciations with their assimilations for granted. Almost none of us attempt to say *natyer* [netjɚ] or *pictyer* [pɪktjɚ]. The same kind of change occurs when we say *wonchu* [wontʃə] for *won't you* [wontju]. Some persons are loathe to accept the assimilation in *wonchu* although they themselves use the same kind of assimilation in *nature*.

Assimilation is illustrated by what has occurred in derivatives of words with the Latin prefix *cum*. The [m] remains in *complicate* and *comfort*, has become [n] in such words as *conspire* and *consign*, and is *ng* [ŋ] in such words as *congregate* and *conquer*. In *complicate* and *comfort*, [m], [p] and [f] all involve the lips. In *conspire*, *consign*, and *contain*, [n], [s], and [t], all involve the tip of the tongue and the gum or alveolar ridge. In *congregate* [ˈkɑŋgrɪˌget] and *conquer* [ˈkɑŋˌkɚ], the *ng* [ŋ], [k], and [g] all involve the back of the tongue and the soft palate. *Dissimilation* is a change where a sound is dropped or changed from the original to make it less like its neighbor. Making two identical or closely similar articulatory movements within a brief time span proves difficult; therefore, to omit or change the sound is easier. The word *turtle* is the result of the change of the final *r* in the original *turture* to *l*. A present-day example is the loss of the first *r* in *library* or in *February*.

Another example of change in onflowing speech is the use of *weak* rather than *strong* forms. The following are examples: When we read the word *to* in a list of words, we pronounce it as *two* or *too*. But when we read *to* in the sentence, "I want to do it," the vowel in *to* is no longer a long o͞o but a short o̅o̅ or even the schwa [ə], the sound in the last syllable of *sofa*. The *to* pronounce like *two* is the strong form, whereas the *to* pronounced like [tə] is the weak form. When we say, "We live in Apartment 2A," we pronounce the *a* to rhyme with *day*. But when we say, "We live in a house," the *a* is the same sound as we use in the last syllable of *sofa*, the schwa. The *a* that rhymes with *day* is the strong form; the one that is the schwa is the weak form. The *a* in *and* in a list of words is pronounced with a short *a*, but the *a* of *and* in the phrase *Mary and John* is likely to be the schwa. The first *a* is the strong form; the second *a*, the weak form. Ordinarily we use the weak forms of pronouns, prepositions, articles, auxiliaries, and conjunctions in conversation, except where we stress a particular word. For example, when we want to stress that *both* Mary and John are going, we may use the strong form of *and*. In strong forms, the vowel is stressed; in weak forms it is unstressed.

CHANGES IN LANGUAGE

Styles of pronunciation change. Many of these changes are obvious. We do not pronounce the *k* in *know, knight*, and *knee*. These words began to lose their *k* sound in the seventeenth century and completed the loss in the eighteenth century. *K* does remain the Germanized pronunciation of such proper names as *Knag* or *Knode*. The seventeenth-century poet Alexander Pope rhymed *join* with *thine*. We know that *join* was then pronounced *jine* [dʒaɪn]. Furthermore, he rhymed *obey* with *tea*. *Tea* was then pronounced *tay* [teɪ]. Changes may occur in the pronunciations within families from one generation to the next. A father and mother may say *erster* [ɜrstɚ] for *oyster* and *boin* [bɒɪn] for *burn*. Their daughter, however, pronounces *oyster* and *burn* the way most of the rest of us do. Here some outside influence, perhaps that of the child's playmates or her teachers, brings about the change.

REGIONAL DIFFERENCES

We have spoken about "prestigious" pronunciations and have indicated that pronunciations, voice, and vocabulary differ in varying speech situations. We have talked about the influence of particular social cultures and subcultures. Another difference exists—that of region. Kenneth Goodman points out that socially acceptable speech varies from region to region and that no dialect of American English has ever achieved the status of some imaginary standard that is correct everywhere and always. He writes:

> It is obvious that a teacher in Atlanta, Georgia, is foolish to try to get her children to speak like cultured people in Detroit or Chicago . . . cultured speech, socially preferred, is not the same in Boston, New York, Philadelphia, Miami, Baltimore, Atlanta, or Chicago. The problem, if any, comes when the Bostonian moves to Chicago, the New Yorker to Los Angeles, the Atlantan to Detroit. Americans are ethnocentric in regard to most cultural traits, but they are doubly so with regard to language. Anybody who doesn't speak the way I do is wrong. A green onion is not a scallion. I live in Detróit not Détroit. I can carry my books to work but not my friends. *Fear* ends with an *r* and *Cuba* does not. Such ethnocentrisms are unfortunate among the general public (Goodman 1967, p. 41).

The educated person from Boston has little difficulty understanding the educated person from Atlanta. The backwoodsman from Minnesota with little education may, however, have difficulty understanding the mountaineer from Tennessee with little education. Differences in speech among the educated are not as wide as those among the uneducated, even though admittedly there are discernible differences in the speech patterns of educated persons of different areas.

The differences among the areas are, however, not too numerous. A New Englander and a Southerner may say *bahn* for *barn*, whereas an Ohioan is likely to pronounce the *r* in the same word. A New

Englander approaches *pahth* for *path*. The Ohioan is likely to use the same vowel in *path* that he uses in *cat*. In the South the *o* in *glory* is usually the same *o* as in *tote*; whereas in some other regions, it may be the *aw* sound in *law*. The vowel in the word *scarce* in the North Central and Eastern areas may be either the vowel found in *hate* or the one in *let*; in the South, for the word *scarce* the vowel in *hat* is heard frequently. In *greasy* and the verb *grease*, the New Englander uses the *s* sound whereas the Southerner uses the *z* sound.

Regional dialect is no real problem for the teacher or for the clinician except when either tries to impose on students an articulatory distinction that is uncommon in the community. Tabbert (1974) notes that such a problem can exist when teachers are using the phonics approach to reading. He cites the example of *knotty* and *naughty* wherein some speakers make no distinction between the vowel sounds in these two words and wherein the resulting sound is a vowel usually made somewhere between the *ah* and *aw* positions, further back in the mouth than *aw* with less lip rounding than *ah*. He indicates that in the *Palo Alto Reading Program* by Theodore E. Glim (New York: Harcourt Brace Jovanovich, Inc., 1968) and in books 3, 4, and 5 of the Roberts English Series: *A Linguistics Program* (New York: Harcourt Brace Jovanovich, Inc., 1970), the *ah* and *aw* phonemes are represented as distinct. Even though in the latter series teachers are forewarned that some Americans have merged the two vowels, they are not given suggestions on how these regional pronunciations should make differences in the use of materials.

When teachers consider regional differences as pronunciation errors and try to correct the pronunciations, they find themselves in trouble. In the first place, the children will have difficulty in differentiating the two sounds themselves and, in the second place, they will not be hearing the differentiation in the community in which they live. The teachers themselves may not make the distinctions except in the classroom and even there, they may be inconsistent. Teachers must accept such regional differences, for no single standard of pronunciation exists in North America.

INFLUENCE OF SPELLING ON PRONUNCIATION

Until the fifteenth or sixteenth century spelling, changing frequently, kept pace with changes in pronunciation. As we look at the following extract from the Prologue to *The Canterbury Tales*, we realize how different our spelling is today. This excerpt is representative of Middle English.

THE PRIORESSE:

Ther was also a nonne, a Prioresse,
That of hir smylyng was ful symple and coy;
Hir gretteste ooth was but by Seint Loy;
And she was cleped Madame Eglentyne.
Ful wel she soong the servyce dyvyne,
Entuned in hir nose ful semely, ...

For the last 400 or 500 years spelling has remained relatively constant while pronunciations have changed. Spelling today, therefore, does not always approximate the pronunciation of words. For example, the *t* sound in *castle* and *whistle*, the *b* sound in *limb* and *comb*, the *w* sound in *write*, the *s* sound in *island*, and the *l* sound in *calm* are not pronounced. The *i* [I] sound is variously spelled as *o* in *women*, *y* in *myth*, and *i* in *linen*.

The discrepancy between sound and spelling has caused some persons to ask that the writing conform to the sounds. Thus, over the years, many attempts have been made to change spelling to reflect the spoken word. Before George Bernard Shaw died, he specified in his will that a considerable sum of money be used for spelling reform. Such systems are frequently proposed, then abandoned. The same discrepancy has caused others to try to make the sound conform to the spelling. Some people today try to pronounce both *p* and *b* in *cupboard* and all the sounds in *indict*. Although the *t* in *often* was dropped, it is creeping back. The same is true of the *l* in *almond*. Some of our American pronunciations as distiguished from British pronunciations show that we have placed some value on spelling. For example, the name *Anthony* in Britain is pronounced with a *t* for the *th* and *secretary* in British English usually has three syllables as compared to our four syllabes.*

INFLUENCE OF DICTIONARIES ON PRONUNCIATION

Long before dictionaries existed, people understood the words that others pronounced. Today, however, lexicographers record pronunciations. One function of the dictionary is to describe the pronunciation of a word, not to dictate or prescribe it. The early lexicographers based their recording of pronunciations not only on the pronunciations of the cultured people of the time, such as statesmen and actors, but also on their own idiosyncracies. Daniel Webster, however, realized that pro-

---

[1] For information on influence of writing on spoken language, see F. W. Householder, *Linguistic Speculation*, Cambridge, England; Cambridge University Press, 1971, ch. 13.

nunciations must be based on the pronunciations of the people. Mencken
says of Webster:

> He was always at great pains to ascertain actual usages and in the course
> of his journeys from State to State to perfect his copyright on his first
> spelling book he accumulated a large amount of interesting and valuable
> material, especially in the field of pronunciation. . . . He proposed there-
> fore that an American standard be set up, independent of the English
> standard, and that it be inculcated in the schools throughout the country.
> He argued that it should be determined not by "the practice of any
> particular class of people," but by "the general practice of the nation..."
> (Mencken 1946, p. 9).

Today, lexicographers try to record accurately the pronunciations
of the educated, cultured members of our country and to keep the
recordings current. They try to inform on the basis of the facts of usage.
When a substantial proportion of the population pronounces a word
in a certain way, they record it.

A pronunciation given in a dictionary is a generalization of the way
many persons say a word. The recording of this generalization differs
from dictionary to dictionary. Dictionaries frequently record more
than one pronunciation. In some instances, the first pronunciation is
the one held to be more widely used; in others, the editor makes no
attempt to show which pronunciation is the more prevalent. At least
one dictionary indicates pronunciations current in regional areas.
Most do not. Some dictionaries record the pronunciations using diacritic markings; others record them with phonetic symbols. Some adopt
for representation the style of formal platform speech; others include
informal pronunciations. Teachers should read the introduction to a
dictionary to learn what its levels and procedures are. They should also
note its date to determine whether the pronunciations recorded are
current.

Dictionaries are useful in assisting us to pronounce unfamiliar words.
When students come across a word such as *esophageal*, the dictionary is an
excellent source of information for pronunciation. But for the usual,
everyday words, students do better to train their ears to listen rather
than to find the pronunciations in the dictionary, for we learn pronunciation largely through imitation. Those desiring to improve their
pronunciations must listen to the speech of the educated, cultivated
members of their communities who have had certain social advantages.
In addition, they must listen to themselves (often with a recorder) so
that they know how their speech differs. If we look up *duty* in the dictionary, we may find the *y* sound before the *u*; however, careful reading of the introduction of the dictionary usually indicates that the word

is pronounced both with and without the *y* sound. Surely to listen and to perceive the differences is more helpful than to use the dictionary. Furthermore, dictionaries give pronunciations of a word as it is used individually. When we speak, however, we rarely speak in single words, but rather in phrases or sentences. The same words used in different phrases with different rhythm, tempo, intonation, and meaning intended by the speaker do not sound alike. For instance, dictionaries usually include the strong forms (stressed ones), not the weak forms (unstressed). The student, whether in elementary or in secondary school, should learn to use the weak forms both in speaking and in reading aloud.

SPEECH STYLES

The particular speaking situation influences the speaker's speech patterns. Joos (1962) notes that people use a wide variety of speech styles—varying from the most intimate to the most formal and that they automatically shift to whatever is appropriate to the social situation. When children play ball in an open field, they speak more loudly than usual, more quickly, often in shorter phrases, and with a quite different choice of language from when they are playing a word game upon which they are concentrating to recall unusual words. As they speak together in the classroom, they are likely to speak more formally, in longer phrases, and be more careful of their pronunciations than they are when they call to each other on the playground. In a school assembly, the child who introduces the speaker speaks still more formally—more slowly, with more stresses, with more careful choice of language. Thus, the continuum goes from very informal speech, often with many nonstandard pronunciations, to formal speech with few nonstandard pronunciations. Labov notes that when subjects in his research answered questions that they formally recognized as part of an interview, their speech was careful. He explains that the situation was not as formal as a public address and was less formal than the speech that would be used in a first interview for a job, but was certainly more formal than casual conversation among friends or family members (Labov 1966, p. 92).

CULTURAL DIFFERENCES

Voice and pronunciation characteristics exist on all kinds of local cultural and subcultural levels. The influence of the social group on both voice and pronunciation is important. When you hear "She roars like a fishwife," you know exactly what the speaker is implying.

Similarly, the influence of the social group on pronunciation is strong. When the child grows up in an environment where all the children say "acrost" [əkrɔst] for *across* and "elem [ɛləm] tree" for *elm tree*, he/she probably uses the same pronunciation.

Improving Pronunciation

The first question is *what* to improve. Teachers are not concerned with regional differences, or with pronunciations that are widely accepted. They are concerned with those characteristics that tend to generate the impression that speech is not prestigious, that it contains many nonstandard pronunciations. These nonstandard deviations, unlike articulatory defects, which are definitely speech difficulties, are not the responsibility of the speech clinician but of the classroom teacher. The ten-year-old boy who substitutes *f* and *v* for the two *th*'s and says *acrost* for *across* is in need of help from the teacher to understand and sometimes to eliminate the nonstandard speech.

NONSTANDARD SPEECH CHARACTERISTICS

Teachers frequently need make but few formal attempts to change nonstandard speech patterns—particularly when the students are participating in communicative situations where there is a kind of standardization of language based on the prestigious dialect of the community. As children and their teachers are thrown together in the classroom, the children's own pronunciations tend to move toward a class standard. Consequently, many of them discard their nonstandard variants. As they share each others' thoughts and feelings in a variety of classroom experiences, their language and speech differences tend to be ironed out.

The guidance of the teacher, however, may be needed in (1) substitution of one sound for another, (2) omission of sounds, (3) addition of sounds, (4) transposition of sounds, and (5) addition of features that are not usually part of a sound.

SUBSTITUTION OF SOUNDS

Nonstandard pronunciation frequently involves the substitution of one sound for another; for example, one consonant may be substituted for another. A common substitution is that of *d* for *th*, as *dem* and *dose* for *them* and *those*. The teacher must remember, however, that many substitutions are made by educated people. For example, many educated speakers pronounce *when*, *where*, and *what* with an initial *w*, though others do use the *wh* sound. Other substitutions frequently used by the educated are *ingcome tax* for *income tax*, *grampa* for *grandpa*, and *pangcake* for *pancake*. The substitution may involve vowels rather than consonants, as when *boyd* is substituted for *bird*. In some areas, this substitution is fast disappearing—perhaps partly because of the humor associated with it. Stories such as the following give a social impetus to drop the substitution:

The child said to the teacher, "Look at the boid on the windowsill."
The teacher remonstrated, "You mean *bird*."
To which the child replied, "Choips like a boid."

Many vowel substitutions are so widely employed that they have become acceptable. *Git* for *get* is heard so frequently that many speakers would not even notice the substitution. Other vowel substitutions are regional. Many Midwesterners use the same vowel in *merry, Mary,* and *marry*. Again these substitutions are so widely used that almost no one would notice them. On the other hand, as *milkman* becomes *mulkman*, as *been* becomes *ben*, the substitution may distract from the message.

OMISSION OF SOUNDS

In informal speech most of us omit many sounds even though they are included in the orthographic representation of the word. For example, the word *clothes* is frequently pronounced *cloz*, omitting the *th* sound. Both the *American College Dictionary* and Webster's *New Collegiate Dictionary* accept these variants. Before a teacher insists on the inclusion of a sound, we recommend consultation of a good, recent dictionary. The following are some of the omissions that probably do not occur in formal speech: *bout* for *about*; *Bufflo* for *Buffalo*; *kunt* for *couldn't*; *ask* for *asked*; *mosly* for *mostly*; *simily* for *similarly*; *reconize* for *recognize*.

ADDITION OF SOUNDS

Sounds are frequently added or inserted. Historically we have added sounds; for instance, *against* was once *agens*. Although dictionaries for years did not recognize the *t* in *often* or the *h* in *forehead*, some dictionaries now include both of these pronunciations. Many speakers pronounce *mince* as if it were *mints* or *dance* as if it were *dants*. The insertion of excrescent [t] makes for easier, more economical pronunciation by all, including the educated. But some additions and insertions are less common in the speech of the educated. Examples of these are *athaletic* for *athletic*; *anywheres* for *anywhere*; *oncet* for *once*; *drownded* for *drowned*; *wisht* for *wish*; *pursh* for *push*.

TRANSPOSITION OF SOUNDS

Children frequently and adults sometimes transpose sounds. Most of us have heard a child ask for psighetti (spaghetti). Here again, dictionaries record that educated persons use some of these transpositions. Kenyon and Knott list both *children* and *childern* and *hundred* and *hunderd*. Transpositions rarely used by educated persons include *prespire* for *perspire*; *plubicity* for *publicity*; *modren* for *modern*; *revelant* for *relevant*; *I akst him* for *I asked him*; *pernounce* for *pronounce*; *tradegy* for *tragedy*; *patrin* for *pattern*; and *osifer* for *officer*.

DISTORTION OF SOUNDS

Sometimes a child approximates a given sound but changes some of the features somewhat. The child may make an *s* so that it cannot be readily distinguished from an *sh*. The problem arises as to how liberal to be in accepting these changes. The first part of the diphthong of *now* is normally a back sound. Many Americans, however, raise the tongue on the first part of this diphthong so that it is in the same position as the vowel in *cat*. Many Americans raise the tongue on the vowel sound in *hat* nearly to the position of the vowel sound in *met*. The teacher must make a value judgment on whether to motivate the child to change the pronunciation of the diphthong in *now* and the vowel in *cat*.

ESTABLISHING PRESTIGIOUS DIALECTS

As noted earlier, some children need to learn to speak standard English as a second language. The work of Shuy suggests methods for this. Other children need to be made aware that to speak well is an economic and social advantage. For this second group, the teacher leads a discussion by asking such questions as: What do we mean by "speaking well?" Who speaks well? Are there various degrees of speaking well? Should we always speak equally well? When do we need to speak particularly well? Where do we need to speak particularly well? How can we help each other to speak well?

As children talk about effective speech, they will not only list "correct" pronunciation, pleasant voices, and saying the sounds "correctly" but they will also include other factors such as sounding friendly, making oneself clear to others, and having others respond favorably. One child said that speaking well was really a way of getting along well with others. This idea, at first rejected by the children, provided the basic impetus for the children's speech work. A teacher can help children to realize that our speech today is a living, changing medium of communication. Children are interested in the idea that pronunciations have changed, that meanings of words have changed, and even that grammar has changed over the centuries.

As children talk about who speaks well, they are really setting up standards against which to compare their own speech. They usually include some of the educated members of the community, some of the well-known broadcasters. Analyzing what makes the speech of a particular broadcaster effective is helpful. Such talk encourages children to listen to the pronunciations of broadcasters and, as a result, often to be critical of their own pronunciations. Many times they imitate some of the pronunciations of broadcasters. One teacher employs a very interesting device to teach the influence of varying speech situations on those involved in them. She uses puppets dressed in various ways—as a king, a queen, a bedraggled beggar. As the children manipulate the puppets, they speak as they think the characters would. This device serves as a basis for a discussion of how people in various walks of life speak differently.

The question "Why do we need to speak well?" is provocative. Some students frankly feel little need to speak well; they say that nobody seems to have trouble in understanding them and that the quality of their speech makes no difference in their relationships with people. Other youngsters, however, consider good speech a valuable asset. One boy said that when he collected for his newspapers he talked carefully. He said he thought his customers might not consider him a good salesman if he spoke carelessly. He also made the point that his attempts at good speech and good manners paid dividends in terms of tips. He ended by admitting that he enjoyed speaking well and being courteous to his customers.

This topic leads naturally into a discussion of the places where acceptable speech is important. Children usually agree that whatever their jobs are going to be, they will have to speak well. This objective is not immediate. Therefore, children must think of present situations where they need good speech. One child said that while he works in his father's shoe repair shop, he must wait on customers with good manners and with good speech so that they will feel right toward him and understand him easily.

In this discussion the teacher's own voice and pronunciations are important. Unconsciously, the child thinks of how the teacher sounds. As children feel warm and friendly toward their teachers, they imitate them, wearing similar clothes, walking like them, and talking like them.

FEEDBACK

Having been motivated to speak well, what do the children do about it? Authorities who discuss change often emphasize the need for three functions: (1) scanning, (2) comparing, and (3) correcting.

In *scanning*, the children receive information through sensory channels about how their speech mechanisms are performing and about the result of the performances, the utterances. In addition, they feel what part of their speech mechanisms work on what other part and are aware of such a factor as the nasal emission of [m]. Children, taught to scan effectively, examine the product of their speech mechanisms carefully.

In *comparing*, children match their speech patterns against the standard they desire to achieve. They examine the dominant features of an utterance and match what they say against what they wish to say. Because there is obviously not time to match every sound before uttering the next sound, they compare key features of entire patterns of sounds rather than individual sounds.

Ogilvie and Rees (1970) use the comparison of expert typists: As you watch expert typists, you can understand the comparison of the back flow of message against a standard pattern. Typists place their fingers on the eight designated keys and proceed to hit the necessary keys to type the words that correspond to the pattern they are following. In their almost automatically controlled typing, a discrepancy between their pattern and the copy can take place. They discover the error through their "feel" that they have hit the wrong key or through the visual inspection of their typed copy. The "feel" is all important for speed in typing. Expert typists often know through "feel" that they are about to make an error; they then correct the error before it actually occurs, thereby maintaining their rhythm and speed. But when the error has occurred, the typist confirms the impression of error through visual inspection and proceeds to correct it. In this instance, the rhythm has been broken. Thus, the corrector function becomes involved. In speech improvement the discrepancies between the desired speech patterns and the actual speech patterns (error signal) are what determine the amount and kind of improvement. Here, too, correcting is involved (Ogilvie and Rees 1970, p. 16.).

The third function, then, is *correcting*, based on information obtained through the child's scanning and comparing. As an adult, you are aware of this function. When you unconsciously mispronounce a word, you correct the mispronunciation by stressing a different syllable. When you utter a sound incorrectly, you change your mechanism to what feels and sounds right. You vary your utterance until no difference exists between the pattern you are producing and the one you want to produce (zero error signal). Children become aware, with your help, of what speech patterns need to be changed, find for themselves patterns they wish to produce consistently, and adjust their mechanisms through hearing, feeling, and seeing so that they produce the desired patterns. They then proceed to practice until the control is automatic.

Typists, as they start to learn to type, find their control far from automatic. They probably begin with *a-s-d-f*-space, semicolon-*l-k-j*-space and practice until an almost automatic "feel" takes over. Just as in typing, an almost automatic "feel" for control of speech is learned. In early childhood, you compared the self-hearing of your own utterances with those around you; as you matched fairly well, those around you rewarded you. The kinesthetic and tactual messages from your placement and from the operation of parts of the articulatory mechanism became vivid and satisfying. Soon the kinesthetic and tactual feedback was so well established that the auditory feedback became secondary. You came to rely almost entirely on the "feel" of the movements of the speech mechanism rather than on hearing.

In helping children to change their speech patterns, you are helping them to substitute conscious control for automatic control. They must match the auditory feedback from their mouths with the auditory patterns of someone else—either you or a tape. They adjust their mechanisms by hearing, seeing, and feeling. You make use of yourself, of tapes, or of other speakers as models.

Having helped the children to find patterns as models, having helped them to make the necessary corrections, you then encourage them to work toward automatic control. Learning to type is often slow and clumsy. Learning to speak differently is also often slow and clumsy. In both instances, practice is essential. You supply the children with phrases, poetry, limericks, and ditties. You teach them to "feel" themselves going through the necessary motions. Eventually, the control becomes automatic.

Unacceptable Vocal Qualities

The teacher is concerned that students' voices serve their communicative purposes as well as they can. The student's voice problems may be serious. The more serious difficulties of voice are discussed in Chapter 12. When a child has a consistently hoarse voice, the teacher may assume that the difficulty calls for specialized help. Many times, however, children's voices are adequate for communicative purposes but they would be more effective if improved. In such instances, the teacher works for improvement taking into consideration four aspects of voice: volume, pitch, quality, and rate of speaking. (See Chapter 12 for correcting significant vocal difficulties.)

LOUDNESS

Childrens' voices should not be too loud or too soft. They should be able to adjust the loudness of their voices to the demands of the room in which they are speaking. Florence always spoke rather quietly. In the classroom, children heard her fairly well although sometimes they had to listen carefully. But when she was to act as mistress of ceremonies in the auditorium, she discovered that the children in the back of the room could not hear her. She had to learn to adjust the volume of her voice to the size of the larger room. She further learned that speaking more slowly and articulating more clearly helped her to be heard. Harry, a ten-year-old, seemed to be yelling. He rarely spoke quietly. He appeared afraid that his classmates would not heed him and felt that when he spoke loudly they listened more attentively. He came from a family where the person who spoke loudest received the most attention. With the teacher's direction Harry came to realize that he was more effective as a personality and easier to listen to when he spoke more softly.

PITCH

Children's voices should be appropriate to their age, sex, and physical maturity. They should express the meaning and emotion of what they desire to communicate. The material on pitch, pages 318–320, is important in consideration of children's pitch. No child's habitual pitch should be changed without careful diagnosis. Many changes in pitch can safely be made, however. Mark's voice tended to be monotonous, for he spoke on one pitch level. Although he was a lively youngster, he had acquired the habit of speaking with little inflection. The school psychologist believed that his monotonous speech was a carry-over from a time when he had had many adjustment problems. These problems were no longer evident, but the monotonous voice was. The teacher helped Mark to make his voice more lively.

QUALITY OF VOICE

Quality of voice refers to the tone that distinguishes one voice from another. The tone differs because of the way the resonating system acts to modify it and because of the particular way in which vocal cords vibrate. The quality may be clear, pleasant, resonant; or it may be breathy, muffled, or nasal. The changing of a consistent quality of voice is discussed in the chapter on voice. Quality, however, is also used to help express a person's feelings and emotions. The teacher can help the child to use a quality of voice that does express feeling. One child, partly because of personality difficulties, always spoke as if he were angry. With the teacher's help, the child began to realize that his attitude toward life tended to be negative rather than positive. With the guidance of the school psychologist and with such classroom work as creative dramatics, the boy changed his tone from one of almost consistent anger to one of friendliness.

RATE OF SPEAKING

Few children speak too slowly. A large number of them speak at too fast a rate. Some are in a hurry to get their words into the conversation. Others tend to run fast, to work fast, and to talk fast. They need to realize that their listeners may miss part of what they are saying because of their speed. One 14-year-old boy sang very well. In fact, he was the best boy vocalist in his school. But when he spoke, he ran his words together and overassimilated sounds so that his listeners missed at least half of what he was saying. The speed with which he spoke affected even the quality of his speaking voice. It became muffled. Yet when he sang he articulated very clearly and the quality of his voice was excellent. As he heard the contrast between his singing and speaking voices on a recording, he diagnosed his own difficulty and proceeded to do something about it.

Teaching the Improvement of Voice

Discussing voice and its part in communication makes children aware of their own voices. Children talk about the kinds of voices they like. Almost inevitably, they will discuss how voice reflects personality. They ask themselves whether certain voices suggest friendliness and kindness or whether voices indicate that the person is bored and irritated. Children also talk about the control of pitch, volume, and speed. The individual child then uses a voice that expresses his/her intended meaning and feeling. A recording of voice is an excellent motivation for children to change their voice. (See Chapter 12 for a detailed discussion of voice).

LOUDNESS

Sometimes children have to be reminded to speak loudly enough to be heard in a classroom. The inability to hear a child justifies interrupting him. One teacher said that he did not like to interrupt Jimmy to ask him to speak louder, because Jimmy was so interested in what he was telling. Jimmy was interested, but at least 16 children in the room were squirming and at least six were talking with one another. They resented the teacher's admonition to them to listen. An early interruption, casually asking Jimmy to speak so that all could hear him, might well have avoided the discourtesy on the part of his audience. Children need to know that rate of speaking and clear articulation are related to ability to be heard. When the teacher insists on each child's speaking loudly enough to be heard, communication is easier. In some instances, the child's speaking too softly may be related to a feeling of insecurity in the room or of general insecurity. Teachers must do what they can to make sure the social atmosphere of the room is conducive to speaking and being heard. If the child is generally insecure, help should be given to modify this situation.

PITCH, QUALITY, AND RATE

Children learn that the rate of speaking and the pitch and quality of their voices show how they feel about what they are reading or saying. Some teachers use puppets or creative dramatics very effectively for this purpose. One child holds the angry puppet who tells the other puppets off. Another holds the sad puppet who speaks slowly of the misfortunes of others. Another holds the gay puppet whose speech is merry. The teacher helps the child to use the pitch, quality, and rate that are most expressive for a particular puppet. The teacher can use creative dramatics for the same purpose. Through setting up particular situations, children realize the importance of pitch, quality, and rate of speaking in their interpersonal relationships. They learn that the expression of different moods and of different meanings requires differences in pitch, quality, and rate.

One teacher uses a single phrase, asking that the children think of as many ways as possible of conveying different meanings with it. One of the phrases is, "Why, Joe and Jill were half an hour late." Children express happiness, sorrow, anger, sarcasm, or sympathy at Joe and Jill's being late. Sometimes they build a story around a particular child's rendition of the phrase.

Summary

All human beings need to communicate. Communicative behaviors and responses to them change from situation to situation, from culture to culture, and even from region to region. The responses, charged with emotional reactions to vocabulary, to pronunciations, and to syntax, can be as varied as happily accepting or hostile, condescending or sympathetic, and interested or apathetic, partly because language and culture are so closely entwined. As children enter school, they bring with them their native language and their attitudes about its particular attributes; at this stage they speak their native language. But at a later date they are encouraged to speak a classroom standard language set by teachers and themselves. The dialect they may learn, sometimes as a second language, is usually representative of the educated members of the community in which they live. Because of school and life demands, children should be instructed at the appropriate stage to acquire this school dialect. Some of the facets involved in setting a Standard classroom English are examined, and specific ways are pointed out to improve both the articulation and voice of the children.

Problems

1. Listen for *y'know* in a classroom discussion. How often did it occur? What do you think motivated its use in some of the particular incidents?
2. What is your reaction to a college professor who says
   a. He don't.
   b. He hardly never.
   c. He done fine?
3. Would you use any of the following phrases? Under what circumstances would you use those phrases?
   a. I wrote a letter.
   b. I put pen to paper and sent it off with a flourish.
   c. I penned a sympathetic note.
4. The word *strategy* is applicable to educational methods. Indicate other uses for the same word. What remains constant in the various uses of this word?
5. *Competencies* and *competence* are used in Chapters 2 and 7. What are the differences and similarities in the two uses of the word?
6. List some of the present-day slang terms for *drunk*.
7. Would you say, "She's a compiler of terminological inexactitudes."? Would anyone say this at any time? If so, when?
8. List ten pronunciations that you have changed over the past few years. Why did you change them?
9. Remember when you met someone from a different region. What were some of this person's pronunciations that were different from yours?
10. Visit a classroom. List either (a) the articulatory errors you hear or (b) the characteristics of the voices that are ineffective in the classroom situation.
11. Indicate the ways in which the teacher of a classroom you have visited helped the children to speak with more pleasant and more effective voices.
12. Read the introductions to two unabridged dictionaries. Tell how the information might prove helpful in your use of the dictionary in the classroom.

13. Listen to your favorite newscaster. What are the characteristics of his voice that made you think him effective?
14. As far as possible, list the influences of parents, school, community, and education upon your own speech.
15. List five sentences, phrases, or words in which assimilation occurs. Indicate the assimilation that may occur.
16. Would you accept the following omissions or transpositions in the pronunciation of the following words?
    goverment for *government*.
    childern for *children*.
    liberry for *library*.
    English (without the *g*) for *English* (with the *g* sound).
    Support your "decision."

References and Suggested Readings

Adler, S., "Data Gathering: The Reliability and Validity of Test Data from Culturally Different Children," *Journal of Learning Disabilities*, **6** (August/September 1973), 429–434.

———, "Dialectal Differences. Professional and Clinical Implications," *Journal of Speech and Hearing Disorders*, **36** (February 1971), 90–99. (Lists five suggestions for the clinician as he/she works with culturally different children.)

———, "Pluralism, Relevance, and Language Intervention for Culturally Different Children," *ASHA*, **13** (December 1971), 719–723.

———, "Social Class Bases of Language: A Re-examination of Socioeconomic, Sociopsychological, and Sociolinguistic Factors," *ASHA*, **15** (January 1973), 3–9.

Allen, H. B., *Readings in Applied English Linguistics*. New York: Appleton-Century-Crofts, 1968. (Contains an excellent discussion of the standards of pronunciation and grammar.)

Bailey, B. L., "Some Aspects of the Impact of Linguistics on Language Teaching in Disadvantaged Communities," *Elementary English*, **45** (May 1968), 570–578. (Reports the findings of linguistic research as related to the teaching of English in schools that serve the disadvantaged. Includes phonology, grammar, language programs. Contains many examples of the speech of the disadvantaged.)

Baratz, J. C., "Language and Cognitive Assessments of Negro Children: Assumptions Are Research Needs." Washington, D.C.: *ERIC* ed. 020518, 1968.

———, "Should Black Children Learn White Dialect?" *ASHA*, **13** (September 1970), 415–417.

Bolinger, D., *Aspects of Language*, 2nd ed., New York: Harcourt Brace Jovanovich, Inc., 1975.

Bronstein, A. J., *The Pronunciation of American English*. New York: Appleton-Century-Crofts, 1960 (Chap. 1 gives the nature of standard speech and explains levels of speech; Chap. 3 talks about regional variations.)

Cohen, S. A., and G. S. Kornfield, "Oral Vocabulary and Beginning Reading in Disadvantaged Black Children," *Reading Teacher*, **24** (October 1970), 33–38.

Eisenson, J., *The Improvement of Voice and Diction*, 3rd ed. New York: Macmillan Publishing Co., Inc.; 1974. (Chap. 10 discusses changing speech patterns.)

Evertts, E. L., ed., *Dimensions of Dialect*. Champaign, Ill.: National Council of Teachers of English, 1967. (Contains a series of articles about social dialects.)

Foerster, L. M., "Language Experience for Dialectically Different Black Learners," *Elementary English*, **51** (February 1971), 193–197.

Frentz, T., "Children's Comprehension of Standard and Negro Nonstandard English Sentences, *Speech Monographs*, **38** (March 1971), 10–16.

Golden, R. L., *Improving Patterns of Language Usage*. Detroit: Wayne State University Press, 1960. (Stresses the importance of speech improvement as self-improvement.)

Goodman, K. S., "Dialect Barriers to Reading Comprehension," in E. L. Evertts, ed., *Dimensions of Dialect*, Champaign, Ill.: National Council of Teachers of English, 1967. (Discusses regional variations.)

———, "Dialect Barriers to Reading Comprehension," in J. C. Baratz and R. W. Shuy, eds., *Teaching Black Children to Read*, Washington, D.C.: Center for Applied Linguistics, 1970, 3–25. (Lists alternatives for school programs.)

Goodman, Y. M., and R. Sims, "Whose Dialect for Beginning Readers?" *Elementary English*, **51** (September 1974), 837–841.

Joos, M., "The Five Clocks," Publication 22, Indiana University Research Center in Anthropology, Folklore and Linguistics, April 1962. (Discusses a wide variety of speech styles, from the most intimate to the most formal.)

Kenyon, J. S., and T. A. Knott, *A Pronouncing Dictionary of American English*. Springfield, Mass.: G. & C. Merriam Company, 1944. (Provides an excellent source for the pronunciation of American English words.)

Krescheck, J. D., and L. Nicolos, "A Comparison of Black and White Children's Scores on the Peabody Picture Vocabulary Test," *Language, Speech, and Hearing in the Schools*, **4** (January 1973), 37–40. (Studies the differences between the scores of black and white children on the Peabody Picture Vocabulary Test. Finds a significant difference and suggests differences may be because of cultural bias.)

Labov, W., *Language in the Inner City: Studies in the Black English Vernacular* (Conduct and Communication Number 3), Philadelphia: The University of Pennsylvania Press, 1972.

———, *The Social Stratification of English in New York City*. Washington, D.C.: Center for Applied Linguistics, 1966. (Indicates the different pronunciations of certain sounds in different strata of society in New York City.)

———, "Some Sources of Reading Problems for Negro Speakers of Nonstandard English," in J. C. Baratz, and R. W. Shuy, eds., *Teaching Black Children to Read*. Washington, D.C.: Center for Applied Linguistics, 1969, 29–67.

LeFevre, C. A., "Language and Self: Fulfillment or Trauma?" *Elementary English*, **43** (March 1966), 230–234. (Decries the ancestral, puritanically rigid adherence to the black and white syndrome of correct and incorrect English.)

Levy, B. B., and H. Cook, "Dialect Proficiency and Auditory Comprehension in Standard and Black Nonstandard English," *Journal of Speech and Hearing Disorders*, **16** (December 1973), 642–649.

Loban, W., "Teaching Children Who Speak Social Class Dialects," *Elementary English*, **45** (May 1968), 592–599. (Tells how to add a second language to teach a prestigious dialect, established usage, and pronunciation.)

McDavid, R. I., Jr., "Variations in Standard American English," *Elementary English*, **45** (May 1968), 561–564. (Considers regional differences.)

Mencken, H. L., *The American Language*, 4th ed., New York: Alfred A. Knopf, Inc., 1946.

Morgan, A. L., "A New Orleans Oral Language Study," *Elementary English*, **51** (February 1971), 222–229. (Studies the phonological, morphological, and syntactical oral language patterns of disadvantaged children of New Orleans.)

Newman, E., *Strictly Speaking*, Indianapolis/New York: The Bobbs-Merrill Company, 1974.

Ogilvie, M., and N. Rees, *Communication Skills: Voice and Pronunciation*, New York: McGraw-Hill, Inc., 1970. (Chap. 1 discusses effect of voice and pronunciation on communication; Chap. 8 discusses speech standards.)

Pillar, A. M., "The Teacher and Black Dialect," *Elementary English*, **52** (May 1975), 646–649.

Quay, L. C., "Language Dialect, Reinforcement and the Intelligence Test Performance of Negro Children," *Child Development*, **42** (March 1971), 5–15.

Ramsey, I., "A Comparison of First Grade Negro Dialect Speakers' Comprehension of Standard English and Negro Dialect." *Elementary English*, **49** (May 1972), 688–696.

Shuy, R. W., "Detroit Speech: Careless, Awkward, and Inconsistent, or Systematic, Graceful, and Regular?" *Elementary English*, **45** (May 1968), 565–569. (Shows the distinction between language differences and value judgments about these differences. Talks about collecting the features of pronunciation, grammar, and vocabulary that set off different social groups, races, age groups, and sexes from each other in Detroit. Tells how to gather this information, analyze it, and evaluate its impact on the teaching of English.)

——, ed., *Social Dialects and Language Learning*, Proceedings of the Bloomington, Indiana Conferences, 1964, Champaign, Ill.: National Council of Teachers of English, 1965.

Tabbert, R., "Dialect Difference and the Teaching of Reading and Spelling," *Elementary English*, **51** (November/December 1974), 1097–1099.

Venezky, R. L., "Nonstandard Language and Reading," *Elementary English*, **47** (March 1970), 334–345. (Contains selected references on specific dialects.)

Williams, F., ed., *Language and Poverty*, Chicago: Markham Publishing Co., 1970.

————, "Psychological Correlates of Speech Characteristics on Sounding 'Disadvantaged'," *Journal of Speech and Hearing Research*, **13** (September 1970), 472–488. (Links language and speech features serving as salient clues in the judgmental process with whatever kinds of evaluations or stereotypes appears in the behavior of listeners.)

————, and R. C. Naremore, "Social Class Differences in Children's Syntactic Performance: A Quantitative Analysis of Full Study Data," *Journal of Speech and Hearing Research*, **12** (December 1969), 778–793. Determines whether statistically reliable social class differences are found in the degrees and types of syntactic elaboration in the speech of selected blacks and whites, males and females.)

4. The Teacher or Clinician As a Communicator

The speech and language clinician and the teacher recognize that children's acquisition of speech and language patterns is not something that exists in a vacuum but in the context of the total communicative act. In this act, children's feelings cannot be separated from their capacity to acquire speech and language and to use them purposefully within their particular environments. To illustrate, both the teachers' and the children's interests, attitudes, appreciations, and values are part and parcel of the communicative act. As children are taught to modify deviant speech and language patterns, the teacher and the clinician alike take into account the elements of the communicative teaching act.

For example, the clinician and teacher may set the objective that the child point to concepts of *big*, *bigger*, and *biggest* in a series of 20 representational pictures. The teacher and clinician may present the concepts by describing the size of three human beings—baby (a big baby), big brother, and father; by throwing to the child three balls— a big one, a bigger one, and the biggest one; finally, by demonstrating with drawings of a big tree, a bigger tree, and the biggest tree. The message has been presented auditorily by having the children listen to the description of the baby, the brother, and the father; tactually, by having the children catch the three big balls; and finally visually, by having the children see the three pictures. The children pay attention, decode the message, and respond in some way to the 20 pictures. One child may elect to be silent; another, to give the wrong response; and still another, to give the right response. The first child may simply wish to withdraw; the second may give the wrong response, because he doesn't understand the message, or because he wishes to annoy the teacher; the third gives the right response, because he is proud of his learning achievement or perhaps because he enjoys pleasing the teacher or impressing his classmates. At this point, the teacher reinforces positively or negatively which reinforcement gives the child encouragement to acquire the comparative and/or superlative concepts. The children are receiving feedback from the teacher and from their own language mechanisms. As noted in Chapter 3, self-feedback in the acquisition of speech and language patterns is particularly important. The process, then, includes the teacher or clinician, the message, the receiver of the message, and the feedback.

The following diagram represents the teaching communicative act:[1]

Teacher or Clinician (Source)	Message	Channel	Receiver
Knowledge	Educational	Seeing	Knowledge
Attitudes	purpose	Hearing	Attitudes
Social milieu and	Structure	Touching	Social milieu and
background	Treatment	Smelling	background
School cultural		Tasting	School cultural
environment			environment
Communication skills			Communication skills

Feedback

The Teacher or Clinician as an Encoder (Source)

KNOWLEDGE

Everyone agrees that teachers should be knowledgeable. When teachers have read widely, thought deeply, inquired judiciously, observed keenly, listened carefully, and appraised completely, they have knowledge and, consequently, a fund of ideas from which to draw. The ideas need not be derived from books, travel, or learned individuals, for some ideas are original. For instance, the teacher may find a picture from which an exciting bit of creative drama can grow, or discover a cartoon that motivates discussion, or may write a poem that depicts the

---

[1] We believe that clinicians are teachers in that they wish to change the speech and language behavior of their students.

school on a snowy day. Or perhaps the teacher may make up a story that is sheer nonsense but well suited to the group. The teacher is a person with wide knowledge and a creative urge, who will continue to acquire a liberal education throughout life. Similarly, clinicians must be knowledgeable. They must know both the theory and practice of their field. They must be able to diagnose accurately, to interpret the diagnostic information clearly, to know when to refer a case, when to handle it, whom to consult. They must be able to plan and carry through a program designed for the speech and hearing handicapped. (Their competencies are discussed in Chapter 2.) Undoubtedly, this intellectual development is important, but, in addition, the teacher and clinician must believe that knowledge is important, that it can be communicated to others, and that it affects the lives of others.

ATTITUDES AND THE TEACHER'S OR CLINICIAN'S SELF-CONCEPT

Effective teaching involves human beings interacting positively. Teachers who believe their students capable of learning behave differently from those who believe them incapable of learning. Furthermore, teachers who feel they are able teachers will try harder to teach children. Teachers who do not feel they are able give up. The teacher, therefore, should possess a positive self-concept, a "fully functioning self," or a "high-level wellness." Since the speech and language clinicians are interacting with either an individual or a small group, their impact is deeply felt. They must believe that their students are capable of learning to communicate and that they are capable of teaching the students to communicate. Like teachers, they should possess positive self-concepts. According to Combs and Snygg, these kinds of teacher are characterized by four general qualities:

1. They tend to see themselves in essentially positive ways. That is to say, they see themselves as generally liked, wanted, successful, able persons of dignity, worth, and integrity.
2. They perceive themselves and their world accurately and realistically. These people do not kid themselves. They are able to confront the world with openness and acceptance, seeing both themselves and external events with a minimum of distortion or defensiveness.
3. They have deep feelings of identification with other people. They feel "at one with" a large number of persons of all kinds and varieties. This is not simply a surface manifestation of "liking people" or being a "hail-fellow-well-met" type of person. Identification is not a matter of polished social graces, but a feeling of oneness in the human condition.

4. They are well informed. Adequate people are not stupid. They have perceptual fields which are rich, varied, and available for use when needed (Combs 1965, p. 70).

Rosenthal and Jacobson (1968) note that the reason usually given for the poor performance of children from a different culture is simply that they are members of a disadvantaged group. They point out that there may be another reason: that the children do poorly in school because that is what is expected of them. Their shortcomings may originate not in their different ethnic, cultural, and economic background but in the teacher's response to that background. Their study, therefore, was devised with this concept in mind: that one person's prediction of another person's behavior somehow comes to be realized. The prediction may, of course, be realized only in the perception of the predictor. But it is also possible that the predictor's expectation is communicated to the other person, perhaps in quite subtle and unintended ways, and so has an influence on actual behavior.

They, therefore, set up a situation whereby teachers would expect certain pupils to show superior performance. The school was one where most of the children came from lower-class families and where the parents were receiving welfare payments, had low incomes, and/or were Mexican in origin. The children were tested with instruments that measured verbal ability and reasoning ability at the beginning and end of the school year. The teachers were told early in the term that certain children were "spurters" who were in reality chosen at random. The results showed that children from whom teachers expected greater intellectual gains showed such gains. The teachers were also asked to describe the classroom behavior of their pupils. The children from whom intellectual growth was expected were described as having a better chance of being successful in later life, and as being happier, more curious, and more interesting than the other children.

The most obvious explanation for these results is that the teachers spent more time with these particular students. But no evidence for this explanation exists. The authors believe that the explanation seems to lie in a subtle feature of the interaction of the teacher and pupils. The tone of voice, facial expression, touch, and posture may be the means by which—probably quite unwittingly—the teacher communicates expectations to pupils. Such effective communication may help children by changing their concepts of themselves, their anticipation of their own behaviors, and their motivation in their cognitive skills. Similarly, clinicians must believe that their children can succeed in changing their speech and language behavior and, furthermore, they must believe in their own role in changing this behavior.

The positive concept that speech clinicians in the schools have of their careers is substantiated by a study on attitudes of speech clinicians in the public schools. Weaver (1968) asked public school clinicians to rank the following professional areas in order of importance: classroom teacher, speech clinician employed outside the school setting, special education teacher, college instructor, and public school clinician. The clincians ranked the classroom teacher first and themselves second. Weaver also asked the respondents to select a level of importance for the work of the speech clinician in the public schools: "Of highest importance," "significant importance," "average importance," "less than average," and "not very important." Forty-one per cent reported a feeling of "highest importance, 52 per cent, of "significant import- ance," 1½ per cent of "average importance," and 1 per cent in the last two categories. The investigation suggests that public school clinicians do have positive attitudes about their contribution to the children in the school system.

Clinicians' attitudes are closely tied to the success of children in modifying their verbal behavior. Clinicians get their feedback from the children themselves and from their supervisors. Clinicians probably all verbalize that they feel warmth, empathy, and respect for their children, but they need to analyze on what level of effectiveness they are be- having. They need to examine both the feedback from the children and from their supervisor. Klevans and Volz (1974) present three levels of interpersonal relationships for clinicians:

Superior Level	*Intermediate Level*	*Minimal Level*
7 6 5	4	3 2 1
Offered empathetic understanding, warmth, and respect to create atmosphere of trust in him and the therapy offered and facilitated sharing of the problem; when appropriate, the clinician shared his own reactions in genuine, self-disclosing, and confronting ways and moved to the problem- solving phase. The clinician was both model and participant in effective interper- sonal relationships.	Created somewhat effective atmosphere; responses indicated a concern for client needs. Imprecise use of "helping skills" reduced effectiveness of responding and problem solving.	Generally unable to establish atmosphere of trust and work jointly with client toward therapy goals; difficulty in relating to client on an open, honest level made him an ineffec- tive model for inter- personal relationships; too much therapy time spent on clini- cian's concerns.

They go on to note that the clinician in the superior category is able to feel warmth, empathy, and respect for the child and to communicate in a way that leads to maximum therapeutic benefits. At the intermediate level of competence, a clinician is aware of the importance of interpersonal skills and does use some of them. Lack of experience and/or training, rather than lack of concern for the children, are the reasons for reduced effectiveness. The clinician at the lowest level may be behaving this way for a variety of reasons, including lack of training, experience, and interest in the children or for personal difficulties in relating to others. Clinicians may become aware of their need to modify their clinical behavior by rating themselves on such scales as these and regarding seriously their supervisors' ratings.

THE TEACHER'S OR CLINICIAN'S SOCIAL MILIEU AND BACKGROUND

A teacher has usually been brought up in a middle-class home and his colleagues and friends generally come from similar backgrounds. But the teacher or clinician may be working with students from either upper- or lower-class homes. The modes of communication in the various social classes differ. Schatzman and Strauss (1966) in a study involving a sampling from 340 interviews of white subjects, 21 to 65 years old, living in Arkansas, compared the oral communication of a group low in income and educational opportunity with one that was decidedly higher in income and educational opportunity. They pointed out differences—not merely in success or failure of communication, or correctness or elaborateness of syntactical structure and vocabulary usage—but in (a) number and kinds of perspectives used in communication, (b) ability to take the listener's role, (c) the handling of classification, and (d) framework and stylistic devices that order and implement the communication.

For example, the description of the catastrophic event by the members of the lower class was a straight, direct narrative of events, whereas the description by members of the higher class was not confined to so narrow a perspective. It involved another person, class of persons, an organization, an organizational role, even the whole town. The members of the higher class described the behavior of others and even included sequence of events as others saw them.

The teacher and clinician need to be aware of the differences between the mode of communication of their social class and that of the class of their students.

CULTURAL ENVIRONMENT OF THE SCHOOL

The students, the faculty, the school administration, and the locale all contribute to the environment of the school. Some schools have rich, stimulating environments: As you enter the school building, you see pictures drawn by inspired young artists, poems written by imaginative young writers; you hear music, other than the ordinary, emanating from a classroom; you feel your muscles tense as you watch young dancers portraying a riot. In this school, children from all social classes have anticipating, eager looks. Or the school can have a well-ordered, tightly run ship look: The poems are beautifully handwritten. The floors are barren of even a scrap of paper. The rooms are neat and tidy. Almost everyone moves in an orderly fashion.

These are but two examples of school environments. Just as individuals have different life-styles, schools can display a variety of postures, moods, and collections of culture. But these affect the communicative processes of the students, of the teachers, and of the clinician.

Clinicians who travel from school to school often have a "favorite" school, the style of which makes clinical speech work profitable. A school with a humanitarian principal, with teachers interested in every child from the gifted to the retarded, with pride in the achievements of each student, with a somewhat permissive attitude but with boundaries firmly established, with an attractive, adequately equipped speech room falls into the category of one clinician's "favorite" school. The principal casually commends the clinician on the ability of a once silent child to communicate with others. A teacher sends a note indicating that one child's mother is ill in the hospital; another, that a child has completed an unusually attractive poster. This school's style fosters effective clinical work.

COMMUNICATIVE SKILLS OF THE TEACHER OR CLINICIAN

The teacher's and clinician's ability to encode messages so that the receivers accept them as intended is important. Choice of vocabulary and syntactic complexity, ability to make information exciting, to make a point clearly, to persuade, to adapt what is said so that students understand and respond, to use appropriate voice and pronunciation, to further interaction by increasing the verbal flow between and among the teacher and students—all these are facets of this ability. Particulary important are the teacher's and clinician's voice and pronunciation, the amount and kind of verbal flow, and vocabulary and syntax usage.

VOICE AND PRONUNCIATION

The teacher's or clinician's voice can be an asset or a liability to purposeful, satisfying communication. When effective interaction between the teacher or clinician and the students takes place, the teacher and clinician seem to have confidence in themselves, their ideas, and their teaching. The voice revealing this confidence is "clearly audible, with a steady rhythm, with a rate slow enough for comprehension but varied so as to express enthusiasm and vigor, with an appropriate pitch and intonation pattern, and with a strong resonant quality" (Ogilvie and Rees 1970, p. 6). The voices of the warm, friendly teacher and clinician, flexible in pitch and loudness, indicate that they have heard their children's comments, value their worth, and anticipate a reaction.

The teacher and clinician may well tape-record a classroom discussion or a clinical session and then listen to discover the kinds of communicative instruments they possess. When the recording gives an impression that is contrary to what they intend, the teachers may benefit by consulting the school speech therapist who often can make suggestions for improvement. For example, one teacher spoke much too rapidly. When she lengthened her vowels and continuant consonants and took more time for pauses, her students were able to perceive a new and different voice quality—seemingly less nasal, less staccato, and much more pleasant. When clinicians find their own voices inadequate, they put into practice their own theory.

Just as the voice may add or detract from the teacher's or clinicians' message, so may pronunciations. Your patterns of pronunciation should not distract your students. If you possess a regional dialect unlike that of those whom you are teaching, your pronunciation may at first be distracting. When your pronunciation represents educated speech, however, the absolute differences are few, and it is rarely found distracting. Just the same, you may perhaps want to adopt some of the pronunciations of the region in which you are working.

VERBAL FLOW

As a clinician or teacher, you may find yourself dominating the verbal flow. When the communicative act is heavily weighted with your performance, the child does not have a chance to use newly acquired language patterns. Shields and Steiner (1973) studied the effect on spontaneous speech of different interpersonal situations. In checking utterance length, they found that certain adult-dominated conversations reduced the child to a respondent position and markedly restricted the length of the child's utterances, whereas other types of adult-child communication facilitated fluent speech.

Similarly, Woolf (1971) advises on verbal flow in speech interview situations. Where clinicians need specific information, the questions are specific such as, "What does Paul like to do best?" But when clinicians want to encourage verbal output, the interviewer says less and uses open-ended probes such as "Tell me about yourself," or "Anything that comes to your mind."

Vocabulary and Syntax

Children generalize syntactical rules and increase their vocabulary as they hear others (including the teacher and clinician) speak. In monitoring their syntax and vocabulary, the teacher and clinician must be careful not to lower their sights too far, for, as noted earlier, young children's reception outdistances their production. Granowsky and Krossner (1970) conducted an experiment involving the taping of kindergarten teachers both in conversation with other teachers and in their classrooms working with their children in the language development sessions. In all cases, the teachers sampled substantially reduced their language production in terms of syntactic structures and vocabulary diversity when talking to their students. In fact, the language production of the teachers was reduced to a level of complexity that was at, or even below, the actual level used by advantaged middle- and upper-middle-class students.

Message

In teaching, the message is usually motivated by the teacher's desire to impart knowledge, to change or confirm an attitude, and/or to instill certain skills—all of which involve behavioral responses on the part of students. The teacher may present information or may use discussion techniques to foster its acquisition. Sometimes the teacher expects the children to make no value judgments based on knowledge. For instance, the scientific principles of the flight to the moon are facts that can be understood in lesser or greater scientific detail depending upon the scientific sophistication of both the encoder and the decoder. On the other hand, the teacher may expect the children to make value judgments that are based on knowledge, as when, having come to understand the present system of electing the president of the United States, the children then debate that system's merits. The teacher deciding whether to involve students in making particular value judgments may ask such questions as: Are my students mature enough to handle this problem? Am I trying to instill my particular bias in them? Is my sole purpose the protection of the status quo? How essential is involvement in the problem for these students?

Many times the acquisition of knowledge and its resulting value judgments changes or strengthens attitudes; it may even motivate the formulation of completely new ones. As high-school students learn more about language patterns they may become much less certain of accepting wholeheartedly a pronunciation such as *status* with a long *a* rather than *status* with a short *a*. They begin to listen for variant acceptable pronunciations and to understand why they hear many pronunciations that differ from the ones they normally use and believe "correct." As they study language they open their minds to the values of accepting descriptive rather than prescriptive attitudes toward pronunciation. Teachers' skill in leading discussion, their source images (involving the respect with which students regard them), and their ability to bring facts to light influence children's acceptance or rejection of attitudes. At other times, the particular environment, the cultural backgrounds, and the social milieu are subtle but dominant influences on certain attitudes. Speech clinicians play an important role in influencing attitudes of the speech-handicapped child. For example, they help the stutterer to accept their stuttering. Their own attitudes about speech difficulties are reflected in the children's attitudes about them and in the teachers' attitudes. As a result, teachers can become more accepting of the speech-handicapped child.

Teachers usually have a set of skills that they wish their students to acquire. They may make sure students understand the prerequisites of the skills, may demonstrate them, and may then provide opportunity for practice. Similarly, clinicians almost inevitably want their children to acquire certain skills. They first motivate the child to accept change as desirable, proceed to explain and demonstrate the needed change, and then provide interesting drill material to effect the change. Finally they give opportunity to use the changed communication in conversation. The ability of the teacher or clinician to decode, and to demonstrate the skills, the ability of the children to encode, and their mental and motor readiness to try the skills are all important in their acquisition. But equally important is the teacher's or clinician's ability to make those skills seem desirable, for the group's attitude in accepting or rejecting their desirability influences their acquisition.

In any of the three purposes, the acquisition of knowledge for knowledge's sake, the making of value judgments, and the acquiring of skills, the teacher and clinician are interested in the "how" of teaching. They use what is commonly called "motivation"—either extrinsic or intrinsic, for they cannot expect their students to react as sponges, soaking up knowledge, or as robots, automatically performing skills. The students must be an intimate part of the process. Affect plays an important role here.

Every message from the teacher has some kind of structure. The structure may be tight, as when the teacher makes the aim clear and then proceeds in a developmental fashion to accomplish it. It is less tight when the teacher presents examples, encourages the students to give examples, and then guides the students to draw inferences leading to the accomplishment of the aim of the lesson. The lesson may have a loose structure, as when it consists of guided conversation used to open avenues of possible investigation or activity. But every lesson possesses some kind of structure.

Similarly every clinic session has a purpose. It may be to improve the child's ability to discriminate between plosive and fricative sounds, to encourage the child to be objective about his/her stuttering, to decrease stuttering symptoms, to improve expressive language in terms of opposites as *hot* and *cold*, to improve ability to hear a particular defective sound. The structure may be tight or loose. In working with some aspects of language development, the structure may be loose as in conversation about growing plants. In other aspects, as when the clinician is teaching the child to build concepts about trucks and their various uses, the structure may be tight.

Today, much of learning is based on systematic instructional goals. We make predictions about the kind of speech and language skills that the child needs to succeed in school and in society. These skills involve decisions about phonology, vocabulary, and syntax. Some clinicians follow the behaviorist tradition; others, the humanistic tradition. Regardless of which of these traditions is to be followed the teacher or clinician should ask four questions:

1. What speech and language behaviors would I like each of my students to possess?
2. What evidence exists for the value of each of these behaviors?
3. What strategies can I employ to help each student attain these speech and language behaviors?
4. What evidence do I use to decide whether the student has attained these goals?

Some of the advantages that have resulted from the discussion of behavioral objectives are that teachers and clinicians now state their goals more precisely than formerly, they question their instructional procedures systematically, and they assess the value and success of their instruction more carefully—often by exact observation of children's speech and language behavior in a variety of situations. Thus, their criteria for goals are based on sound theory and research, their strategies are carefully planned in the light of these goals, and their evaluation of the progress of the child is achieved thoughtfully.

OPERANT CONDITIONING

Messages in the speech and language curriculum of schools and in speech and hearing rehabilitation have been significantly influenced by: (1) behavioral objectives, the result of the Bloom Taxonomy (Bloom 1956) and (2) the Skinnerian approach (Skinner 1968). As a result, many clinicians are now moving away from a games approach, because this approach is often not consistently systematic in establishing goals, criterion for them, or in evaluating their achievement (see Van Hattum 1969, p. 278). Many clinicians are, on the other hand, moving toward operant conditioning with its emphasis on positive and negative reinforcement (McReynolds 1970; Stark 1971; Baker and Ryan 1971). The following are two examples involving language therapy.

Fygetakis and Ingram (1973) describe the language rehabilitation through behavior modification techniques of a five-year-old girl with a badly reduced language system but with a normal intellectual potential (according to the Stanford-Binet and the Columbia Mental Maturity Scale). The program involved presenting an optimum set of sentences to enable the child to move from one level of language production to another level and to help her establish her own rule system. The child made progressively closer approximations to the target construction by imitating increasingly longer units of the model sentences. Once the child was able to repeat the entire construction, the model sentences were systematically faded out as the program progressed, and she then formulated her own sentences showing that she had established the necessary rules.

This instruction was based on two premises: (1) that children develop language normally once they begin to improve in language skills, a concept different from that which argues that linguistically deviant children have different linguistic rule systems, and (2) behavior modification techniques provide a setting conducive to attending behavior and learning in a distraction-free environment.

Leonard (1975) similarly described a modeling procedure to teach specific linguistic structures to language-handicapped children. This procedure, too, based on normative aspects of language learning, uses a problem-solving set to emphasize the structural relationship of modeled utterances. It does not mean, however, that the modeling procedure merely repeats occurrences and happenings in the child's daily life. The child responds to visual stimuli and, in turn, produces the appropriate utterances. After he has produced three such utterances in succession, he goes on to produce appropriate unmodeled utterances in response to novel stimuli. After research, Leonard felt justified in employing shaping sequences that parallel the normal child's development of linguistic forms. This article suggests the sequencing in detail.

Both of these examples involve *operant conditioning*. Girardeau and Spradlin (1970, p. 7) define operant conditioning as follows: "Operant behavior is at first controlled by consequences delivered on some contingency basis. Response → Contingency → Consequence. The response may be brought under the control of the stimuli that precede it and the precise ordering of these antecedent stimuli is important." They illustrate operant conditioning with this diagram:

Program of materials	Specific materials or stimuli	Speech and language behavior	Contingency	Consequence
Certain order of pictures	Pictures involving *th* sounds	Correct responses	Every time	Verbal praise by the clinician

Again, the listeners play an important role in this communicative act. The chances of successful verbal behavior are low in the absence of an audience that does not reinforce, or in the presence of one that punishes (Yoder 1970).

In operant conditioning, reinforcement plays an important part in the children's acting on the message and changing their verbal behavior. Assuming that the teacher and clinician have selected the speech behavior to be modified intelligently, and have chosen the strategies to achieve the modification wisely, they now must make sure that the behavior will persist in most environments. They, therefore, reinforce positively the behavior with material offerings, such as bits of fruit, tokens to be changed for toys, opportunities to play a game, or verbal approval; or they may reinforce behavior negatively with such acts as the removal of annoying noises or objects. Without reinforcement little learning takes place.

Channel

Children usually receive the messages in the classroom through seeing and hearing. They receive, interpret, and evaluate the ideas presented by the teacher and by their classmates. Because the classroom is traditionally a verbal community, listening is particularly important. Children must listen carefully rather than attend to their own affairs. As the message conveys graciousness, children listen courteously. As it conveys information, they listen thoughtfully and carefully; as it conveys persuasion, they listen critically.

The teacher or clinician does well to remember that learning can be achieved through channels other than hearing—that looking at pictures showing night and day, pantomiming answering the phone or the actions of a bully, feeling a smooth stone as contrasted with a rough stone, or tasting a bitter lemon and a sweet orange all add another dimension of communication to the purely verbal one. Not all modalities are integrated. Often a student possesses a primary modality such as pantomimic action that is a favored one. The teacher or clinician then does well to make use of this particular modality—to further communication—to hasten the acquisition of knowledge, attitudes, and skills.

Receiver (Decoder)

Children's knowledge, their attitudes, including the effect of their own self-concept, their own social milieu and background, their cultural environment provided by the school, and their communication skills all affect their ability to understand. These factors also affect the teachers' or clinicians' responses, which are directly motivated by feedback from the children.

KNOWLEDGE

The basic understandings that the child brings to school either facilitate or hinder acquisition of further understandings. Some children bring to school understandings far beyond their years. For example, a seven-year-old when asked, "What does *secure* mean?" responded with: "When the bad guy is put in prison's he's secure; he can't get out." After a pause, she added, "When my brother glues two pieces of his airplane together, they're secure." Other children bring less understanding. Another seven-year-old, when asked the same question, responded with: "Scure . . . Scure . . . Scure . . . Sewer . . . Sewer. The guy in the sewer."

The gap between these two seven-year-olds represents a gap in knowledge already acquired—probably not only in the meaning of this word but in the meaning of many more words and, furthermore, in ideas and concepts. And in all likelihood, the gap extends to the phonological, morphological, and syntactic aspects of language.

Most children in the primary grades are limited in their cognitive language development. Five- and six-year-olds perceive and talk about persons in their immediate environment, about the color, size, shape, and number of objects rather than their use. Children of this age, as a rule, do not analyze, synthesize, or reason inductively or deductively. Because of such cognitive limitations, the speech of children in the early grades reflects their egocentric stage, and, consequently, communication involving problem solving other than by implication is difficult. As children reach the third grade, however, their cognitive ability increases so that they become more aware of communication as a speaker-listener activity. As they mature in their cognitive-linguistic abilities, they prepare their messages with the listeners in mind—giving them appropriate forms and symbols to convey meanings and feelings to a particular audience to attain the communicative purpose they desire.

SOCIAL MILIEU AND BACKGROUND

The children's own social milieu and background may make decoding easier or more difficult. They may have been brought up in a home full or devoid of books, music, trips, and stimulating conversation. Or their particular milieu may have certain inbred attitudes. In his study, "Communication Processes Among Immigrants in Israel," Eisenstadt lists among reasons that immigrants disattached themselves from formal elites:

1. Growing disillusionment about the elites' ability to assure them of various amenities and rights accruing to them in a new social system.
2. Doubts as to the elites' prestige position within the new social system.
3. The feeling of attachment to the old ways blocks their achievement of full status within the new society (Eisenstadt 1966, p. 587).

Similar feelings existing in ethnic groups in today's schools directly influence communication in the classroom.

ATTITUDES

Children's self-concepts affect their ability to communicate. The teacher's and clinician's influence are important, for their evaluation of the child affects the child's self-concept. Davidson and Lang (1960, pp. 107–108) found that children's perception of their teacher's feelings correlated positively and significantly with their self-perception.

Furthermore, language and self-concept are inexorably entwined: Language is an inherent part of the classroom culture—for it is a tool that the child uses in thinking, in communicative acts, and in social intercourse. Erwin and Miller (1963, pp. 107–108) say that language is the greatest force for socialization that exists, and that at the same time it is the most potent single factor in the development of individuality. Language reflects self and self reflects language. Affect related to attitudes engendered by environment and by the teacher influences both the development of a positive self-concept and language. The emergence of the development of language in and out of the classroom may signify emergence and growth of self.

CULTURAL ENVIRONMENT OF THE SCHOOL

The school environment has an effect on the verbal behavior and on the emergence and growth of self. When the school teaches material that has personal meaning for the student, and when it helps the child to become personally involved with ideas, with the school's program and with other children, the child will become more effective in communication. As the curriculum is rich in motivating acquisition of knowledge and skills, as it develops imagination, and as it adapts to its students, language ability improves.

COMMUNICATION SKILLS

Lastly, children must be learning to participate in this verbal environment—recognizing purposes of communication, achieving these purposes effectively, listening to and responding to others in a communicative situation. They learn to express themselves in different ways in different situations, to gauge the particular language needs of a particular situation. Consequently, they need to find their own identities to bring their images of themselves close to reality. The classroom ideally should be a place where each child can find a sense of personal worth in life through communication and contribution to the society of the classroom. Eventually, children need to recognize standard and nonstandard usage so that their decoding can be encoded by all members of society—inside and outside the classroom.

Feedback

The teacher receives feedback from the children that they do not understand the message or do not want to respond to it. The teacher then restructures the message. Children receive feedback from their own mechanism. This feedback is explained in some detail in Chapter 3. Children also receive feedback from the teacher—verbal or non-verbal. A smile may indicate a successful performance. Bryant and Ainsfeld (1969) demonstrated the value of feedback in testing children's knowledge of English pluralization rules. They evaluated two methods of testing kindergarten children for knowledge of English pluralization rules, one using feedback as to the correctness or incorrectness of responses, and one that did not use any feedback. The results clearly indicated that the feedback produced a substantial learning effect, resulting in fewer mean number of errors.

The feedback from teacher to students, however, must be realistic, for the children's concepts of their achievement and effort may mislead them. They may think that they are speaking, reading, and writing well, whereas they may not be doing any of these well enough to fill out a job application or to interview for a job upon their graduation from high school. A study (Blakeslee 1975) reported in *The New York Times* of one group of minority students strongly rebuts the notion that in this instance the blacks and Mexican-Americans did poorly in school because they had low aspirations and low self-concepts that were buttressed by teachers. The study showed that students who were the lowest achievers in the schools reported getting the most praise from their teachers. They had been led to believe that they were doing satisfactory work. The teachers, heaping praise on these students are, the study notes, unwillingly "killing them with kindness." They found that the students were receiving assignments that were "not sufficiently challenging" and were at the same time, receiving unrealistic grades. The study suggests that major changes are needed to improve achievement.

Circular Speech Communication Model

Steck et al. (1973) report on a study that indicates a circular speech communication model: Teacher → Child → Teacher → Child. The results tended to show that clinicians felt rewarded by certain kinds of children's behavior. Appropriate responses, evidence of motivation, independent learning, and compliance to clinicians' requests seemed to provide the most rewarding forms of client behavior. In other words, a reciprocal reinforcement process is at work. This study concludes with two concepts: (1) that some clinicians will tend to hear more responses as appropriate or correct than occur because an inappropriate or incorrect response is as punishing to the clinician as to the child, and (2) clinicians should be aware of their responses to the child's behavior and should monitor them carefully. In this instance, the child may not be working to achieve specific goals in speech and language behavior but rather to attain the approval of the clinician. The clinician is working toward self-satisfaction. The feedback is built into the model but may affect not the child's speech and language change but rather behavior designed to please the clinician.

Thus, the amount of knowledge, the attitudes, the social milieu and background, the schools' cultural environment, and the communication skills of the teacher, the clinician, and the students will all influence the effectiveness of the communication activity. The message may have different purposes tied to the students' behavioral consequences, different structures, and different treatments. It may not only be heard, but seen, touched, smelled, or tasted. The receivers' attitudes about both the teacher and the clinician, the message, and the channel influence the success or failure of the communicative processes. The teacher and the clinician are made aware of these attitudes through feedback. Feedback is a way of monitoring a system that signals correct and incorrect operations, sometimes even before the incorrect operation occurs. This permits and facilitates correction. The teacher and clinician will recognize its importance, for they can most accurately communicate when they are truly responsive to the reactions of their students.

Problems

1. Visit three classrooms. In terms of the communication model cited in this chapter, analyze the communicative situation.
2. Visit two classrooms. Indicate what you consider to be the effect of the teachers' voices on their students.
3. Visit a speech therapy session. Indicate what channels were used in the therapy procedures. What other channels might have been used and how?
4. Describe the "culture" of the elementary school that you attended.
5. Listen to any teacher. Give the indications of the kind of self-concept you think he or she possesses as indicated by his or her verbalizations.
6. Visit a classroom from a lower socioeconomic area. Describe how you would have to modify your middle-class values in teaching this group—both in terms of language and in terms of social customs.
7. Visit a classroom. List the reinforcement techniques used by the teacher.
8. Analyze some of the feedback you have received in any discussion.

References and Suggested Readings

Baker, R. D., and B. P. Ryan, *Programmed Conditioning for Articulation*, Monterey, Calif., Monterey Learning Systems, 1971.

Blakeslee, S., "Study Rebuffs a View of Minority Learning," *New York Times*, October 15, 1975, p. 48.

Bloom, B. S., ed., *Taxonomy of Educational Objectives, Handbook I: Cognitive Domain*, New York: David McKay Co., Inc., 1956.

Borus, J. F., S. Greenfield, B. Spiegel, and G. Daniels, "Establishing Imitative Speech Employment Operant Techniques in a Group Setting," *Journal of Speech and Hearing Disorders*, **38** (November 1973), 533–541. (Gives advantages of group therapy using operant techniques for four language-disabled children.)

Bryant, B., and M. Ainsfeld, "Feedback Vs. No-Feedback in Testing Children's Knowledge of English Pluralization Rules," *Journal of Experimental Child Psychology*, **8** (October 1969), 250–255. (Evaluates two methods of testing kindergarten children for knowledge of English pluralization rules: one using feedback as to the correctness or incorrectness of responses and one that does not use any feedback.)

Cazden, C., V. John, and D. Hymes, eds., *Functions of Language in the Classroom*, New York: Teachers College Press, 1972.

Combs, A. W., ed., *Perceiving, Behaving, Becoming: A New Focus for Education.* 1962 ASCD Yearbook, Washington, D.C.: Association for Supervision and Curriculum Development, 1962. (Gives a concept of teaching based on Rogerian psychology.)

Combs, A. W., *The Professional Education of Teachers*, Boston: Allyn and Bacon, Inc., 1965. (Chap. 6 describes the self of the effective teacher; Chap. 7 explains the purposes of teachers.)

Davidson, A. H., and G. Lang, "Children's Perceptions of Their Teachers' Feelings Toward Them," *Journal of Experimental Education*, **29** (December 1960), 107–108.

DeCecco, J. P., *The Psychology of Language, Thought, and Instruction*, New York: Holt, Rinehart and Winston, Inc., 1967. (Contains readings on language, thought, and culture, language and social class, language and learning, and language and problem solving.)

DeVito, J., *The Psychology of Speech and Language: An Introduction to Psycholinguists*, New York: Random House, Inc., 1970, chap. 4. (Deals with communication theory.)

Eckroyd, D. H., *Speech in the Classroom*, 2nd ed., Englewood Cliffs, N.J.: Prentice-Hall, Inc., 1969. (Covers the development, uses, and techniques of effective speech in terms of both teacher and student.)

Egolf, D. B., and S. L. Chester, "Nonverbal Communication and the Disorders of Speech and Language, "*ASHA*, **15** (September 1973), 511–517. (Discusses the various facets of nonverbal communication in regard to the message of the clinician.)

Eisenson, J., J. J. Auer, and J. V. Irwin, *The Psychology of Communication*, New York: Appleton-Century-Crofts, 1963. (Chaps. 9, 11 deal with communicative process; Chaps. 14, 15 deal with factors in group discussion. Chaps. 19, 20, and 21 deal with personality and speech.)

Eisenstadt, S. N., "Communication Processes Among Immigrants in Israel," in A. G. Smith, ed., *Communication and Culture*, New York: Holt, Rinehart and Winston, Inc., 1966, pp. 576–587.

Erwin, S., and W. Miller, "Language Development," in *Child Psychology*, 62nd Yearbook of National Society for Study of Education, Chicago: University of Chicago Press, 1963, pp. 107–108.

Flanders, N. A., *Analyzing Teaching Behavior*, Reading, Mass.: Addison-Wesley Publishing Co., Inc., (Gives rules for a systematic analysis of what is happening as the teacher teaches. Teaching is seen as a learned behavior and through its analysis the teacher can make conscious changes.)

Fleming, F. L., "Creative Communication in the Elementary Grades," *Elementary English*, **48** (May 1971), 482–488. (Defines convergent and divergent thinking. Suggests ways of developing creative language abilities.)

Fygetakis, L., and D. Ingram, "Language Rehabilitation and Programmed Conditioning: A Case Study," *Journal of Learning Disabilities*, **6** (February 1973), 60–64.

Ginsburg, H., and S. Opper, *Piaget's Theory of Intellectual Development: An Introduction*, Englewood Cliffs, N.J.: Prentice-Hall, Inc., 1969.

Girardeau, F. L., and J. E. Spradlin, "An Introduction to the Functional Analysis of Speech and Language," in F. L. Girardeau and J. E. Spradlin, eds., *A Functional Analysis Approach to Speech and Language*, Washington, D.C.: *ASHA Monograph*, **14** (January 1970), 1–8.

Granowsky, A., and S. Granowsky, "Teachers as Models for Children's Speech," *Elementary English*, **41** (May 1972), 667–668. (Discusses teachers as language models—particularly in regard to vocabulary and syntax.)

Granowsky, S., and W. Krossner, "Kindergarten Teachers as Models for Children's Speech," *Journal of Experimental Education*, **38** (1970), 23–28. (Studied language production of seven kindergarten teachers and found that their language production was reduced to a level of complexity that was at, or even below, the actual level used by advantaged middle- and upper-middle-class students.)

Klevans, D. H., and H. B. Volz, "Development of a Clinical Evaluation Procedure," *ASHA*, **16** (September 1974), 489–491.

Knapp, M., *Nonverbal Communication in Human Interaction*, New York: Holt, Rinehart and Winston, Inc., 1972.

Leonard, L. B., "Modeling as a Clinical Procedure in Language Training," *Language, Speech, and Hearing Services in the Schools*, **6** (April 1975), 78–85. (Advises teaching specific language structures to language-handicapped children making use of a problem-solving set to emphasize the structural relationships of modeled utterances.)

————, "A Preliminary View of Information Theory and Articulatory Omissions," *Journal of Speech and Hearing Disorders*, **36** (November 1971), 511–517. (Suggests that therapy be based on items that contain much information for the child. This therapy assumes that the listeners in a child's environment are, at least in part, responsible for the child's articulatory behavior.)

McClean, J. E., "Extending Stimulus Control of Phoneme Articulation by Operant Techniques," in F. L. Girardeau and J. E. Spradlin, eds., *The Functional Analysis Approach to Speech and Language*, Washington, D.C.: *ASHA Monograph*, **14** (January 1970), 24–47.

McReynolds, L. V., "Contingencies and Consequences in Speech Therapy," *Journal of Speech and Hearing Disorders*, **35** (February 1970), 12–24. (Discusses some of the types of consequent events used to modify behavior, how they function to change behavior, and how they can be used in therapy.)

Minskoff, E. H., "Remediating Auditory Verbal Learning Disabilities: The Role of Questions in Teacher-Pupil Interaction," *Journal of Learning Disabilities*, **7** (August-September 1974), 406–413. (Classifies four types of teacher questions: cognitive-memory, convergent thinking, divergent thinking, and evaluative thinking.)

Muma, J. R., "The Communication Game: Dump and Play," *Journal of Speech and Hearing Disorders*, **40** (August 1975), 294–309. (Describes in detail the communication game—dump and play operations in a clinical setting.)

Ogilvie, M., and N. Rees, *Communication Skills: Voice and Pronunciation*, New York: McGraw-Hill, Inc., 1970, chap. 1. (Notes the effects of voice and pronunciation on communication.)

Reger, R., "What Does 'Mainstreaming' Mean?" *Journal of Learning Disabilities*, **7** (October 1974), 513–515. (Makes clear the different concepts of "mainstreaming" in terms of the degree of integration of the handicapped child with the normal child.)

Rogers, C. R., *On Becoming a Person*, Boston: Houghton Mifflin Company, 1961. (Makes the perceptual viewpoint of psychology clear.)

Rosenthal, R., and L. F. Jacobson, "Teacher Expectation for the Disadvantaged," *Scientific American*, **128** (April 1968), 3–7.

Ross, R. S., "Fundamental Processes and Principles of Communication," in K. Brooks, ed., *The Communication Arts and Sciences of Speech*, Columbus, Ohio: Charles E. Merrill Publishing Co., 1967, pp. 107–128. (Explains communication perception process.)

Schatzman, L., and A. Strauss, "Social Class and Modes of Communication," in A. G. Smith, ed., *Communication and Culture*, New York: Holt, Rinehart and Winston, Inc., 1966, pp. 442–455.

Schultz, M. C., "The Bases of Speech Pathology and Audiology: What Are Appropriate Models?" *Journal of Speech and Hearing Disorders*, **37** (February 1972), 118–122. (Considers interaction of patient and clinician and the appropriate models for speech and hearing.)

Shields, M. M., and E. Steiner, "The Language of Three-to Five-Year-Olds in Preschool Education," *The Journal of Educational Research*, **15** (February 1973), 97–105. (Examines a sample of spontaneous speech for developmental features and for the effect on language of different interpersonal situations.)

Shriberg, L. D., "The Effect of Examiner Social Behavior on Children's Articulation Test Performance," *Journal of Speech and Hearing Research*, **14** (September 1971), 659–672. (Studies interpersonal variables in the clinical process.)

————, F. S. Filley, D. H. Hayes, J. Kwiatkowski, J. A. Schatz, K. M. Simmons, and M. E. Smith, "The Wisconsin Procedure for Appraisal of Clinical Competence (W-PACC): Model and Data," *ASHA*, **17** (March 1975), 158–165. (Describes a systematic way of supervising and appraising clinical competence.)

Silberman, C. E., *Crisis in the Classroom*, New York: Random House, Inc., 1970. (Describes contemporary American education. Includes references to interaction analysis, earlier internships, and sensitivity training.)

Skinner, B. F., *Science and Human Behavior*, Englewood Cliffs, N.J.: Prentice-Hall, Inc., 1953.

————, *Verbal Behavior*, Englewood Cliffs, N.J.: Prentice-Hall, Inc., 1957.

Stark, J., "Current Clinical Practice in Language," *ASHA*, **13** (1971) 217–220.

Steck, E. L., J. W. Curtiss, P. J. Troesch, C. A. Binnie, "Clients Reinforcement of Speech Clinicians: A Factor-Analytic Study," *ASHA*, **15** (June 1973), 287–289. (Explores the possibility that certain behaviors consistently reward and others punish speech clinicians who offer therapy.)

Van Hattum, R. J., *Clinical Speech in Schools*, Springfield, Ill.: Charles C Thomas, Publisher, 1969. (Describes the operation of a speech and hearing therapy program in the public schools.)

Weaver, J. B., "An Investigation of Attitudes of Speech Clinicians in the Public Schools," *ASHA*, **10** (August 1968), 319–322. (Examines the attitudes of school clinicians toward the role of their profession in the school setting and toward ASHA.)

Winitz, H., "Problem Solving and the Delaying of Speech as Strategies in the Teaching of Language," *ASHA*, **15** (October 1973), 583–586. (Describes a set of language training principles that have been developed and that reflect the fact that children are able to solve problems of grammatical structure because mothers are skillful in presenting language stimuli.)

Woolf, G., "Informational Specificity: A Correlate of Verbal Output in the Diagnostic Interview," *Journal of Speech and Hearing Disorders*, **36** (November 1971), 518–526. (Examines the influence of the clinicians' verbalizations on the clients' verbal output.)

Yoder, D. E., "The Reinforcing Properties of a Television Presented Listener," in F. L. Girardeau, and J. E. Spradlin, eds., *A Functional Analysis Approach to Speech and Language, ASHA Monograph*, **14** (January 1970), 10–18.

5. The Mechanisms for Speech

In the discussion on the development of language later in this book, we emphasize that speech—the capacity to acquire language by listening and to produce language by "word of mouth"—is a form of behavior that is peculiar and specific to human beings. Despite this assumption, it is difficult to localize and identify the unique anatomical structures that make speech, as a form of behavior, possible. Students of speech and language who are concerned with such matters attribute the behavioral achievement of language to differences in the nervous system between human beings and other living beings. Within the nervous system, the greatest difference is in the brain. Primates such as the chimpanzees come closest to human beings in regard to anatomical structures that serve speech. The chimpanzees also come closest to human beings in regard to their capacity to use symbols that parallel if not approximate those used in human oral linguistic systems.

The following review of the mechanisms for speech, their structure and their manner of functioning, is intended to provide an understanding of normal speech functioning and what, on occasion, may go wrong when children have problems and deficiencies in acquiring proficient speech.

Voice Production

The human voice-producing mechanism functions in a manner that is roughly comparable to that of a musical wind instrument. The wind or horn instruments employ (1) reeds or the lips of the blower as vibrators or noisemakers; (2) air blown over or through the reeds as the source of energy to set the reeds in vibration; and (3) an elongated tube to reinforce the sound produced by the "vibrating" reeds. The human voice-producing mechanism employs laryngeal folds (vocal bands) for vibrators, air that might otherwise have served only normal respiratory purposes for a source of energy, and the cavities of the larynx, pharynx (throat), mouth, and nose as reinforcers or resonators. These cavities,

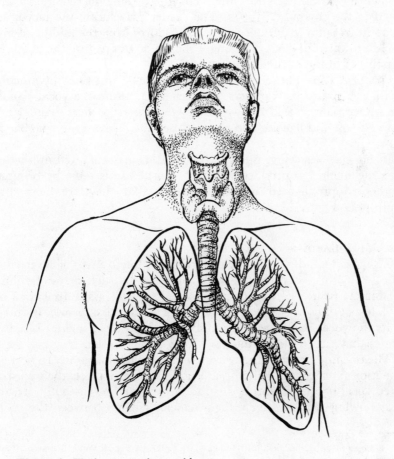

Figure 1. The larynx, trachea, and lungs.

if we include the trachea or windpipe, may be directly compared to a curved, elongated tube of a wind instrument. The human "elongated tube" is considerably more modifiable than that of any wind instrument, however, and so is capable of producing a wide variety of laryngeal tones that may be modified in respect to pitch, quality, loudness, and duration. The arrangement of the parts of the voice mechanism is indicated in Figure 1.

THE LARYNX

The larynx, commonly referred to as the voice box, is located in the neck between the root of the tongue and the trachea. The outer and largest part of the larynx consists of two shield-shaped cartilages fused together along an anterior line. Together, these fused shields are known as the thyroid cartilage. The reader may locate the larynx at this point by running his/her index finger down from the middle of his/ her chin toward his neck. The finger should be stopped by the notch at the point of fusion of the cartilages.

From each side of the larynx, folds of muscle tissue lined by mucous membrane appear as transverse folds that constitute the vocal bands. The upper pair of folds (the paired ventricular or false bands) are relatively soft and flaccid, and not as "movable" as are the true bands below.

In normal breathing, the true vocal bands are separated in a letter V arrangement. To produce voice, the vocal bands must be brought together (approximated or adducted) so that they are close and parallel (see Figure 2).

The Vocal Bands

The vocal bands or vocal folds[1] are small, tough strips of connective tissue, which are continuous with comparatively thick strips of voluntary muscle tissue. Viewed from above, the vocal bands appear to be flat folds of muscle with inner edges of connective tissue. In male adults the vocal bands range from about $\frac{7}{8}$ inch to $1\frac{1}{4}$ inches; in adult females they range from $\frac{1}{2}$ inch or less to about $\frac{7}{8}$ inch.

The opening between the vocal bands is called the glottis. In normal phonation (vocalization) the breath under pressure meets the approximated vocal bands and forces them to move apart. As a result, a stream of air flowing with relatively high velocity escapes between the vocal

---

[1] Unless otherwise specified, all references are to the true vocal bands. These may also be referred to as the vocal folds or vocal cords.

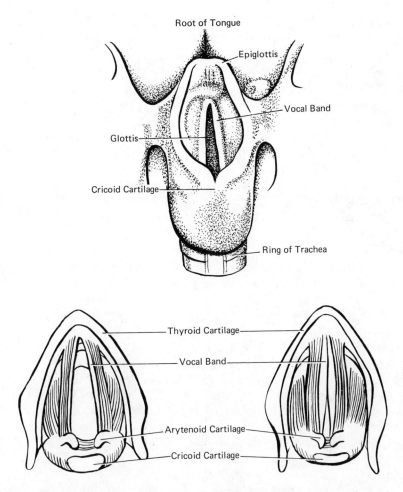

Figure 2. The larynx from above and behind. Below, the vocal bands, in position for breathing (left) and for vocalization (right).

bands, which continue to be held together (approximated) at both ends. The reduction in pressure beneath the bands, together with the reduced air pressure along the sides of the high-velocity air stream, aided by the elasticity of the bands themselves, brings about recurrent closures after successive outward movements of the bands. Thus vocalization is maintained. If the action or position of the vocal bands fails to produce a "complete" though momentary interruption in the flow of air, the result is a kind of noise or voice quality we identify as breathiness or hoarseness. Figure 2 indicates the position of the vocal bands as they are approximated and ready to be set into motion by the pressure of the air beneath them.

LOUDNESS

The loudness of the voice is directly related to the vigor with which air is forced from the lungs through the larynx, though not to the total amount of air that is expended. Pressure and velocity depend, in part, upon the size of the glottal opening and the length of time the glottis is open. Loudness is, in effect a result of the pressure of the released pulsations produced by the movements of the bands. Vocal tones are reinforced in the larynx, in the tracheal cavity immediately below the larynx, in the cavities of the throat and mouth, and in the nasal cavities.

PITCH

The fundamental pitch of a vibrating body varies directly with its frequency of vibration. Thus, the greater the frequency, the higher is the resultant pitch. Vocal pitch is a product of factors related to the condition of the vocal bands. The primary factors are the mass or thickness of the bands, their length, and the elasticity of the bands (tension) in relationship to their mass and length. In the process of phonation the vocal bands elongate as they increase in tension. By the same process, the bands are reduced in mass per unit area. The overall effect of the modification of mass-tension factors is to produce a higher rather than a lower pitch when the bands are set into motion. In general, the greater the tension, the higher is the pitch. If tension is held constant, with greater length or mass, the pitch is lower. If length and mass are held constant, the tension of the vocal bands is greater, and the pitch is higher.

Women tend to have higher pitched voices than men because usually they have shorter and thinner vocal bands than men. Our voices become lower in pitch as we mature because maturation is accompanied by an increase in the length and thickness of the vocal folds.[2]

The changes in pitch that we are able to produce under voluntary control take place, as we have indicated, largely by modifications in the degree of tension of the vocal folds. Through these modifications, we are capable of producing tones with ranges of pitch. The ranges may vary somewhat for singing and speaking. Good speakers may

---

[2] The average fundamental frequency for male voices is 128 cycles (Hz) per second; it is between 200–256 Hz for adult female voices.

have a range of about two octaves. Poor speakers may have narrower ranges. For most nonprofessional speakers it is probably more important to have good control of a one-octave range than poor control of a wider range. For each individual speaker it is important that voice be produced within the pitch range that is easiest and most effective for him. The range will include the optimum pitch level—the level of pitch at which the individual is able to produce the best quality of tone with least expenditure of effort. This is considered later in the discussion of optimum pitch.

THE ARYTENOID CARTILAGES

The vocal bands are attached at their sides to the wall of the thyroid cartilage. At the front, the bands are attached to the angle formed by the fusion of the two shields of the thyroid cartilage. At the back, each of the bands is attached to a pyramidal-shaped cartilage known as the arytenoid. The shape and muscular connections of the arytenoid cartilage enable them to move in ways that make it possible for the vocal bands to be brought together for vocalization, partly separated for whispering, or more widely separated for normal respiration. The arytenoids can pivot or rotate, tilt backward, or slide backward and sideways.

THE CRICOID CARTILAGE

The arytenoid cartilages rest on the top of the first tracheal ring. This ring, which has an enlarged and widened back, is known as the cricoid cartilage.

The movement of the vocal bands is brought about by the muscular connections of the bands to cartilages, and by the interconnections of the cartilages. Two types of action are important for vocalization. One is for the closing and opening of the bands (adduction and abduction) and the other is for changing the length and tension of the approximated bands to bring about changes in pitch.

THE CHEST CAVITY

The larynx, with its intricate structure of cartilages and muscles, provides the vibrator for phonation. The source of energy that sets the vibrators into motion is found in the chest cavity.

The chest (thoracic) cavity comprises a framework of bones and cartilages that includes the collarbone, the shoulder blades, the ribs, the breastbone or sternum, and the backbone. The diaphragm, as may be noted in Figure 3, constitutes both the floor of the thoracic cavity and the ceiling of the abdominal cavity. The lungs and the trachea

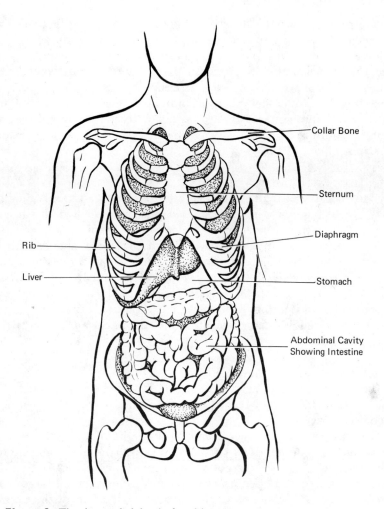

Figure 3. The chest and abdominal cavities.

are within the chest cavity. In the abdominal cavity directly below are the digestive organs, which include the stomach, the intestines, and the liver.

THE LUNGS

The lungs consist of a mass of air sacs that contain a considerable amount of elastic tissue. The lungs expand or contract, and so are partly filled or partly emptied of air as a result of differences in pressure brought about by actions of the muscles of the ribs and abdomen, which expand and contract the thoracic cavity. When the muscles of the ribs and abdomen and the downward action of the diaphragm expand the chest cavity, air is forced into the lungs by the outside air pressure. When the ribs and the upward movement of the diaphragm and abdominal muscles act to contract the chest cavity, air is forced out of the lungs. Through these actions, inhalation and exhalation take place.

THE DIAPHRAGM

The diaphragm is a double-domed muscular organ that separates the thoracic and abdominal cavities. The right half of the diaphragm rises somewhat higher—is more dome-shaped—than the left. When the capacity of the chest cavity is increased, air enters the lungs by way of the mouth, nose, throat, and trachea. In this part of the respiratory cycle—inhalation—the diaphragm is actively involved. The contraction of the diaphragm and its downward action serve to increase the volume of the chest cavity. In exhalation, the diaphragm is passive. It relaxes and returns to its former position because of the upward pressure of the abdominal organs. In the modified and controlled respiration necessary for phonation and speech, the muscles of the front and sides of the abdominal wall contract and press inward on the liver, stomach, and intestines. These organs in turn exert an upward pressure on the diaphragm, which transmits the pressure to the lungs and so forces air out of the lungs. Throughout the respiratory cycle, the diaphragm remains roughly dome-shaped. The height of the dome, as may be observed from Figure 4, is greater after exhalation than after inhalation.

Although the diaphragm is passive during exhalation, it does not relax suddenly and completely. Because the diaphragm maintains some degree of muscular tonus at all times, pressure upon it produces a gradual rather than an all-at-once relaxation. Gradual relaxation makes it possible for a steady stream of breath to be created and used to set the vocal bands in vibration. Pressure exerted by some of the abdominal muscles on the diaphragm supplies the extra amount of energy needed for setting the vocal bands in vibration. Without such pressure, exhalation would be passive, and sufficient only for normal respiratory purposes.

Breathing for Phonation. Normal respiration for a person without pathology or anomaly of the respiratory mechanism requires no special thought or effort. Breathing for phonation is different from normal respiratory breathing in at least two respects: (1) the ratio cycle of inspiration to respiration is modified so that there is a considerably longer period for exhalation than in casual breathing; (2) a steady

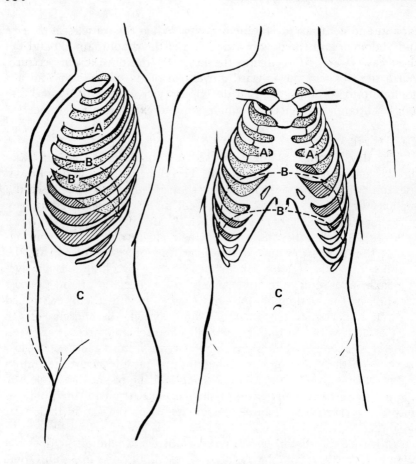

Figure 4. Action of the diaphragm and abdomen in breathing.
A. The chest cavity or thorax.
B. The diaphragm "relaxed" when exhalation is completed.
B'. The diaphragm contracted as in deep inhalation.
C. The abdominal cavity. The abdominal wall is displaced forward as the diaphragm
   moves downward during inhalation.

stream of air must be created and controlled at the will of the speaker
to ensure the initiation and maintenance of good tone. This type of air
flow is usually most easily accomplished by controlling the abdominal
musculature and by using small amounts of air rather than by inhaling
large amount of air. Attempts at deep inhalation tend to be accompanied by exaggerated activity of the upper part of the chest. This type
of breathing (clavicular) frequently promotes unsteadiness. The result
may be a wavering tone and a strained voice quality. Clavicular breathing tends to produce excessive neck and throat tensions, and so prevents

free and appropriate reinforcement of vocal tones in the cavities of the larynx and throat. Adequate breath supply is difficult to maintain, and the speaker needs to inhale more frequently than in abdominally controlled breathing.

THE RESONATING CAVITIES

The important resonating cavities for the human mechanism are those of the larynx, throat (pharynx), mouth (oral or buccal cavity), and nose (nasal cavity). To a lesser but not insignificant degree, the part of the windpipe below the larynx also serves as a resonating cavity. The principal cavities may be located by an examination of Figure 5.

The resonating cavities serve two functions in voice production: (1) they permit us to reinforce or build up the loudness of tones without resorting to constant energetic use of air pressure; and (2) through modification in the tension and shape of the cavities of the mouth, the nasopharynx, and the nasal cavity, we produce changes in the quality of vocal tones. For example, nasality may result when sound is permitted to enter and be emitted through the nasal chambers. This, however, is not the only cause of nasality as a voice quality.

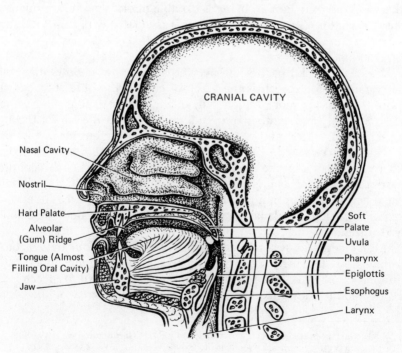

Figure 5. Head section showing principal resonators and organs of articulation

We have little control over the larynx as a resonating chamber. We have most control over the oral cavity and considerable control over the pharynx. The speech sounds we identify as vowels are produced by modifications in the size and shape of the oral cavity. Those sounds we recognize as consonants are produced as a result of changes of the organs of articulation, the lips included, within the oral cavity.

THE NERVOUS MECHANISM

Primates such as the apes have oral and respiratory mechanisms that approximate and parallel those of human beings, but with one important exception. The exception is that the nonhuman primates do not have a nervous system capable of the fine and specialized perception of those auditory events that constitute the signals and symbols of oral language. Nor do their systems permit, even on a reflexive level, the production of the variety of sounds that is normal for the infant and young child. Most apes are relatively quiet unless they are agitated. The chimpanzee, the subject of considerable study and training for its possible capabilities for learning a language system, is notably a very quiet animal.[3] So if we proceed on the assumption that, until proven otherwise, only the human being is capable of oral speech, we ought to consider what is unique about him that is associated with this capability.

THE CEREBRAL CORTEX

The very special part of the nervous system that endows man with the capability for speech is the cerebral cortex, the outer layer of the brain. The ten or more billion cells of the cortex enable man to perceive, analyze, and synthesize events that come to the cortex through the sensory avenues, and to determine appropriate output in the light of what was received. Particular areas of the cortex are related to different kinds of intake and output. For the purposes of this chapter, there is no need for us to go into detail about cerebrocortical functions. The diagram of the brain (Figure 6) shows some of the areas of specialization in which particular language functions are normally controlled or localized.

Man's cerebral system is significantly different from that of other primates in that the two hemispheres have become functionally different (see Figure 7.) Most important for us in regard to speech is the recently gained knowledge that the left temporal area of the cortex

---

[3] See References at end of chapter to articles by R. A. Gardner and B. T. Gardner and J. D. Fleming on the recent achievements of chimpanzees to learn to use visual sign-symbol systems.

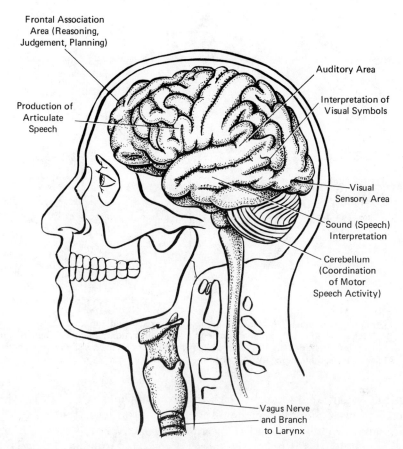

Frontal Association
Area (Reasoning,
Judgement, Planning)

Production of
Articulate
Speech

Auditory Area

Interpretation of
Visual Symbols

Visual
Sensory Area

Sound (Speech)
Interpretation

Cerebellum
(Coordination
of Motor
Speech Activity)

Vagus Nerve
and Branch
to Larynx

Figure 6. Localization of some brain functions in relation to speech.

processes speech events for almost all right-handed persons and for a majority of left-handed persons, whereas the right temporal cortex processes auditory intake that is not speech, for example, musical, mechanical, and other environmental noises. By virtue of this specialization, we may say that the left brain (cortex) is for speech listening. Because those of us who do not have severe impairment in hearing learn to speak by imitating what we hear, the left brain is also for talking. Damage to the left temporal cortex impairs the capacity for auditory perception of speech and so results in serious delay in the onset and development of language. Damage to a child or an adult who has acquired language will usually result in a breakdown of language function. Fortunately for the child below the age of 12, his cerebro-

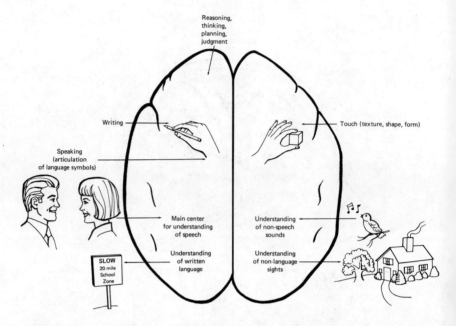

Figure 7. The two hemispheres of the brain cortex showing special areas related to language (left half) and non-language areas (right half). Although the hemispheres are virtually twins in superficial appearance, they have different functions. As may be noted from the diagram, many of the functions are related as to modality of intake.

cortical system at this stage seems to have sufficient plasticity for the alternate or nondominant hemisphere to take over the language functions normally controlled by the left or dominant hemisphere. Unfortunately, this is not so for most adults. Impairments of language function associated with brain damage are known as aphasias. We discuss the aphasic child in Chapter 16.

Problems

1. What determines the range of pitch of a musical instrument? What part of the violin reinforces the sounds of the vibrators? What are the essential differences between the sounds of a violin and those of a cello?

2. Is deep breathing necessary for most speech purposes? Why should clavicular breathing be avoided?

3. Read pages 344–346 of Van Riper and Irwin, *Voice and Articulation* (Englewood Cliffs, N.J.: Prentice-Hall, Inc., 1958). What do these authors recommend as the best techniques to control breathing for vocalization? How do their recommendations compare with those of this text?

4. What are the functions of the resonating cavities in phonation?
5. Over which resonators do we have the most control? Over which do we have the least control?
6. What is nasality? What is denasality? Is nasal reinforcement always to be avoided? What is the effect of a "stuffed" nose?
7. What cavities does the diaphragm separate? What is the shape of the diaphragm during exhalation? How does the shape of the diaphragm change during inhalation? How are these changes achieved?
8. What is a syrinx? What are the essential differences in sound making between birds and most mammals? How does a parrot manage to sound as if he is speaking? What is the source of the whistling of dolphins?
9. Male and female vocal bands overlap in range of length, yet it is usually easy to distinguish the voices of low-pitched females from high-pitched males. Why?
10. What is cerebral dominance? How is cerebral dominance related to language functioning? Where are nonlanguage auditory events perceived?
11. Read a recent article on animal language. Is any animal coming close to human beings in learning (acquiring) a language system merely by exposure rather than by being directly taught? What modality seems to be most feasible in teaching language to chimpanzees? Why?
12. Read an article on dolphin communication. Do you think that dolphins have a symbol-language system? Why?

References and Suggested Readings

Denes, P. B., and E. N. Pinson, *The Speech Chain: The Physics and Biology of Spoken Language*, Baltimore: The Williams & Wilkins Co., 1963, chaps. 2–7. (An introductory but authoritative discussion of the mechanisms for spoken language.)

Eisenson, J., "The Left Brain Is for Talking," *Acta Symbolica*, **2** (1971), 33–36. (A discussion of why the left hemisphere is dominant for language functioning.)

————, *Voice and Diction: A Program for Improvement*, 3rd ed., New York: Macmillan Publishing Co., Inc., 1974, chap. 2. (A more detailed but basic consideration of the mechanisms for speech than in the present chapter.)

Fleming, J. D., "Field Report, The State of the Apes." *Psychology Today* (January 1974), 31–50. (An overview of recent accomplishments in teaching sign language and other symbol systems to chimpanzees. Includes an explanation of why chimpanzees are not able to learn to use an oral (word-of-mouth) language system.)

Gardner, R. A., and B. T. Gardner, "Early Signs of Language in Child and Chimpanzee," *Science*, **187** (February 1975), 752–753. (An updated explanation of how two chimpanzees are learning to use signs by exposure to deaf persons who use the American Sign Language.)

Moore, P., *Organic Voice Disorders*, Englewood Cliffs, N.J.: Prentice-Hall, Inc., 1971. (Chaps. 1–3 deal with the mechanisms for voice production. Brief, clear scientific exposition.)

Palmer, J. M., and D. A. La Russo, *Anatomy for Speech and Hearing*, New York: Harper & Row, Publishers, Inc., 1965, chap. 8.

6. The Production of Speech Sounds

In this chapter we explain how consonants, vowels, and dipthongs are usually produced. We recognize that the described positions are merely the conventional ones and that, because our mechanism is adaptable, we produce sounds in ways other than the conventional ones. We further attempt to show characteristics that are shared by a number of sounds, for to recognize likenesses in sounds is important in understanding the development of speech sounds and in the correction of speech sounds. The teacher needs this information to understand children's speech patterns, and the clinician needs it to work with children who have articulatory problems.

Most of this discussion of sounds is based on the writings and research of articulatory phoneticians who work primarily in the discipline of speech communication. You may have studied the production of sounds in a linguistics course or in a course dealing with acoustic phonetics. We have included, however, a brief explanation of terms used in research dealing with distinctive features and have included a summary of a distinctive feature scheme, because some of the recent articulatory therapy discussion is based on distinctive feature concepts.

Relationship of Spelling to Sounds

It is hardly necessary to impress the readers of this text with the realization that American English, or British English for that matter, does not consistently represent the same sound with the same alphabet letter. The teacher who has had any concern with teaching children to read has on numerous occasions had to explain that many words are pronounced in a manner that is only remotely suggested by their spellings. Perhaps the teacher has been aware that we have 40 or more sound families in our spoken language. If not, the teacher has surely known that we have 26 letters, many of which represent more than one sound, and some of which, according to given words, represent the same sound. So the child has been instructed to memorize the pronunciation and spelling of such words as *though, enough, through,* and *cough* as well as the varied ways in which the sound *sh* is represented in the words *attention, delicious, ocean,* and *shall.* Vowel sounds, too, have their inconsistencies so that before children at school are too far along in their careers they become aware that the sound of *ee* in *see* may be represented differently in words such as *eat, believe, receive, species,* and *even.* Later, they may be able to accept without too much consternation the spellings of words of foreign derivation such as *subpoena* and *esprit.*

Phonemes

If the teacher has had a course in phonetics, the concept of the phoneme may have been established. A phoneme is a distinctive phonetic element of a word. It is the smallest distinctive group or class of sounds in a language. Each phoneme includes a variety of closely related sounds that differ somewhat in manner of production and in acoustic end results, but do not differ so much that the listener is more aware of difference than of similarity or sameness. So, for example, the *t* of *tin* is different from the *t* of *its, spotted, button,* and *metal,* and from the *t* in the phrase *hit the ball,* but an essential quality of *t* is common in all these words. Despite differences we have a phoneme *t.*

In this text, phonemes are represented by the symbol of the International Phonetic Alphabet (IPA).

Note that phonetic symbols represent pronunciations as they are made. The same sound and its phonemic variants are represented by a single symbol. This is not the case with diacritic symbols, which, for some vowels and diphthongs, require several representations for the same phoneme.

The Common Phonemes of American English

Key Word	IPA Symbol

CONSONENTS

	Key Word	IPA Symbol
1.	*p*at	[p]
2.	*b*ee	[b]
3.	*t*in	[t]
4.	*d*en	[d]
5.	*c*ook	[k]
6.	*g*et	[g]
7.	*f*ast	[f]
8.	*v*an	[v]
9.	*th*in	[θ]
10.	*th*is	[ð]
11.	*s*ea	[s]
12.	*z*oo	[z]
13.	*sh*e	[ʃ]
14.	trea*s*ure	[ʒ]
15.	*ch*ick	[tʃ]
16.	*j*ump	[dʒ]
17.	*m*e	[m]
18.	*n*o	[n]
19.	si*ng*	[ŋ]
20.	*l*et	[l]
21.	*r*un	[r]
22.	*y*ell	[j]
23.	*h*at	[h]
24.	*w*on	[w]
25.	*wh*at*	[ʍ] or [hw]

VOWELS

	Key Word	IPA Symbol
26.	f*ee*	[i]
27.	s*i*t	[ɪ]
28.	t*a*ke	[e]
29.	m*e*t	[ɛ]
30.	c*a*lm	[ɑ]
31.	t*a*sk	[æ] or [a] depending upon regional or individual variations
32.	c*a*t	[æ]
33.	h*o*t	[ɒ] or [a] depending upon regional or individual variations
34.	s*a*w	[ɔ]
35.	*o*bey, s*ew*	[o] or [ou]
36.	b*u*ll	[ʊ]

Key Word	IPA Symbol
37. b*oo*n	[u]
38. h*u*t	[ʌ]
39. *a*bout	[ə]
40. upp*er*	[ɚ] by most Americans and [ə] by many others
41. b*i*rd	[ɝ] by most Americans and [ɜ] by many others
	DIPHTHONGS
42. s*igh*	[aɪ]
43. n*oi*se	[ɔɪ]
44. c*ow*	[aʊ] or [ɑʊ] depending upon individ- ual variations
45. m*ay*	[eɪ]
46. g*o*	[oʊ]
47. ref*u*se	[ɪu] or [ju] depending upon individ- ual variations
48. use	[ju]

* If distinction is made in pronunciation of words such as
what and *watt; when* and *wen.*

If you wish to memorize the phonetic symbols, it may encourage you to know that 16 of the consonant symbols are taken from the English alphabet. They are: p, b, t, d, k, g, f, v, s, z, m, n, l, r, h, and w. IPA symbols for vowels, however, vary considerably from alphabetic representations.

Morphemes

The speaker combines phonemes meaningfully to produce what the linguist calls *morphemes*. A morpheme is a minimal unit that carries meaning and is made up of one or more phonemes. Lloyd and Warfel note that "written sentences break up into words, but spoken sentences break up into morphemes" (Lloyd and Warfel 1956, p. 61). When the speaker combines morphemes in meaningful ways, he produces phrases and sentences, or what the linguist calls *utterances*. This example may illustrate: The word *hit* is a combination of the phonemes [h], [ɪ], and

[t]. This combination [hɪt] is a morpheme, for it cannot be broken into a smaller form with meaning. The word *lemon* constitutes a morpheme for neither the syllable [lɛm] or [ən] carries meaning. In the plural form [lɛmənz], the added [z] is a morpheme in itself for it is a minimal unit that does carry meaning.

In this chapter, although we are primarily concerned with phonemes, we wish to emphasize the influence of one sound upon another in context. The following discussion is concerned with how sounds are produced and a description of the parts of the speech mechanism that are employed in articulation.

Articulatory Mechanism

Speech sounds are produced when the breath stream that comes from the lungs by way of the trachea and larynx is modified in the mouth before leaving the body. Breath may be modified by movements of the lips, teeth, jaws, tongue, and the soft palate (roof of the mouth). Most American-English sounds are produced as a result of lip and tongue activity and resulting contacts with other organs of articulation. The front part of the tongue (tip and blade) and the part of the mouth at or near the upper gum ridge is the "favored" area for articulatory contact for American-English speech sounds. The sounds *t, d, l, n, s, z, sh* [ʃ], *zh* [ʒ], *ch* [tʃ], and *j* [dʒ] are all produced by action of the anterior tongue and contact at or close to the upper gum ridge.

As can be seen in Figure 8, the upper gum ridge or alveolar process is the area directly behind the upper teeth. Immediately behind the alveolar process is the hard palate. Posterior to it is the soft palate or velum. The uvula is the most posterior part of the "roof of the mouth."

The tongue lies within and almost completely fills the oral or mouth cavity. The tongue, from the point of view of articulatory action, may be considered as being divided into tongue tip, blade, front (mid), and back, as indicated in Figure 8.

The lips act as articulators for the production of the sounds *p* and *b*. The sound *m* is produced with closed lips. The sounds *f* and *v* are usually produced as a result of action involving the lower lip and upper teeth. The various vowel and diphthong sounds are produced with characteristic lip and jaw movement, though the lips do not make any articulatory contacts for these sounds. The production of American-English sounds is considered later in somewhat greater detail.

Speech sounds may be emitted either through the mouth or through the nasal cavity. In the absence of specific pathology, the speaker is able to determine the avenue of sound emission. Most American-English

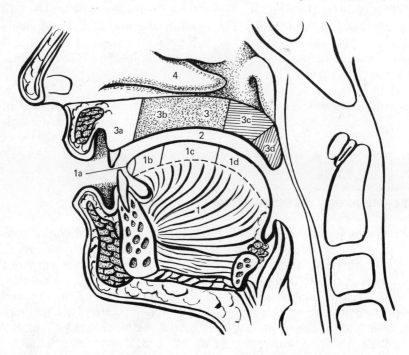

Figure 8. Diagram showing parts of the tongue in relationship to the roof of the mouth.

1. Tongue	3. Palate
1a. Tongue tip	3a. Gum or alveolar ridge
1b. Blade of tongue	3b. Hard palate
1c. Front or mid of tongue	3c. Soft palate
1d. Back of tongue	3d. Uvula
2. Mouth (oral) cavity	4. Nasal cavity.

sounds are emitted through the mouth. The sounds *m, n,* and the consonant that is usually represented in spelling by the letters *ng* are emitted through the nasal cavity.

Sounds usually are categorized as (1) consonants, (2) vowels, and (3) diphthongs. A consonant is a sound that results from the action of articulating agents somehow interrupting the expiring breath, with the vocal bands sometimes vibrating, sometimes not. A vowel is a sound with little or no stoppage of the breath stream, whose quality comes from the vibration of the vocal bands and from the shape and size of the resonating chambers in the throat and mouth. Diphthongs are combinations or rapid blends of two vowels—usually beginning with one vowel and gliding into another.

Consonants

As you say *pat*, *bat*, and *mat*, you hear three distinct words, because the first consonant in each of these three words is different. However, as you say the three words, you find that in each instance you have made the sounds with your two lips. Another likeness exists in [p] and [b]. In these sounds, you have held the sound briefly and quickly released it. [p] and [b] are called *stops*. How, then, do [p] and [b] differ? [p] is made without voice, [b], with voice. How, then, do [b] and [m] differ? Both sounds are voiced but [p] is held and quickly released without nasal emission, whereas [m] is continued and is emitted nasally. Thus, the manner of production of [m] results in acoustic features that enable the listener to distinguish it from [p].

From this discussion we can then classify the consonant sounds according to (1) manner of production, (2) place of articulation, and (3) the vocal component.

MANNER OF PRODUCTION

Stops

When you say the [p] and [b] in *pat* and *bat*, you use your lips but you also make the sounds by compressing the breath and suddenly releasing it. These sounds are therefore called stops. Other stops are [t], [d], [k], and [g].

Continuants

All other sounds are continuants, which in turn are classified as [1] frictionless consonants or *semivowels* and (2) fricatives. The continuant [m] that you hear in *mat* is emitted nasally by lowering your velum and by directing the air through the nose. The other two nasal sounds are [n] and [ŋ] as in *sing*. The lateral [l] and the glides are also classified as semivowels. [l] is made with the sound being forced over two sides of the tongue. The glides, [r] as in *run*, [j] as in *yell*, [w] as in *won*, and [ʍ] as in *what*, are made by the movement of the articulatory agents from one position to another. All these sounds are frictionless. Other continuant sounds called fricatives, however, have a frictionlike quality, which is caused by the release of sound through a narrow opening between the organs of articulation. A stream of breath is maintained with some pressure to make the sound continuous. These sounds are [f], [v], [s], [z], [h], [θ] as in *thin*, [ð] as in *this*, [ʍ] as in *what*, [ʃ] as in *she*, and [ʒ] as in *treasure*.

AFFRICATES

Lastly, American-English sounds include affricates or the consonantal blends, as [tʃ] in *check* and [dʒ] in *jump*. Thus, each sound achieves some of its characteristic acoustic quality by its manner of production.

PLACE OF ARTICULATION

The classification of consonants just given was according to manner of articulation. Consonants may also be classified as to which articulators are used and the position they are in during the act of sound production. The following is a classification of consonants as to position of articulators:

1. *Bilabial.* Sounds are produced as a result of the activity of the lips. The sounds [p], [b], [m], [ʍ], and [w] are bilabials.

2. *Lip-teeth* (*labiodental*). Contact is made between the upper teeth and lower lip for the production of labiodental sounds. The sounds so produced are [f] and [v].

3. *Tongue-teeth* (*linguadental*). Contact is made between the point of the tongue and the upper teeth or between the point of the tongue in a position between the teeth. The *th* sounds [θ] and [ð] may be made either postdentally or interdentally. Most mature speakers are likely to produce these sounds postdentally.

4. *Tongue-tip gums* (*lingua-alveolar*). The region of the mouth at or near the gum ridge is the "favored place" for the articulation of American-English sounds. The sounds [t], [d], [n], and [l] are produced with the tip of the tongue in contact with the upper gum ridge. The sound [r] is most frequently produced with the tongue tip turned back slightly away from the gum ridge. The sounds [s], [z], *sh* [ʃ], *zh* [ʒ], *ch* [tʃ], and *j* [dʒ] are produced with the blade of the tongue making articulatory contact a fraction of an inch behind the gum ridge.

5. *Palatal.* The sound *y* [j] is produced with the middle of the tongue initially raised toward the hard palate. The sounds [k] and [g] are usually produced with the back of the tongue in contact with the soft palate. In some contexts [k] and [g] may be produced with the middle of the tongue in contact with the hard palate. The reader may check his place of articulation for the [k] in *car* compared with [k] in *keel.* He may also wish to compare the [g] of *get* with the [g] of *got.*

The sound of *ng* [ŋ] is most likely to be produced with the back of the tongue in contact with the soft palate.

In some contexts, the sound [r] is produced with the middle of the tongue raised toward the palate. Some persons produce the [r] of *rose* and *around* in this manner.

6. *Glottal.* One American-English sound, [h], is produced with the breath coming through the opening between the vocal folds and without

modification by the other articulators. The [h] is referred to as a glottal sound.

VOCAL COMPONENT

A third classification of sounds is according to the presence or absence of voice. Consonants produced without accompanying vocal-fold vibration are referred to as *voiceless* or *unvoiced*; those produced with accompanying vocal fold vibration are called *voiced*. The voiceless consonants of American-English speech are [p], [t], [k], [ʍ], [f], *th* of *th*ink [θ], [s], *sh* [ʃ], and [h]. The voiced consonants are [b], [d] [g], [m], [n], *ng* [ŋ], [v], *th* of *th*is [ð], [z], *zh*, [ʒ], [w], [r], y[j], and [l]. A resumé of the multiple classification of American-English consonant sounds is presented in the chart that follows.

Production of American English Consonants

Involvement of Articulatory Agents

Manner of Production	LIPS (BI-LABIAL)	LIP-TEETH (LABO-DENTAL)	TONGUE-TEETH (LINGUA-DENTAL)	TONGUE TIP ALVEOLAR RIDGE (LINGUA-ALVEOLAR)	TONGUE AND HARD PALATE (LINGUA-PALATAL)	TONGUE AND SOFT PALATE (VELAR)	GLOTTIS (GLOTTAL)
Voiceless stops	p			t		k	
Voiced stops	b			d		g	
Voiceless fricatives	ʍ	f	θ	s*	ʃ†	ʍ¶	h
Voiced fricatives		v	ð	z*	ʒ†		
Nasals	m			n		ŋ	
Lateral semivowel				l			
Glides	w				r‡ j	w¶	
Voiceless affricate					tʃ		
Voiced affricate					dʒ		

　* In [s] and [z], the channel is narrow.
　† In [ʃ] and [ʒ], the channel is broad.
　‡ The tongue tip in many instances is curled away from the gum ridge to the center of the palate.
　¶ In [ʍ] and [w], both the lips and the back of the tongue are involved.

Distinctive Features of Consonants

If we apply the term *distinctive features* to the system just described, we base our distinctions on the differences in consonants on manner of production, place of articulation, and the vocal component. For example, let us contrast [p], [b], and [m]. The feature distinguishing [p] and [b] is the vocal component. On the other hand, [m] has three features to distinguish it from [p]: it possesses voice, is made with nasal resonance, and is a continuant, whereas [p] does not possess these three characteristics.

The term *distinctive features* as applied in the literature refers to features presented as binary contrasts. The feature is present [+] or absent [−]. If we put the distinguishing features of [p], [b], and [m] as just discussed in this form it would appear as:

Distinctive Features of /p/, /b/, and /m/

	Voice	Nasal	Continuant	Labial
[p]	−	−	−	+
[b]	+	−	−	+
[m]	+	+	+	+

So far we have been talking about strictly articulatory features. But in describing systematic phonemes, a more general categorization is used. This categorization is appropriate in describing the phonological rules of the languages of the world. As noted previously distinctive features are binary in form; that is, each feature is present [+] or absent [−]. This structure can be helpful in noting the rules of phonology. An example from assimilative processes (see Chapter 4) follows: Assimilative processes are at work in the word *small*. Normally [m] possesses the feature [+voicing]. But the [m] in *small* is preceded by [s] with its feature [−voicing] and this [m] then changes its feature to [−voicing], because of the influence of the feature of [−voicing] in [s]. Or where an unvoiced sound as [t] in *better* is surrounded by two sounds [ɛ] and [ɚ] with the feature [+voicing], the [t] tends to change the [−voicing] feature to [+voicing].

The following scheme used in articulatory therapy based on distinctive features mixes the criteria from both articulatory and acoustic phonetics. Its origin is hybrid; for example, *high* is a physiologic term, whereas strident refers to *quality*. The terms used in this scheme[1] and their definitions follow:

Terms Used in Distinctive Feature Analysis

Term	*Characterized by*
Consonantal	Interference of breath stream and abrupt movements of formants.
Vocalic	No interference of breath stream and steady or slow moving formants.
High	Front or back of tongue being raised from neutral position.
Low	Front or back of tongue being lowered from neutral position.
Back	Back of tongue being retracted from neutral position.
Anterior	Production in the front position of mouth, tongue, or lips.
Coronal	Involvement of the tip or blade, which is raised from neutral position.
Continuant	Partial obstruction of air stream, which continues to flow.
Voicing	Accompanying vocal fold vibration.
Nasal	Lowering of the velum with the air stream passing through the nose.
Strident	High degree of turbulence or noisy sound where articulated.
Sonorant	Absence of any interference with flow of glottal sound.

Distinctive Features of Various Phonemes

Feature	p	b	t	d	k	g	tʃ	dʒ	f	v	θ	ð	s	z	ʃ	ʒ	m	n	y	r	l	j	h	w	ʍ
Consonantal	+	+	+	+	+	+	+	+	+	+	+	+	+	+	+	+	+	+	+	+	+	−	+	−	+
Vocalic	−	−	−	−	−	−	−	−	−	−	−	−	−	−	−	−	−	−	−	+	+	−	−	−	−
High	−	−	−	−	+	+	+	+	−	−	−	−	−	−	+	+	−	−	+	−	−	+	−	+	+
Low	−	−	−	−	−	−	−	−	−	−	−	−	−	−	−	−	−	−	−	−	−	−	+	−	−
Back	−	−	−	−	+	+	−	−	−	−	−	−	−	−	+	+	−	−	−	−	−	−	−	+	−
Anterior	+	+	+	+	−	−	−	−	+	+	+	+	+	+	−	−	+	+	−	−	+	−	−	+	+
Coronal	−	−	+	+	−	−	+	+	−	−	+	+	+	+	+	+	−	+	−	+	+	−	−	−	−
Continuant	−	−	−	−	−	−	−	−	+	+	+	+	+	+	+	+	−	−	−	+	+	−	+	+	+
Voicing	−	+	−	+	−	+	−	+	−	+	−	+	−	+	−	+	+	+	+	+	+	+	−	+	−
Nasal	−	−	−	−	−	−	−	−	−	−	−	−	−	−	−	−	+	+	+	−	−	−	−	−	−
Strident	−	−	−	−	−	−	+	+	+	+	−	−	+	+	+	+	−	−	−	−	−	−	−	−	−
Sonorant	−	−	−	−	−	−	−	−	−	−	−	−	−	−	−	−	+	+	+	+	+	+	−	+	−

Some authors use [č] for [tʃ]
[j] for [dʒ]
[š] for [ʃ]
[ž] for [ʒ]
[y] for [j]

---

[1] See, for example, the schemes in L. V. McReynolds and K. Huston, "A Distinctive Feature Analysis of Children's Misarticulations," *Journal of Speech and Hearing Disorders*, **36** (May 1971) or H. Winitz *From Syllable to Conversation* (Baltimore: University Park Press, 1975).

Such a scheme is but the beginning of distinctive feature articulatory generalizations. More research and study will likely bring about refinement in the categories and in their descriptions. For example, in the literature we find questioning of the assignment of the feature *stridency* to [f] and [v] but not to [θ] and [ð]. Bolinger calls this assignment "rather arbitrary" (Bolinger 1975, p. 80).

Parker (1976) contrasts the two theories of distinctive features (generative and phonemic), emphasizing that the two theories are conceptually different. He notes that the phonemic theory is more widely advocated in speech science than the generative theory. But he believes that the generative theory has several advantages over the phonemic theory in working out a general theoretical framework within which distinctive features and parameters of speech production (production features) can be put into perspective.

From your newly acquired knowledge of the presence or lack of voice, the articulatory agents involved and the manner of production of consonants, examine the following changes and indicate what happens. For example, *tense* often becomes [tɛnts]. The insertion of [t], which is made with approximately the same articulatory agents as [s] and [n], takes place because the morpheme becomes easier to utter with the [t] inserted. Why, then, does *something* become [ˈsʌmpˌθɪŋ], tenth [tɛntθ] and *dance* [dænts]?

1. As you say *tackle* and *gargle*, the [k] and [g] are exploded laterally. Explain why.
2. As you utter *at the store* and *add the numbers*, the [t] and [d] are made with the tongue on the teeth rather than on the alveolar ridge. Why?
3. In *let out the dog, little, city mouse, cutting the grass*, [t] takes on some of the voiced characteristics of [d]. Why?
4. In *grandmother* and *handsome*, speakers frequently omit [d]. What characteristic of the [n] influences the omission of [d]?
5. In *campfire* and *obviate*, the [f] and [v] are made by some speakers with both lips, causing the sounds to become labial fricatives. Why does this happen?
6. In rapid speech, you are likely to omit [θ] in *fifth* and *seventh*. Explain in terms of the place of articulation.
7. Why in the speech of one individual do two pronunciations of *with* occur—*with Dan* [wɪð dæn] and *with Tom* [wɪθ tɑm]?
8. Why, in terms of the articulatory agents involved, does *Captain* become [kæpm̩]?

Vowels

Whereas consonants are important because they help bring intelligibility to the message, vowels through their variables of quality, pitch, time, and loudness bring emotion and feeling to the message. The word *no* printed singly carries some meaning as a written symbol, but *no* spoken singly carries more meaning and feeling. Spoken with loudness and a downward inflection, it conveys one kind of meaning and feeling; spoken softly with a rising inflection, it carries another kind of meaning and feeling.

Vowels are more variable than consonants; neighboring sounds influence vowels more than consonants. And the effect of the continuing movement of the vocal articulators during the utterance of a vowel in a word or phrase makes for differences both in acoustic results and articulatory movements. Although we describe vowels according to the previous discussion, you must remember that these characteristics are based on norms and that many individual variations exist.

Vowel sounds share the following characteristics in their manner of production: (1) All vowels are voiced, unless for special purposes the entire speech content is intentionally whispered; (2) all vowels are continuant sounds in that they are produced without interruption or restriction of the breath stream; (3) changes in tongue and jaw position are primarily responsible for the distinctive differences in vowel phonemes. To a lesser degree, lip activity accounts for some of the difference in articulatory activity and in acoustic end result.

PLACE OF PRODUCTION

All vowel sounds require activity of the tongue as a whole. It will be noticed, however, that each of the American-English vowels is produced with one part of the tongue more actively involved than the remainder of the tongue. For example, in the production of the vowel of the word *me*, the tip of the tongue remains relatively inactive behind the lower teeth while the front of the tongue is tensed and raised toward the hard palate. In changing from *me* to *moo*, we may note that the front of the tongue is relatively relaxed while the back is tensed and elevated toward the roof of the mouth. The vowel of *me*, because of its characteristic tongue activity, is considered to be a *front vowel*; similarly, the vowel of *moo*, because of the back of the tongue activity, is considered to be a *back vowel*.[2]

HEIGHT OF TONGUE

Now, let us contrast the production of the vowels of *me* and *man*. Both of these are produced with front of the tongue activity, but the tongue is higher for the vowel of *me* than it is for the vowel of *man*. Similarly, the tongue is higher for the back vowel of *moon* than it is for the vowel of *mock*. In the words *mirth* and *mud*, where middle-of-the-tongue activity is characteristic, we may also note that the vowel of *mirth* is produced with the tongue higher in position than it is in *mud*. The difference in height of tongue position, however, is not as great as for the other pairs of words.

Thus, far, we have seen that vowels differ somewhat in individual production according to the part of the tongue that is most actively involved and the height of the tongue. We may also have noted that the change in the height of the tongue is likely to be accompanied by a change in the position of the lower jaw. That is, the jaw drops as the tongue drops, in going from a "high" to a "low" vowel. A third aspect of vowel production is now considered.

MUSCLE TENSION

If we compare the vowels of *tea* and *tin*, we should be able to sense that the tongue is more tense for the vowel of *tea* than it is for the vowel of *tin*. Similarly, the vowel of *moot* is produced with more tongue tension than the vowel of *mock*. Further analysis will show that the differences in tension are not confined to the muscles of the tongue. The muscles of the chin also differ in degree of tension. A third muscle difference may be felt by observing the changes in the position of the apex of the larynx—the "Adam's apple." When the tongue and under part of the chin are tense, the apex of the larynx is elevated and moves toward the front of the chin as it does in the act of swallowing. When the tongue and the under part of the chin are relatively relaxed, the larynx drops back to its normal position of rest as in quiet breathing.

On the basis of our discussion thus far, we may arrive at a threefold classification for vowel sounds.

---

[2] In some contexts, the positions we have described may be more theoretic than real. The descriptions may sometimes be more accurate for the isolated vowel than in the flow of speech. Nevertheless, we think that when a child has difficulty in producing the vowels of English, training that follows these descriptions should be helpful. The reservation about tongue positions also holds for the other features of vowel production.

1. Vowels differ as to place of production. They may be produced either in the front of the mouth, with the front or blade of the tongue most active; in the middle of the mouth, with the midtongue most active; or in the back of the mouth, with the back of the tongue most active.
2. Vowels differ as to height of tongue position.
3. Vowels differ as to degree of muscle tension.

Front Vowels		*Midvowels*		*Back Vowels*	
	PHONETIC SYMBOL		PHONETIC SYMBOL		PHONETIC SYMBOL
meet	[i]			boon	[u]
milk	[ɪ]			book	[ʊ]
may	[e]	Mirth	[ɜ] or [ɝ]	boat	[o]
men	[ɛ]	about	[ə]	ball	[ɔ]
mat	[æ]	upper	[ɚ]	bog	[ɒ]
ask*	[a]	mud	[ʌ]	balm	[ɑ]

* When the speaker compromises between the vowels of *mat* and *balm*.

LIP ROUNDING

A fourth feature that distinguishes some vowels from others, especially when the vowels are produced as isolated sounds, is lip-rounding. Back vowels, with the exception of the *a* of *calm*, are produced with the lips somewhat rounded. The vowel of the word *pool* is most rounded. There is lesser rounding for the vowels in *pull*, *boat*, *ball*, and *cot*. For persons who do not distinguish between the vowels of *cot* and *calm*, there will be no lip-rounding for either.

In the lists of words in the preceding section, the first column contains front vowels, arranged in order of highest to lowest tongue position. The second column contains midvowels, and the third column contains back vowels, arranged in the same order.

The tongue positions for the vowels of these words are shown in Figure 9. The dotted area represents the high points of the tongue.

DEGREE OF STRESSING

Vowels with greater stress tend to be longer than those with less stress; in fact, the stressed vowel often becomes diphthongized. Where [e]

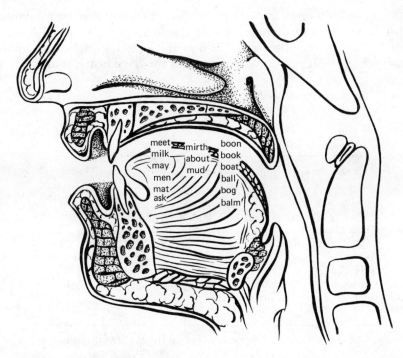

Figure 9. Representative tongue positions for American-English vowels. In actual speech there is considerable individual variation from these positions according to speech context.

is stressed as uttered in the list of words, *vague, day, rain*, it is diphthongized. But when it is not stressed, as in the first syllable of *vacation* and in the last syllable of *mandate*, it is not dipthongized. Context is also important in the degree of stress. When you say, "Give me Kay's address," you are likely to use the monophthongal [e]. But when you say, "Are you meeting Kay?" you are likely to use the diphthongal [eɪ]. A second example involves [o]. When you say *obey*, the [o] not being stressed is usually [o], whereas in *row*, the [o] being stressed is usually [oʊ]. When you stress *throw* in "Throw it out," the [oʊ] is diphthongal. But when you do not stress *throw* in "Did Johnny throw away today's paper?" the [o] tends to be the monophthongal [o].

Defective Vowel Production

Defects of vowel production do not occur as frequently as those for the production of consonants. The intensity of the vowels and possibly the visible aspects of their articulation help to make it comparatively easy for most children to learn to produce them accurately. Difficulties are sometimes experienced by the child who has hearing loss in the low-pitch ranges. A child exposed to foreign language influences may also experience some difficulty in the production of American-English vowels. We should be careful not to confuse defective vowel articulation with differences in vowel production on the basis of regional variations.

From our discussion of vowels, we can hypothesize that vowel phonemes will never contrast in voice but that they *will* contrast in such features as where the tongue is raised or bunched, whether it is high or low in the mouth, and whether the vowel is rounded or un-rounded and lax or tense. Some of these features coexist. No front vowel is rounded; back vowels tend to be rounded.

On the basis of the characteristics of vowels just discussed (height of tongue, raising or bunching of tongue) explain what has happened in the following changes. For example, *Patricia* is sometimes pronounced with an [i] not an [ɪ] in the second syllable. The [ɪ] used by most speakers has been raised to become [i].

1. Why does *keel* become [kɪəl]?
2. What happens as *milk* is pronounced [mʊlk]?
3. The final sound in *Monday, Tuesday, Wednesday* is usually pronounced [ɪ]. How in this different from the final sound being pronounced [e]?
4. Southerners sometimes pronounce *pen* and *pin* alike. In terms of the characteristics just discussed, what is happening?
5. What has occurred in these changes?
   [frʌm] for *from* in *from the farm.*
   [e haʊs] for *a house*
   [ði dɔg] for [ðə dɔg].
   [rʊf] for [ruf].
   [tʊrɪst] for [turɪst].
6. In *tomato salad* and *I bought a tomato*, what is the change in the last sound in *tomato*?
7. Some Southerners say [ra:t] for [raɪt]. What change has occurred?

Diphthongs

Diphthongs, like vowels, are produced as a result of modifications in the size and shape of the mouth and position of the tongue while vocalized breath is being emitted without obstruction of the breath stream. Diphthongs are voice glides uttered in a single breath impulse. Some diphthongs, such as the one in the word *how*, are blends of two vowels. Most diphthongs originally—as far as the history of the language is concerned—were produced as "pure" vowels but "broke down" to what is now a strong vowel gliding off weakly to another vowel lacking distinct individual character. The diphthongs in the words *name* and *row* are examples where the first element is emphasized and readily recognizable and the second element is "weak" and somewhat difficult to discern.

The following list of words includes the most frequently recognized diphthongs in American-English speech. Most phoneticians would limit the *distinctive* diphthongs to those in the words *aisle*, *plough*, *toil*, and *use*.

aisle	*bay*
plough	*hoe*
toil	*dear*
fair	*sure*
fort	*use*

Problems

1. Distinguish spelling representation from sound representation:
   a. Pick out all words with the sound [ɪ] as in *hit* in *Women are undependable. Their so-called stability is but a myth.*
   b. List as many different spellings for these sounds as you can think of: [i] as in *tree*, [eɪ] as in *jail*, [aɪ] as in *try*.
2. Note slight differences within these groups of phonemes:
   [k] *cool, key*
   [t] *stop, tape, rat*
   [p] *paid, spray, apt*
   [ʌ] *but, cut.*
3. Note the similarities and dissimilarities in terms of articulatory agents involved, manner of production, and vocal components in the final sounds of *tank, tack; rat, race; lamb, can; taps, tabs; cough, five; truth, bathe; call, car.*
4. The following are pronunciations of other cultures as reported in various articles. What are the changes from a phonetic standpoint?
   duty [dʒutɪ]
   forget you [fəgɛtʃu]
   have [hæb]
   chicken [ʃɪkən]
   record [rɛkət]
   them [dɛm]

    man [men]
    set or sat [sɑt]
    ice [is]
    pig [pɪɪg]
    storm [tɔrm]
    lets [lɛs]
    lumber [lʌmɚ]
    children [tʃɪrən]

On the whole do the preceding substitutions make more phonetic sense than the following:

    cat [tæk]
    squirrel [gɝˑdl]
    run [bʌn]
    look [lik]
    Sam [ræt]
    mule [mel]

What substitutions would make sense in the preceding words?

5. Why, in teaching [s], would you use the phrases *can sing* and *right song* rather than *bath soap*? The explantion is a phonetic one.
    Why, in correcting the substitution [f] for [θ], would you use the phrase *right through the door* rather than *come through the door*?
    Why, in correcting the substitution of [w] for [l], would you use the phrase *the cat's long hair* rather than *blow long and hard*?
    Why, in correcting the substitution of [w] for [r], would you use the phrase *turn red* rather than *barn door*?

6. A child makes the following substitutions:
    [t] for [k] as in [tæt] for [kæt]
    [f] for [θ] as in [bof] for [boθ]
    [d] for [g] as in [do] for [go]
    [θ] for [s] as in [θi] for [si]

Chart these substitutions in terms of distinctive features. Note changes in features and whether there is any consistency in the change of features in the four substitutions.

References and Suggested Readings

Amerman, J. D., R. Daniloff, and K. L. Moll, "Lip and Jaw Coarticulation for the Phoneme [æ]", *Journal of Speech and Hearing Research*, **13** (March 1970), 147–161. (Investigates the extent of coarticulation and the synergy of two articulatory gestures, lip-rounding and jaw-lowering, for the vowel [æ].)

Bolinger, D., *Aspects of Language*, 2nd ed., New York: Harcourt Brace Jovanovich, Inc., 1975, chaps. 3 and 4.

Bronstein, A. J., *The Pronunciation of American English*, New York: Appleton-Century-Crofts, 1960.

Chomsky, N., and M. Halle, *The Sound Patterns of English*, New York: Harper & Row, Publishers, Inc., 1968.

Denes, P. B., and E. N. Pinson, *The Speech Chain*, New York: Bell Telephone Laboratories, 1963, chap. 4. (Outlines anatomy and physiology of speech production.)

Harms, R. T., *Introduction to Phonological Theory*, Englewood Cliffs, N.J.: Prentice-Hall, Inc., 1968. (Introduces the student to generative phonology.)

Ladefoged, P., *Preliminaries to Linguistic Phonetics*, Chicago: University of Chicago Press, 1971.

LaRiviere, C., H. Winitz, J. Reeds, and E. Herriman, "The Conceptual Reality of Selected Distinctive Features," *Journal of Speech and Hearing Research*, **17** (March 1974), 122–133.

Lehmann, W. P., *Descriptive Linguistics: An Introduction*, New York: Random House, Inc., 1971, Chap. 2. "Articulatory Phonetics," Chap. 3. "Acoustic Phonetics."

Liberman, A. M., K. S. Harris, H. S. Hoffman, and B. G. Griffith, "The Discrimination of Speech Sounds Within and Across Phonetic Boundaries," *Journal of Experimental Psychology*, **54** (November 1957), 358–368.

———, K. S. Harris, P. Einas, L. Lisker, and J. Bastian, "An Effect of Learning on Speech Perception: The Discrimination of Duration of Silence with and Without Phonemic Significance," *Language and Speech*, **4** (October–December 1961), 175–196.

Lloyd, D. J., and H. R. Warfel, *American English in Its Cultural Setting*, New York: Alfred A. Knopf, Inc., 1956.

McReynolds, L. V., and K. Huston, "A Distinctive Feature Analysis of Children's Misarticulations," *Journal of Speech and Hearing Disorders*, **36** (May 1971), 155–156.

Menyuk, P., "The Role of Distinctive Features in Children's Acquisition of Phonology," *Journal of Speech and Hearing Research*, **11** (March 1968), 138–146.

Parker, F., "Distinctive Features in Speech Pathology," *Journal of Speech and Hearing Disorders*, **41** (February 1976), 23–39.

Thomas, C. K., *An Introduction to Phonetics of American English*, New York: The Ronald Press Company, 1958.

Winitz, H., *From Syllable to Conversation*, Baltimore: University Park Press, 1975, chap. 2. (Describes in some detail distinctive features and their role in articulation therapy.)

7. Development of Language

As indicated earlier, we consider speech—the capacity to learn an oral/aural code—to be a specific function of the human species. The particular code acquired is, of course, a learned function. Almost all human beings acquire speech, or learn a given language code, because they are born with the capacities for this particular type of learning. Spoken language is a system of symbols, a code, which normally is produced by articulatory activity that associates sounds (utterances) and meaning in particular ways.

Children may be said to be speaking, to be using an oral/aural linguistic system[1] when they demonstrate by their productions that their utterances conform to the conventions of other speakers in their environment. These conventions include the acquisition of a phonemic or sound system, a morphemic system (the combination of sound elements into words), a semantic system (acquisition of vocabulary), and a syntactical system (the combining of words into "strings" or formulations that approximate the utterances of the mature members of their culture).

---

[1] Deaf children who learn to use a visible code or sign system are an exception in regard to the use of the oral/aural code. A visible code is, however, acceptable within our definition of speech. We believe that the American Sign Language (ASL) meets the criteria for a symbol-linguistic code. The SEE System (Signing Exact English) adds English morphemes to ASL and so brings the sign system closer to a full-fledged morphemic language. [G. Gustason, D. Pfetzing, and E. Zawolkow (*SEE: Signing Exact English*, Rossmoor, Calif.: Modern Signs Press, 1972.]

Criteria for Language Acquisition

Sometime between the last quarter of the first year and the middle of the second year of life, the vast majority of children begin to speak. The acquisition of speech, the development of language,[2] is a continuous process throughout life. Normally, comprehension precedes production and exceeds production from the beginning to the end of life. We may, however, consider the following to be the criteria for the establishment of sufficient competence in comprehension and production to permit us to identify a child as one who has acquired language. Children may be said to be speaking:

1. When they understand—decode and derive meanings from—a conventionalized system of audible and/or visible symbols.
2. When, without specific and direct training, they can understand verbal formulations to which they never before have been specifically exposed. Children are then *listening creatively*. They understand what people say based on past understandings of what people have said.
3. When they can produce verbal formulations, new utterances that they never before have tried, and have the utterances understood by others. Children are then *talking creatively*.

Criteria (2) and (3) reveal that the child is capable of generalizing from the specific words and utterances individually learned "directly" to the comprehension and production of an indefinite number of new utterances. In a very real and important sense, the child has become a

---

[2] We recognize that language is described by linguists according to hypotheses about competencies shared by a specific language community and that speech represents the performance of an individual user of the language. Speech, therefore, often provides the bases for linguistic research. We also recognize that a child may *know* the linguistic rules but may not be able to use them in speaking. In other words, there may be a discrepany between the actual speech output and the potential force for speech proficiency. In this chapter, describing the child's acquisition of linguistic proficiencies, we are not primarily concerned with abstract concepts of language but rather with the individual speaker's verbal output. We are, therefore, not making distinctions between the cognitive competence and the speech output.

linguistic generalizer and generator. Children indicate that they have learned the rules of their language, and are applying these rules—the conventions of older and presumably proficient speakers—to what they hear and what they want to say. Children are likely to make many errors that are products either of overgeneralizing or of correct generalizing where a linguistic system has exceptions, for example, saying *sheeps* and *childs* as plurals for *sheep* and *child* or *foots* as plural for *foot*. Children may make errors because they have not really caught on to the rules but are moving in that direction. Such errors are good positive indicators that a given child is linguistically normal, and has become a verbal being and a member of a verbal culture.

Although children begin to speak because they are born with the capacities for this achievement, their accomplishments as verbal beings will vary with a variety of innate and environmental factors. The *onset of speech* appears to be unrelated to the particular language a child will speak, only roughly to his /her level of intelligence (unless the child is severely subnormal), or to the talkativeness of members of the family or other key persons in the environment, providing, of course, that these persons *do* talk. An individual child's proficiency as a speaker, including language development, is determined by a number of factors that we consider later.

THE FUNCTIONS OF LANGUAGE

Primarily, the function of language is to permit the child to behave like a human being in the variety of ways in which human beings behave. More specifically, language is used for talking to and with others, to signal needs, intentions, feelings, and thoughts. Language is also used for self-talking (thinking), and for controlling and directing one's own behavior, as well as for controlling and directing the behavior of others. Language is used for deception and even for self-deception, for saying many nothings to avoid a vacuous existence and to becoming an accepted, socialized, and civilized human being. Language is used to disarm or delay nonverbal hostility, and for engaging and instigating hostility. In time, the maturing child will learn that not only does man have a way with language but that language has a way with man. Not too long after the child acquires a command of language he begins to appreciate that language has a command of him.

In the discussion that follows we consider the levels or stages of language development and some of the correlated maturational factors in these stages.

Language Developmental Stages

PRELINGUAL STAGES

Before a child speaks first words—produces verbal signals with intended meaning—the girl or boy normally goes through a series of stages in vocalic and articulatory productions that are characteristic and universal[3]. That is, regardless of the particular language a given child will begin to use during the second year of life, children are almost all likely to engage in some amount of vocal "behavior" that is peculiar to human infants. We assume, even though it is not clearly established[4] that these stages are necessary precursors for later speech sound production. In our review of the stages we speculate as to their implications for later language acquisition.[5]

UNDIFFERENTIATED CRYING

Babies cry, and parents, especially if they are new in this role, wonder why. Although we offer no philosophic speculation as to the reason for the early cries, we do know that babies enter the extrauterine world with a cry. Should a baby fail to do this, the attending physician is likely to give him a sharp slap on his tender backside to elicit such a cry. Perhaps the cry is a reflexive expression of the pain that comes initially with the baby's having to take care of its own breathing. If we cannot say positively that the child cries because of discomfort, we can certainly observe that the child cries when uncomfortable. In any event, the birth cry and the crying during the first few weeks of life are considered reflexive manifestations of discomfort. The cries are *undifferentiated*, in that the adult ear cannot distinguish or associate the nature of the discomfort with any features of the crying. The crying may be described as nasal, shrill wailing. It is essentially the same whether the child is hungry, thirsty, cold, in pain, or needs a change of linen. Students in infant crying may recognize differences. Most of us cannot.

---

[3] For an expanded exposition of this concept see N. Chomsky, "The Formal Nature of Language," in E. H. Lenneberg, *Biological Foundations of Language* (New York: John Wiley and Sons. Inc., 1967), pp. 397–442.

[4] E. H. Lenneberg, *Biological Foundations of Language* (New York: John Wiley & Sons, Inc., 1967), pp. 140–141. A psychologist concerned with the development of language behavior, reports that some children have begun to speak without going through the prelingual stages normal to almost all children.

[5] Our discussion is about children born after a normal, full-term pregnancy without any pre-, para-, or immediate postnatal factor to suggest any abnormality.

We regard the first cry, and the subsequent undifferentiated crying, as reflexive expression of physiological (chemico-neuro-muscular) internal ongoings. The occurrence of crying indicates that for the time being the respiratory and laryngeal mechanisms are functioning normally. The child is responding normally to internal changes. The child can approximate the vocal bands, and they can be set into action as air on intake and breath on output is forced between them. If there are any identifiable sounds in reflexive crying, they are likely to be nasalized vowels.

We should point that our observations about the child's crying are based on assumptions relative to the changes that take place when an adult does something because the child is crying. Thus, we conclude that the child who stops crying after being fed must have cried initially because he was hungry, or that the child who stops crying after being given additional covering must have cried because he was cold. These may well be likely cause-and-effect changes in behavior. It is possible, nevertheless, that the child's cessation of crying may be the result of being handled and receiving some direct human physical contact. The actual cause of the child's crying may not, however, have been alleviated. Perhaps that is why the child so quickly resumes crying when the adult leaves him.

COMFORT SOUNDS

A few children may vocalize during noncrying periods in states we consider comfortable, for example, after a feeding and burping. Most infants are silent, awake or asleep, when they are not crying. Comfort sounds become considerably more evident during the second and third month. This is also the period of differentiated crying and more generally of differentiated vocalization.

DIFFERENTIAITED VOCALIZATION

Beginning in the second month, most children become differentiated vocalizers, when crying or when otherwise engaged in sound production. In regard to crying, most mothers can tell when a child is hungry, not just because the child is crying when the mother thinks it is time to be hungry, but because the cry sounds characteristically different at such a time than when there is evidence that a diaper change is needed or that the child is cold. There is a crescendo pattern to the child's hunger cry that is not present under other discomfort conditions.

The differences in crying constitute an early signal system for parents. Parents who tune in are able to make associations between a kind of condition and a form of vocalization. We are not suggesting that the child has any intention or awareness about the vocalization. The productions are still reflexive. However, because the infant's neuromuscular system has matured, the unwitting evocations become increasingly differentiated. The child is a reflexive producer, but those who attend may become interpreters of varying states. Differentiated vocalization thus permits a one-way communication for the sensitive listener-respondent, usually the mother.

Cooing, gurgling, and "squealing," and sounds that approximate consonants are soon added to the vowel-like sounds in the child's inventory of sound production. Lenneberg (1967, p. 128) observes that beginning at 12 weeks of age, vowel-like (cooing) sounds may be sustained for 15–20 seconds. The infant is well on his way to becoming a proficient sound maker. At this stage, the infant is an internationalist in sound making. The products are by no means restricted to the language or languages of the home. We may, according to our prejudices, recognize front vowels in the child's squealings, and mid- and back vowels, *ah*, *uh*, and *oo*, in the child's cooing. We may also identify sounds that suggest *m*, *b*, and *g* and *k*.

By 16 weeks of age, the child begins to make definite responses to human sounds and sound makers. The child, on hearing a voice, turns toward the speaker. The infant's eyes begin to scan and search for the sound maker. If the child is engaged in vocalization, the initial response is likely to be an interruption of the effort. On making visual "contact" with the other speaker, the child may then respond by smiling or cooing. Vocal play may be maintained by an interchange of sound making between the child and another vocalizer. The evidence is strong that infant vocalization is reinforced by the presence and stimulation of an adult. Research on the sound making of children brought up in orphanages as well as on their early true speech development [Goldfarb (1954), Lenneberg (1967, p. 137), and Van Riper (1972, p. 56)] reveals that these children engage in less sound play than do those of peer age who are brought up in homes and receive parental attention.

It is possible to overwhelm the child by too much stimulation. Some children respond to adult efforts by ceasing their own vocalization. The wise adult can be guided by what needs to be done by observing the effects of what is done. If the child responds to adult sound play by more vocalization then the play should be continued. If the child stops vocalization, then the adult should cease too. We are not suggesting that the adult should refrain indefinitely from stimulating the child. The effort should certainly be resumed at a later time, and the results observed. A 16-week-old child may welcome stimulation that was rejected a week or two earlier or even an hour or two earlier. Few normal children will long deprive adults or themselves of the enjoyment of vocal interchange.

The first three months take the infant from undifferentiated, reflexive crying to differentiated vocalization. Even the objective observer may conclude that the child's sound play, the cooing, gurgling, and more discernible oral products, is fun. There are, however, some silent children who cry very little and with no suggestion of feeling or enthusiasm. Though some of these ultimately will become adequate if not loquacious speakers, a few will be among the small number who will grow up as nonverbal children. These, whom parents retrospectively recall as "very good" infants, whose cries were token whimpers, may later be identified as autistic children. Not only in their failure to respond to human speech, but in other aspects of their behavior, they are essentially silent and nonrelating children. They rarely smile in response to stimulation that produces smiles or laughter in most children.

BABBLING

The period from three to six months of age is one characterized by a considerable increase in vocalization that includes identifiable sounds that are used in speaking. Some of these sounds, and combinations of sounds, are reduplicated. So we may hear "ga-ga" and "ug-ug" and "bah-bah." There is also a marked increase in the child's responses to the nonverbal behavior of members of the environment. The child may squeal with apparent pleasure at the sight of mother, or when given a toy, or when picked up for play by a parent. The child may respond with crying to loud sounds, or any suggestion of "No" or scolding in the voice of someone from whom warmth and friendliness are usually expected. By six months of age most children have reached the prelingual stage we designate as babbling.

We consider babbling an exceedingly important stage in speech development. Innate drives toward vocalization and sound play may be reinforced or discouraged. Environmental factors—the influence and effects of external stimulation—become determinants of what the child will be doing as a future sound maker. The child seems to be aware that sound making is pleasurable, both as an accomplishment in itself and as a technique for giving pleasure to others. We agree with Lewis (1959) that the primarily innate forces that bring the child to babbling will be enhanced and sustained by the nature of his environment. The child needs a favorable climate, with attentive but not overwhelming adults, to sustain him in his continued speech development.

By about the sixth month, differences in the vocalizations of deaf and hearing children may be discerned by a sophisticated listener. For the most part, these differences are more readily apparent in the deaf child's responses to the vocalization of others than in his own spontaneous efforts. The deaf child now seems to have a more limited repertoire of sounds than does his peer who can hear. Lenneberg (1964, p. 154) observes:

> the total amount of a deaf child's vocalization may not be different from that of a hearing child, but the hearing child at this age will constantly run through a large repertoire of sounds whereas the deaf children will be making the same sounds sometimes for weeks on end and then suddenly change to some other set of sounds and "specialize" in them for a while. There is no consistent preference among deaf children for specific sounds.

The voice of the deaf child in spontaneous utterance is no different from that of the hearing child. In response to inner drives, the deaf child's voice is as true an indicator of feelings as is the voice of the hearing child. The internal physiological mechanisms that create the neuromuscular state for vocalization are the same for the deaf child as for the one with normal hearing. So, too, the product is of the same variety. It is only when the deaf child's voice is part of a voluntary effort that differences appear and the high-pitched, poorly modulated voice of the deaf begins to be heard.

LALLING

By eight months of age, most children engage in a considerable amount of self-imitation in their sound making. We can begin to hear clear "ga-ga," "da-da," and "ma-ma" utterances, often accompanied by intonation patterns that resemble those in the child's home. The child's voice will make it quite clear to the listener that something is wanted *now*, or that the child is pleased or displeased with what is going on at the moment. During this stage of development the child is not as random a sound maker as in infant babbling. The child makes fewer sounds, but has better control of the oral products. The child is listening to and monitoring the oral products produced, and so is able to control them. Sound replication is an expression of such control. Some of the sound combinations such as "da-da" and "ma-ma" resemble words. However, parental pride to the contrary, very few children who say "ma-ma" at eight months of age assign any meaning to their utterance. But many children do associate sound and meaning at eight months of age, and parental pride may not always be misplaced. Most children need a few months before they really mean what they utter. Part of this time is devoted to responding to what they hear with their own echolalic, imitative utterances.

Deaf children are not likely to enter spontaneously into the lalling stage. All too frequently, without the ability to hear and to feel the results of their articulatory play, they tend to become silent children. When provoked or extremely uncomfortable, deaf children may make sounds as in the babbling stage. However, it is possible for some deaf children to progress from babbling to lalling if they can see themselves in a mirror when they are engaged in sound play. In more than one way reflexive action may produce reflective behavior. If deaf children can be motivated to keep their oral mechanisms in shape, they can also be motivated to listen and so continue to use their residual hearing. Virtually no deaf child is "stone deaf."

ECHOLALIA

Echolalia is a normal stage in language development that occurs, as we have indicated, after the lalling stage. The echolalic child is an imitator of others and not, as in the lalling stage, almost exclusively a self-imitator. The imitative effort more often begins to approximate the sounds and the words the child hears. Thus, the child may mimic both the manual gesture and the syllables "bye-bye" without understanding the meaning of either. The child may utter "ma-ma" or "da-da" or even "baby" without any intended meaning. Vocal intonations are also imitative, so that it is difficult for many parents to believe that the child's utterances are parrotlike and not true speech.

In another sense, however, the baby is developing speech. We may note an increasing amount of differential behavior to specific utterances directed to the child. An appropriate gesture may be made when the child hears "bye-bye." We may also observe anticipatory action such as reaching when the child is asked "Do you want your dolly?" When, perhaps between 10 and 12 months of age, and not uncommonly before the age of 15 months, the child says "doddy" or "da da" or just "da" when presented with a doll, we do have the onset of speech.

Some children seem to become arrested at the echolalic stage. Such children include the severely mentally retarded (intelligence quotients below 50 or 60) and the autistic. However, some autistic children may be able to mimic long strings of words with accurate articulation and vocal intonation. They sound as if they are talking except that they give no indication of expecting anything in particular to happen as a result of what they seem to have said.

Deaf children do not go beyond the early lalling stage unless extraordinary measures are taken to make maximum and effective use of their residual hearing and their ability to see what people do when they speak.

IDENTIFICATION LANGUAGE

By the beginning of the second year and usually by 15 months of age, most children have words to identify objects, persons, and some satisfying events in their environment. However, because echolalic utterances are likely to continue, one-year-old and post one-year-old children will seem to speak some words for which they have no apparent meaning. Their first words—ones with apparent meaning—are likely to be reduplicated syllables, such as "dada" and "mama." The child may now be able to obey verbal "commands," such as pointing to the nose, ears, and so on, in response to directions. "Show me your nose," "Where is baby's nose?" and so forth.[6] The child may also play "Peek-a-boo," or bang a cup when an adult says "cup." In these situations the child's utterances, as well as the nonverbal actions, are used to identify events. Unless somewhat on the precocious side, the child is not likely to be using words to bring about an event, to get the doll or a bottle of milk, or to call for mother when any one of these is not in view.

TRUE SPEECH: ANTICIPATORY LANGUAGE

By the middle of the second year, most children are able to use language to bring about an event, to get something or someone not physically in view and/or to "command" something or someone in view. During this stage the child's utterance may be accompanied by a change in "motor set" that is consistent with an appropriate reaction to what is expected to happen. Thus, the child not only says "up" but gets ready to be picked up. When the child says "mama," the words are accompanied by looking to the door through which mother is supposed to make her appearance. Words at this stage have a "magical" power for the child. Words are a way of getting people to do one's bidding, of satisfying one's needs physically and psychosocially.

Between 18 and 24 months of age most children have productive vocabularies of from three to 50 words, and much larger comprehension vocabularies. They are definitely "with it" linguistically, and ready for more complex verbal behavior.

---

[6] Many children are able to respond to verbal commands while still in the echolalic stage and a few can do so in the latter part of the lalling stage.

The child's single-word utterances are, in effect, sentences. The meaning of the utterance is indicated by the manner of intonation. Thus, "mama," depending on intonation, may mean an empiric "Mother, come here!" or "Where is mother?" or even, "Mother, I've had enough of you now." Similarly, "cup" may mean "Fill it up" or "I've had my fill of it." If we accept intonation as a form of syntax, then we may consider that the child's variously intoned words are complete sentences, which may have as many meanings as adults regularly give to the word forms "yes" or "no" or "uh-uh."

Children who later will be designated as severely intellectually retarded may not go beyond the stage of identification language, even though they may have a small vocabulary for naming (identifying) some objects and persons in their environment. A few retarded children may develop single-word or two-word utterances to bring about events, but growth of vocabulary is slow, both for comprehension and production of language. Retarded children have fewer words than their normal age peers, and fewer meanings for the words they know. Moderately intellectually retarded children will shadow the linguistic development of normal and bright children. Severely retarded children (those with intelligence quotients below low-grade idiocy) may be totally nonverbal or almost completely so.[7]

Some children are slow in onset but not at all slow in their understanding of speech. These children may not say their first words until they are two years of age, and a few, happily a very few, do not speak until they are 30 months old. These children go through the prelingual stages on schedule and show that they understand what is said to them in games they play with adults. They can even carry out spoken directions to "fetch and carry" and yet make no verbal responses of their own. Some of these children come from families of late talkers, especially on the father's side. Most of these children catch up quickly once they begin to talk. They do manage to give their parents, and more particularly their grandparents, a difficult and anxious time. Just why these children are well within normal range for understanding

---

[7] Here we may be dealing with circuitous thinking, with the effect as well as the cause of retarded onset of language. A child of three or more who has not begun to speak may get less stimulation than a normal child. If the severely retarded child is institutionalized, he may indeed never get around to speaking. E. H. Lenneberg *in Biological Foundations of Language* (New York: John Wiley & Sons, Inc., 1967), p. 154–155, reports on a population of 54 mongoloid children who were raised at home (age range six months to 22 years). These children were observed over a period of from two to three years. At the end of the study period, 75 per cent of the children had reached a stage of at least identification language. The children had small vocabularies and could execute simple verbal commands. Lenneberg notes that progress in language development was noted only in the children who were below 14 years of age.

speech and yet slow to start speaking remains a mystery. It is, however, important to distinguish these children from others who are both slow to talk and slow to understand what others say to them.

SYNTACTIC SPEECH

By two years of age the child is likely to have a vocabulary of between 50 and 100 words. Some children may be able to name all the familiar objects in their environment. The most distinctive achievement is the combination of words from their inventory into phrases that, though lacking in the conventional markers of syntax, nevertheless constitute sentences. The form of the words used may be two nouns—for example, *cup* and *milk* to mean "Give me a cup of milk" or "I want milk" or, in the adult usage, an adverb + noun, for example, "more milk" with the meaning apparent. Lenneberg (1967, p. 293) points out that it makes little sense to try to determine whether the child's vocabulary has a preponderance of nouns and some adjectives and a few conventional verbs that function as sentences. Any of the child's words may be used contextually to indicate a variety of meanings. Frequently one word is used recurrently as a pivot (Braine 1963), so that we get such phrases as "here cup," "here shoe," "here doll," as well as "doll here" and "kitty here." We may also have such phrase-sentences as "more milk" and "more up." The significant of this accomplishment is that the child is developing a sense of word combination, which in time will be modified by conventional word order and markers of syntax.

At two years of age an increasing number, perhaps 50 per cent, of the child's utterances are sufficiently intelligible to be comprehensible to persons who are not members of the child's family. Of great significance is the ability of most two-year-old children to combine words into novel sentences of their own making. These sentences begin to follow the grammatical rules of the language of older members of their environment but are not word-for-word replications. Many two-year-old children now speak creatively in that they are formulating sentences based on their individual word inventories, yet are obedient to the rules or conventions of the syntax of their language. At first, the "syntax" may be just one of word order. So , from "baby up" a child may go to "dolly up" or "mommy up." Some children will begin to show an ability for transformations, if only one of word order. Thus, we may hear "up baby," "up mommy," and "up ball."

When children achieve a vocabulary of 50 or so words, some of which are commands as well as labels, they are likely to begin to combine words into two word phrase-sentences such as the type just indicated. Then, as children progress and build up their word inventories and increase the length of their spontaneous utterances, syntactical features become incorporated into their phrase-sentences and later into more clearly identifiable sentences. Interestingly, there is a fair amount of regularity as to the syntactical features that accompany the increases in length of children's utterance. Thus, correlations have been worked out between Mean Length of Utterance (MLU)[8] and syntactical structure based on samples of normal children's early speech.

Ingram and Eisenson (1972, 148–188) provide samples of five basic levels beyond the single word stage of syntactic constructions in the language acquisition of young children. These levels are based on an investigation by Ingram. Language samples[9] were taped and analyzed for mean length of utterance and for syntactical constructions employed in spontaneous speech. The five levels closely parallel the five stages of language development presented by Roger Brown (1973) in his book *A First Language.*

Some examples of the constructions in the Ingram-Eisenson levels include

---

Level I—Average Utterance Range 2.0—2.5 Words*

hit ball	kick box
big girl	small cat
John candy	Mary cookie
boy walk	girl eat
that kitty	that mommy
doggy hear	kitty there
put in truck	look in box
in small box	in big house
hit it	throw it
it walk	it jump

* Note that child constructions at level I do not include grammatical markers. So we have *it walk* and not *it walks.*

---

[8] Mean Length of Utterance (MLU) can be determined by taking a sample of a child's spontaneous utterances and dividing the total number of words spoken by the number of utterances. Thus, if the sample consists of 100 utterances and the total number of words is 300, the MLU is 3. A second and more frequently used method is to add the total number of words and the total number of morphemes and divide this number by two for a word-morpheme count. Then, divide this total by the number of utterances. So 300 words + 450 morphemes divided by two = 375, divided by 100 (number of utterances) gives us an MLU of 3.75.

[9] Tyack and Gottsleben (1974) have published a manual on the technique of language sampling.

Level II—Average Utterance Range 2.5—3.0 Words

boy drink water

throw small can

kick Tom ball

this ball

on table

put on box

on red table

Bobby put on table

a boy

the cat

boy eat a cookie

boys (plural contrast with singular)

hit ball

mommy wear shoes

boy eating

boy catching ball

Bobby put in box

Mary eating cookies

What that

Where girl run

girl eat candy

kick big ball

See Mary doll

that doll

in truck

put on table

on green box

Mary sit on chair

a doll

the doll

Mary see the ball

girls

eat candies

boy hold books

girl swimming

girl riding bike

Dick jump on box

girls feeding birds

Where boy

Where boy go

Level III—Average Utterance Range 3.0—4.0 Words

boy open door

put kitty in box

going (gonna) eat cookie

Mary put doll in wagon

John is boy

Bobby is here

Man is big

But ball in box

gonna throw balls

Baby is crying

Man is pulling wagon

put the box on table

boy and girl

at home

Go to school

Girl is at home.

Boy run to house.

She eat cookie.

He hold her.

She is here.

He is in wagon.

She gonna (going to) drink milk.

They carry cookies to mommy.

Girl gonna go to school.

Boy is running to school.

What is that?

Where that?

girl feed cat

sit dog on chair

going (gonna) ride bike

Mommy put baby in bed

Cathy is girl

baby is there

Dolly is small

Put candies in box

gonna eat candies

Girl is jumping

Mommy is driving car

throw the ball in box

baby and mommy

at park

Go to park.

Mommy is at store.

Girl run to school.

They play ball.

She carry him.

He is there.

She is in car.

He gonna eat cookie.

They carry ball to park.

Boy gonna kick ball in park.

Man is walking to store.

What the girl doing?

Where the mommy going?

Dog is running.   Baby is eating.
I put the ball in box, OK?   I eat cookies, ok?

Level IV—Average Utterance Range 4.0—5.0 Words

The mommy hold the boy.
The doggy dig the hole.
The girl put a candy in the box.
The boy throw the red ball.
The mommy gonna feed the baby.
The big dog runs.
Tommy is a boy.
That is a dog.
The boy is in a wagon.
Tommy goes to school with Billy.
That is Bobby('s) ball.
That is her cat.
That is Billy('s) dog.
The ball hit Tommy.
You and I laugh.
Daddy see us.
You and I eat cookies.
The dog is running.
This is a bird.
The man is big.
You are laughing.
John eats a candy.
Mommy drives a car.
I see the girl's bike.
The bird has to fly.
I have to (hafta) run home.
What's this?
What is the man reading?
Will Tommy run?
Will the mommy see the baby?

Level V—average utterance age 5.0—6.0 words

The girl won't run.
The boy can't go.
The baby won't drink the milk.
The airplane flies over the house.
The ball is under the table.
The dog is near the wagon.
The kitty climbs up the tree.
The dog is running.
The baby cried.
The boy jumped.
This is their wagon.
This is our car.
The girl reads the book that she likes.
Won't the dog run?
Who is driving the car?
Who is sleeping on the bed?

TRANSFORMATIONS

We indicated earlier that when children "realize" that they can say either "up baby" or "baby up" they have learned a simple transformation, or two ways of communicating essentially the same meaning. How the child learns this way we do not know. Nor do we know how a child learns that when asked "Do you want candy?" the answer may be simply "yes" or, more rarely, "No." It may also be "Yes, I (or me) want candy?" Now we have an example of a nominal transposition, another kind of transformation. The *you*, if the child is normal, is replaced by *I*. (It may also be replaced by *me*, but either *I* or *me* represents a transformation.) A question form is reconstructed into a simple declarative statement. Later the child will learn that one may say either "Bobby held mother's hand" or "Mother's hand was held by Bobby." Again, the meaning of the two sentences is essentially the same. Perhaps, less similar are the sentences "Johnny kicked Mary" and "Mary was kicked by Johnny." Some children feel that when "Johnny kicked Mary" the pain was greater that when "Mary was kicked by Johnny." However, the underlying meaning if not the full impact continues to be the same.

Most transformations involve the use of grammatical forms and structures that permit children to understand new meanings and, in turn, to express new meanings. These include how to make distinctions between singular and plural; to use tense endings to indicate the present, past, and future; and to deal with the hypothetical in the past as well as in a possible future. They also learn to make negative statements and to ask questions. The first questions children ask are those that may be answered by "Yes" or "No." Later they learn to ask questions that begin with interrogative (*wh*) words—*where, what, who, why, when,* and *how.*

In the later stages of syntactic acquisition, children learn to combine two or more single statement sentences into a single complex sentence. So the sentences "John is my big brother. He will take me to the zoo tomorrow." may become "John, my big brother, will take me to the zoo tomorrow." Also, sentences such as "The girl sees the bird. The bird is flying." may become "The girl sees the bird that's flying."

We are avoiding a discussion of the theory of transformational grammar at this point. We believe that the kinds of transformational forms that children learn *and understand* are associated with their cognitive (intellectual) state. A child will have no use for future tense without an ability to project from present to future, or to use a subjunctive "If I were" form without a capacity to deal with the hypothetical. Some of these forms, however, may be used on an imitative basis, without true comprehension. So, we may have performance (production) without understanding. It is probable, as Carol Chomsky (1969) has found, that children still have much to learn about syntax beyond the age of five and quite likely up to and a bit beyond the age of ten.

The student interested in the theory of transformational grammar may find relevant discussions adapted to child language acquisition in Bloom (1970), McNeill (1970), Dale (1972), Cazden (1972), and Jacobs and Rosenbaum (1968).

COMMUNICATIVE INTENT

By two-and-a-half years of age most children include functional words— prepositions, articles, and conjunctions—in their utterances. In other respects, too, their formulations approximate those of the older speakers to whom they are exposed. They begin to speak grammatically, or agrammatically, usually depending upon how those in their surroundings speak. Three- to four-word sentences are frequent. Between the age of two-and-a-half and three years, the child's increase in vocabulary is likely to be greater proportionately than for any other equal time period in his life. Between 24 and 30 months of age, the child's intention to communicate, to speak with the expectation both of being understood and responded to, becomes clear. If the child is not understood, frustration may be evidenced. Fortunately, the normal three-year-old not only shows control of syntax but control as well of most of the sounds of his language. So-called infantilisms, such as "wawa" for "water," decrease. The child's phonemic or articulatory proficiency is usually good enough for most of what is produced to be readily intelligible.

Literally, the three-year-old speaks as a self, using "I" in contexts that a few months before contained "me." The child understands and distinguishes between "I," "we," "me," and "you." The three-year-old can usually transform the "you" of a question addressed to him or her, for example, "Do you want a cookie?" to "I want a cookie." Interestingly, autistic children, even when they begin to speak, are slow to make the distinction and transformation of "you" to "I" or "me." Characteristically, autistic children refer to themselves in the manner in which they are addressed. Thus, "Do you want a cookie?" is likely to be answered by "You want a cookie," or by a repetition of the entire sentence.

THREE TO FOUR—THE EMERGENCE OF AN INDIVIDUOLECT

No attempt is made here to discuss, in any detail, the language development of children beyond the age of three. Most children beyond this age progress with giant strides in their ability to use conventional syntax. For the most part they have both the words and the word structures to express their thoughts and they can suit their actions to their words. Yet this is the age of considerable hesitation and repetition in speaking. These disfluencies, we think, suggest that some children have thoughts or the beginnings of thoughts for which they have no adequate verbal formulations. On the other hand, some post three-year-olds will talk quite glibly and use both words and structures that makes it evident to a discerning and critical listener that the youngsters do not really know what they are saying.

In general, we may conclude that children in the three-to four-age range who began to speak by 15 months of age are well along the way to adult syntactic proficiency. However, as previously noted in the reference to Chomsky's (1969) findings, a child of this age still has a way to go. Perhaps by age ten, children will have reached adult proficiency in their syntactical usage.

Although the language development of four-year-olds is far from completed, in many ways they are mature speakers. Most show clear evidence of having developed individual rhetorical styles, and have favorite words and favorite ways of turning phrases. Some are glib and others are on the quiet side. Four-year-olds speak for themselves and about themselves as *selves*. Each is an individual and each, in manner of speaking, is developing an *individuolect*.

Acquisition of Sounds: Phonemic Development

Thus far in our discussion we have emphasized the lexical (vocabulary) and syntactic aspects of language development. Neither, of course, can take place without the acquisition of the phonemic or sound system of the linguistic code. Many children take longer to establish completely proficient control of the sounds of their language than to acquire a vocabulary of 1,000 words or more and much of the syntax of their system. As infants engage in sound play, many sounds are produced that will not be controlled voluntarily and articulated intentionally until the child is six or seven years of age. Children also show great variability in their phonemic proficiency. Some, especially girls, may arrive at an almost adult level of control by age four or five. Most children, however, need at least a year or two longer before they arrive at this level of proficiency.

Children's errors in phonemic production are not random. Children make their words out of the sounds they are able to control. These, as we have noted, begin with vowels, nasals, and labials (lip sounds). The young child also engages in reduplication. So, with the few sounds under control, the child builds a word inventory. Words such as *mama* present no problem. A *kitty* is, however, likely to be pronounced *kicky* because the child can usually produce a /k/, before he/she can a /t/. So the child substitutes one stop sound for the other and, economically, uses the same sound twice. The production of *bummy* for *bunny* may be explained by the fact that /m/ is a bilabial, as is /b/. The child beginning a word with one bilabial finds it easier to include a second /m/ rather than to introduce a tip-tongue nasal /n/. How would you explain *doddy* for *doggy*?

CHARACTERISTICS OF EARLY PHONEMIC DEVELOPMENT

Though some children are laws unto themselves, most follow well established tendencies in their speech sound (phonological) development. Following are some general observations of typical "errors" or, more appropriately, *characteristics of early child speech sound production*.[10]

Weak Syllable Deletion. Many children delete an unstressed (weak) syllable in a polysyllabic word. So, the word *elephant* may be pronounced as *elfant* or *hefant*. Even shorter words, such as *belong* and *away*, may be reduced to bong [bɔŋ] and way [wei].

Syllable Repetition. Words such as *cracker* and *paper* may become kaka [kæ kæ] and paypay [pei pei]. Dada [dædæ] or [dada] for *daddy* is an early example of syllable repetition. We should, of course, not confuse this with the syllable or sound repetition (disfluency) that characterizes much early child speech.

Cluster Simplification. Many children do not achieve control of cluster (sound blend combinations) until age five or six, and some do not do so until age seven. English has many sound clusters, such as *bl*, *pl*, *cl*, *cr*, *gr*, *dr*, *st*, and triple clusters, such as *str*, *sks*, and *sts*. Some of these, such as *sts* and *sks*, continue to be troublesome even for adults. Young children tend to simplify sound clusters by dropping out one or more of the sounds, almost always those not yet under comfortable control, and retaining the sound under control. So, the word *cracker* shows both cluster simplification and syllable repetition when the child pronounces it as [kæ kæ]. The pronunciation of *please* as *pease* [piz] and *spoon* as *poon* [pun] are examples of cluster simplification.

---

[10] These observations are based on an article by D. Ingram, "Phonological Rules of Young Children," *Journal of Child Language*, 1974, 49–64.

Assimilation. Assimilation is the tendency for one sound to be modified in production as a result of proximity to another sound. Young children show a general tendency to produce (substitute) a sound under control for one not yet controlled. So we may hear *doddy* for *doggy* if the *d* is under control. Later we may get *goggy* if the *g* is controlled. Finally, when both the *d* and *g* are secure and controlled in any position within a word, we get *doggy*. Similarly, *kitty* may go from *kiky* [kiki] to *titty* [titi] before it becomes a more mature *kitty*.

Phonemic Discrimination and Production

Differential Sound Perception. If we are tuned in to infant sound production and base our judgments on the first words infants produce, we might come to the conclusion that most infants hear (perceive and differentiate) very few sounds. First words such as *mama, dada, ba-ba* (a form of bye-bye), *doddy* (dolly), *up, mow* (more), *nuh nuh* (no-no) require the production of either a nasal plus a vowel or a stop plus a vowel. Yet there is evidence that even in the first two or three months of life, infants respond differentially to consonants as close together acoustically and in manner of production as /b/-/p/, /m/-/n/, and /k/-/g/. Infants also respond differentially to the different vowel sounds.[11] How do we account for differential reactions in the first months of life and so limited a productive phonemic inventory when the child begins to talk, a year or so later? One explanation is that reflex or conditioned noncognitive responses call for different nervous system capabilities than do cognitive responses. Another possible explanation is that though ultimately our perceptions and productions become intimately related, initially we can perceive differences we cannot produce. So, children may reject an adult's pronunciation of *wawa* for *water* though maintaining that pronunciation for a while themselves.

What, then, do children perceive—differentially and cognitively process—of the speech sounds they hear? Do they follow basic principles or rules? Is there a chronological order or expected sequence in their speech sound discrimination? The answer to each of these questions is "Probably, yes." However, we should not expect invariable or slavish observation on the part of children. Individual exceptions are always

---

[11] Eimas and his associates in "Speech Perception in Infants," *Science*, **171** (1971) found that infants from one to four months of age responded differentially when exposed to voiced and voiceless cognate sounds such as /b/ and /p/.

possible, especially for children who present problems in language acquisition.

Shvachkin (see Slobin 1967) studied phonemic perception in early childhood (11 to 23 months of age). Specifically, Shvachkin investigated Russian children's comprehension of words that differed by a single phoneme. On the assumption that speech sound (phonological) discrimination as well as speech sound production remain the same regardless of the language the child is acquiring, we can apply Shvachkin's observations to a child learning English.[12] The following pattern then emerges:

Pattern of Phonemic Development (Distinctions)

1. The presence or absence of consonants in syllables: [bɑk] and [ɑk], [vek] and [ek].
2. Stop and fricative sounds with sonorants (nasals, vowel-like consonants): *b–m, d–r, g–n, v–y/j/.*
3. Nasal and liquid sounds: *m–l, m–r, n–l, n–r, n–y, m–y.*
4. Intranasal distinctions: *m–n.*
5. Intraliquid distinctions: *l–r.*
6. Fricative and nonfricative: *z–m, v–n.*
7. Labial and nonlabial: *b–d, v–z.*
8. Stop and fricative: *b–v, d–z, k–f.*
9. Lingual and velar: *d–g, t–k.*
10. Voiceless and voiced cognates: *p–b, t–d, k–g, f–v, s–z.*
11. Blade and groove sibilants: s–sh /ʃ/, z–zh /ʒ/.
12. Liquid and glide: *r–y, l–y.*

PRODUCTION

Production, as we suggested, follows perception and discrimination for the sounds of a language system. Articulatory development has been a subject of considerable study for many years. Rather than review "older" studies, we confine our considerations to a few studies published since the middle 1950s. The older studies generally found later ages for articulatory control than do more recent ones. Though it is possible that our population is changing and that children are becoming almost as precocious as their grandparents believe, it may

---

[12] R. Jakobson, in *Child Language, Aphasia and Phonological Universals* (The Hague: Mouton & Company, 1968), p. 46, states without reservation: "Whether it is a question of French or Scandinavian children, of English or Slavic, of Indian or German ... every description based on careful observation repeatedly confirms the striking fact that the relative chronological order of phonological acquisitions remains everywhere and at all times the same."

also be that our standards of proficiency are more lenient. Though lenient, they may nevertheless be more realistic. The table that follows, based on Templin's data (1957, p. 43), summarizes her findings for the phonemic development of children ages three to seven. This table should be compared with the next one that presents data for children ages two to four. The Prather, et al. (1975) observations begin at an earlier age than Templin's. Templin could have made similar observations for children below age three. However, though we find age differences that indicate earlier age for phonemic proficiency, order of development is generally and impressively the same. Note also the correspondence in order for the pattern of phonemic distinctions and the Templin and Prather observations for sound production.

Speech Sound Proficiency Based on Templin's (1957) Data and Criteria of 75 Per Cent Correct Production

Sound	Age	Sound	Age
m	3	r	4
n	3	s	4.5
ng	3	sh	4.5
p	3	ch	4.5
f	3	t	6
h	3	th	6
w	3	v	6
y	3.5	l	6
k	4	th(voiced)	7
b	4	z	7
d	4	zh	7
g	4	j	7

In a more recent statement, Templin (1966) states that "Cross-sectional normative studies have quite consistently shown that seven- to eight-year-old children can satisfactorily utter all the phonemes of English." Fry (1966) observes that "The rate of speech development varies greatly among individual children, but in the normally hearing child one can expect that by five to seven years of age the phonemic system will be completely and fairly well established."

Sander (1972) argues that the "older" criteria for mastery (proficiency) for speech and control were arbitrary and, as we have suggested, possibly unrealistic. Sander considers that a realistic criteria may be one as correct articulation for a sound in two of three word positions. He also considers 50 per cent of correct performance to be a

Comparison of Order of Sounds (Articulation Development) in Children *

Ages Two to Four Years

SOUND	AGE PRATHER, HEDRICK, KERN	TEMPLIN	SOUND	AGE PRATHER, HEDRICK, KERN	TEMPLIN
m	2	3–0	s	3	4–6
n	2	3–0	r	3–4	4–0
h	2	3–6	l	3–4	6–0
p	2	3–0	ʃ (sh)	3–8	4–6
ŋ(ng)	2	3–0	tʃ (ch)	3–8	4–6
f	2–4	3–0	ð (voiced th)	4	7–0
j(y)	2–4	3–6			
k	2–4	4–0	ʒ (mea*s*ure)	4	7–0
d	2–4	4–0	dʒ (*j*ump)	4+	7–0
w	2–8	3–0	θ (voiceless th)	4+	6–0
b	2–8	4–0			
t	2–8	6–0	v	4+	6–0
g	3	4–0	z	4+	7–0

* Adapted from E. M. Prather, D. L. Hedrick, and C. A. Kern, "Articulation Development in Children Aged Two to Four Years," *Journal of Speech and Hearing Disorders,* **40** (1975), 179–191.

more reasonable expectation than 75 per cent correct performance. The following order of speech sound development is presented in the following table based on Sander's lenient and perhaps more realistic criteria.

Again, note that the order of sounds is essentially the same as for Templin's observations, and the general correspondence with pattern for phonemic discrimination (distinction).

Order of Consonant Sound Proficiency Based on Sander's (1972) Criteria

Age	Sounds
2	h, m, n, w, b, p, t, k, g, ng, /ŋ/, d
3	f, y /j/, s, r, l
4	ch /tʃ/, sh /ʃ/, j /dʒ/, z, v
5	voiceless th /θ/, voiced th /ð/
6	zh /ʒ/

SPEECH READINESS

A review of the semantic and syntactic acquisition (see the table that follows on Maturational Milestones), indicates that the child makes great spurts at particular periods in his life, for example, the great (proportionate) increase in vocabulary at about 30 months of age; the development of syntax at about three years; the control of consonant clusters (blends) between five and six years of age. These may be considered periods of readiness in which basic skills are incorporated and the child then becomes ready for the next stage of development. Perhaps even more striking is the universal onset of speech, regardless of what language the child will speak, between 15 and 18 months of age. We indicated at the opening of this chapter that we consider speech to be a specific function of the human species. Children are born with the potential to speak if the opportunity is provided. The opportunity, so far as the onset of speech is concerned, is exposure to persons who speak. The rate at which children progress from their beginnings is determined by a combination of innate factors such as the integrity of the child's neurological and sensory systems, native intelligence, *and* cultural-environmental factors, which, for the most part, are those that exist *within* each *family*. We now consider some of these factors.

Maturational Milestones: Motor Correlates and Language Development*

Age	Speech Stage	Motor Development
12–16 weeks	Coos and chuckles	Supports head in prone position; responds to human sounds by turning head in direction of sound source
20 weeks	Consonants modify vowel-like cooing; nasals and labial fricatives are frequently produced	Sits with support
6 months	Babbling, resembling one-syllable utterances; identifiable combinations include *ma, da, di, du*	Sits without props using hands for support
8 months	Lalling and some echolalia	Stands by holding on to object; grasps with thumb apposition
10 months	Distinct echolalia, which approximates sounds heard;	Creeps efficiently; pulls to standing position; may take a

Age	Speech Stage	Motor Development
	responds differentially to verbal sounds	side step while holding on to a fixed object
12 months	Reduplicated sounds in echolalia; possible first words for identification; responds appropriately to simple commands	Walks on hands and feet; may stand alone, may walk when held by one hand, or even take first steps alone
18 months	Has repertoire of words (between three and 50); some two-word phrases; vocalizations reveal intonational patterns; great increase in understanding of language	Walks with stiff gait; may build two-block tower; begins to show hand preference
24 months	Vocabulary of 50 or more words for naming and for bringing about events; two-word phrases of own formulation	Walks with ease; runs, can walk up or down stairs, planting both feet on each step
30 months	Vocabulary growth proportionately greater than at any other period in life; speaks with clear communicative intent; conventional sentences (syntax) of three, four, and five words; articulation still includes many infantilisms; good comprehension of speakers in his surroundings	Can jump; stand on one foot; good hand and finger coordination; can build six-block tower
36 months	Vocabulary may exceed 1,000 words; syntax much like that of older persons in his surroundings; most of his utterances are intelligible to older listeners	Runs proficiently; walks stairs with alternating feet; hand preference established
48 months	Except for articulation (phonemic production) the linguistic system is essentially that of the adults in his surroundings. He may begin to develop his own "rhetorical" style of favorite words and phrases	Can hop on one foot (usually right); can throw a ball to an intended receiver; can catch a ball in his arms; can walk on a line

*Adapted from E. H. Lenneberg, *Biological Foundations of Language* (New York: John Wiley & Sons, Inc., 1967), pp. 128–130.

NEUROMUSCULAR SYSTEM

Children's nervous systems must be capable of doing their bidding and of providing them with feedback as to what and how well they are doing. Their nervous systems must be adequate to make them sensitive to the sights and sounds in their environment, and to permit them to make differential responses to different conditions. They must not only be able to hear but to discriminate between speech sounds and other auditory events. It is possible, as we learn later in our discussion of brain-damaged children in Chapter 16, for a child to be able to discriminate, perceive, and make appropriate responses to nonspeech signals and yet not be able to perceive speech as a different form of sounds. Such a child may hear, and yet not learn to speak, for what the child hears does not include the auditory perceptual capacities necessary for speech.

Cerebral-palsied children are, as a total special population, markedly retarded in speech development. Those cerebral-palsied children who are also mentally retarded by virtue of their brain damage are likely to be retarded in all aspects of speech development. In a study of the articulatory proficiency of cerebral-palsied children, Irwin (1952, pp. 269–279) found that these children at five and a half years of age are at a proficiency level equivalent to that of the 30-month-old child. The problems of some cerebral-palsied children are further complicated by hearing loss of both a peripheral and a central nature. Central hearing loss, as a consequence of damage to the auditory area of the brain, makes it difficult for the child to perceive speech differentially from other audible environmental events.

THE AUDITORY SYSTEM

As previously suggested, the auditory system must permit the reception as well as the perception of speech events. That is, the speech signal must reach the brain (reception) and be processed differentially in the brain (perception). Children with hearing loss severe enough to impair reception are slower in speech development than hearing children. Deaf children are those whose receptive impairment is so severe that they cannot learn to speak through the auditory mode. However, some mildly or moderately hearing-impaired children, especially if their impairment is recognized early in life, may speak quite competently if given appropriate attention and training. The perceptually impaired (aphasic-dyslogic child) is considered at some length in Chapter 16. Later (Chapter 14) we consider in more detail the implications of hearing loss on speech.

CEREBRAL DOMINANCE AND LATERALITY PREFERENCE

Human motor development is characterized by the preferential use of a paired organ, hand, foot, eye, or ear. This preference is an expression of laterality. Most of us are right-handed and right-footed *and* right-eyed. That is, given an opportunity to reach or grasp, to hop or stand on one foot, to view something with one eye, we are likely to use the same organ for the task—the one on the right side of the body—with great consistency. About 7 to 10 per cent of us are left-sided. However, mixed preference, that is, the combination of right-handedness and left-eyedness, is quite common. A small percentage of us are ambilateral, that is, there is less consistency as to which hand will be used for reaching, or grasping, or executing some task that requires only one hand, or where one hand exercises a skill with the aid of the other hand. Among the ambilateral we have some who are also *ambidextrous*, who are equally skilled with either member of paired organs. Usually such skill is expressed in manual (hand) skills. Ambilaterality does not imply ambidexterity. Among children who are intellectually and maturationally retarded, we have a considerable amount of ambilaterality accompanied by ambi-nondexterity. The truly ambidextrous are a chosen few, most of whom are probably innately left-handed (sinistral) and who have developed more dexterity in the use of the right hand than innately right-handed persons are likely to develop in the use of the left.

The expression of laterality—let us use "hand preference" as an indicator of such expression—parallels critical stages in the development of speech. By 18 months of age, when most children have uttered their first true words, they have also begun to indicate hand preference. By three years of age, when syntax becomes acquired, hand preference, foot preference (standing or hopping on one foot), eye preference, *and* ear preference are also normally established. These laterality expressions mean that one hemisphere of the brain is dominant or controls a function.

Speech, however, employs paired organs for intake as well as output.[13] We listen with both ears, and take in visual events with both eyes. However, as we have seen, the perceptual appreciation of language events, the interpretation of what we hear or what we read, is normally processed in the left hemisphere for at least 95 per cent of right-handed persons and 60 per cent of left-handed persons. We may generalize

---

[13] For example, the tongue consists of two halves, which receive nervous innervations from both hemispheres of the brain.

therefore that *the vast majority of human beings have cerebral dominance for language behavior in the left hemisphere.* Such dominance is normally established by three years of age (Kimura 1967). Cerebral dominance is delayed in the moderately and severely mentally retarded and in brain-damaged children. Nonspeech events, the noises of our environment, and the perception of music are normally processed in the right hemisphere. Thus, as we indicated earlier, it is possible for a child to respond appropriately to the barking of a dog, or the ringing of a bell, and even to listen to music, and yet not be able to make the discriminations and perceptions that are necessary to understand and acquire speech. This very special capacity—the processing of speech signals— is associated with cerebral dominance and the functioning of the temporal lobe of the left cerebral hemisphere.

INTELLIGENCE

The factor of intelligence is so intimately related to language development that we must be careful to avoid circuitous thinking. There is little doubt that intelligence is positively related to vocabulary growth and, perhaps to a lesser degree, also to syntactic competence (sentence length and complexity). Templin's study (1957, p. 117) is representative of most findings. She reports a correlation of .50 between intelligence and vocabulary growth in young children. Virtually all verbal intelligence tests for children, for example, the Stanford-Binet and the Wechsler Intelligence Scale for Children, include a vocabulary test as part of the scale because of the established relationship between lanuage development, as measured by vocabulary, and intelligence.

One of the by-products of being born with good native intelligence is the likelihood that one's parents, and other members of the family, may also be intelligent, and provide an environment where proficient language usage will stimulate and encourage more of the same. Further, we have a likelihood that such a background will have books as well as parents for reading, for storytelling, and for the other social advantages that go along with good language development.

SEX

Though studies vary in their findings, we may accept as a general observation that up to age eight or nine, girls are somewhat more advanced than boys of like age in overall language development. McCarthy (1954, pp. 492–630) reports such an advantage for girls over boys. Templin (1957), based on much the same procedures for collecting data as McCarthy, found smaller differences than those detected in earlier studies. Templin notes that whereas on overall language competence girls do tend to be somewhat superior to boys, the differences for specific language achievements are not consistent and are usually not great enough to be statistically significant. Girls do seem to be about a half year ahead of boys in articulatory proficiency. Boys, however, may exceed girls in word knowledge. Templin explains her findings of reduced differences between the sexes on the basis of changes in child rearing during the past few decades. We have changed from bringing up little girls as girls and little boys as boys to a single standard in child care and training (Templin 1957, p. 147). This observation is supported by the findings of Winitz (1969) on a study of the language development of kindergarten children. Winitz found no significant differences between the sexes in regard to such language measures as length of response, the number of different words used, the structural (syntactic) complexity of the child's utterances, vocabulary skill, and articulatory proficiency.

ENVIRONMENTAL FACTORS

It is not possible to disassociate factors, such as intelligence, both child and parental, parent-child relationships, and "talkativeness" of key members in a family setting, from other presumably nonlinguistic aspects and influences on a child's language development. Cazden (1972, pp. 130–136) reviews some of the pertinent literature on environmental influences on early child language development. She summarizes the indirect effects as follows (p. 130):

"Non linguistic aspects of the child's environment can be influential in at least three ways: differences in who speaks to the child, differences in the characteristics of the context or situation in which the conversation takes place, and differences in attitudes of the speaker toward language and toward the child."

Cazden cites investigations that indicate that families differ in the amount of talking directed to the young child compared with speech between parents or directed to older siblings. Mothers usually do considerably more talking to a young child than do fathers. Cazden also observes (pp. 105–107) that talking directed to infants, whether by parents or older siblings, tends to be more simplified in syntactic structure than adult-to-adult talking. Thus, the young child may have fewer and less complicated constructions to decode.

Our inclination is to emphasize the importance of the home and the relationship of members of the family within the home as the most important factors for language acquisition in the early stages. Children's potentialities for language development, from onset until the time they begin to spend more of their working hours away from home than at home, are nurtured by key members of the family. The key members may be older siblings or grandparents. Usually, parents are the key members, and mothers the dominant ones and the most significant influences on the child's language development. If we consider an individual child, born without physical or sensory disability or any primary emotional handicap, the following assumptions are positive for normal onset and development of language.

1. The mother has normal maternal drives and enjoys and wishes to interact with the child. Similarly, the father has a normal paternal drive and parallel wishes.

2. The parents enjoy talking to the child even if in the prelinguistic stage of language acquisition, they may be talking *at* the child. In any event, when the child indicates readiness, the parents will provide opportunity for interaction whether it be for sound play in responding to early verbal demands, or later by answering questions with relevant answers, or extending a child's remarks without overelaborated explanations.

3. These assumptions imply an underlying one that the child will have an older speaker or speakers with whom to identify and whose speech, in time, will be decodable.

4. The home is not so noisy, either human or electronic (radio and television included), that the child cannot hear and attend to the parent or other key family members.

Given a home where these assumptions prevail, the great likelihood is that the child will start speaking by 15 months of age. If these assumptions do not prevail, development of language, both qualitatively and quantitatively, may be delayed. We believe that unless the child's environment is grossly abnormal, initial onset and acquisition of speaking is less likely to be delayed than is the child's subsequent language development. Parents who have little or no time to talk to their infants, and who provide no surrogate for language stimulation, cannot expect normal language development from their children. We have interviewed fathers who admitted that they had no real interest in their infant children until their little ones began to talk. Fortunately, most mothers do not share this attitude. Fortunately, also, this attitude on the parts of fathers is becoming rare.

Bilingualism

A bilingual child is one who is exposed to *two different language systems* before either has become firmly established. Bilingualism should not be confused with *bidialectism*, which refers to exposure to two dialects of the same language. This may be any two regional dialects of American English or Black English and one dialect of American English. It may also mean any two dialects of British English as well as a dialect of British (regardless of geographic area) and American English.

Some bilingual children are exposed to and acquire two languages simultaneously. These children are brought up in homes where two languages are spoken, or are brought up in an environment where one language is spoken in the home and another is spoken outside of the home. Other bilingual children are exposed to and learn one language, presumably in the home, and then a second language, either in the home or at an early (preschool or primary school) age outside of the home.

What are the effects of bilingualism, either simultaneous or sequential, on language development? Unfortunately, our information is relatively sparse. Many reports on bilingual children are biographical and deal with exceptional homes and so, presumably, potentially exceptional children. On the other hand, some reports lack objectivity because they are generated to prove, rather than to find out, what factors, other than sociopolitical ones, are related to the acquisition and development of language in children who are brought up in bilingual environments. Many questions and issues involved in bilingualism are objectively reviewed by Cazden (1972, pp. 175–181), who says in her closing statement: "In the United States ... through its influences on children, teachers, and parents—bilingual education can affect both speech behavior and attitudes toward language...."

Early studies, such as Smith's (1949), indicated that bilingual children had below age expectancy vocabularies in English. The children studied were of Chinese ancestry who lived in Hawaii. Smith also observed that for only two fifths of the 30 Hawaiian children in the study did the combined vocabularies of words they knew in Chinese as well as in English exceed the age norms. When words of the same meaning in both languages were subtracted from the combined Chinese and English vocabulary, only one sixth of the children exceeded the norm.

Smith's study is an "older" one, and her findings may have been influenced by social factors as well as by educational opportunity. For much of the Western world, English is a second if not a first language. We have no evidence to indicate that children in Switzerland or in India or in Israel who learn English as a second language (usually but not invariably sequentially) suffer from any ill effects on their first language.

Our position is that the vast majority of children can learn two languages either through simultaneous or sequential exposure, and that such children are likely to be the richer, linguistically and culturally, for this achievement. On the other hand, if a child is slow in language acquisition and reveals confusion as a result of bilingual exposure, the family should make a choice as to which language the child is to be exposed and to hear. "To hear" means the language that is directly addressed to the child. If even overhearing a second language produces delay or confusion, then as far as possible a child should hear only one language.

Most Americans, unfortunately, are so accustomed to a monolingual environment that they tend not to know the extent of bilingualism around the world. Much of the Southwestern part of the United States is bilingual, as is much of Eastern Canada. Pertinent issues of bilingualism are considered by Macnamara (1967)[14] and by Ervin-Tripp (1973).[15]

Social Class (Socioeconomic Level and Social Linguistic Status)

What can we project and predict about language development in relationship to the social class and socioeconomic status of the family? On an individual basis for a family, or even for a given child, expectations should be made with caution and reservation. Especially in a mobile and rapidly changing society, social status is not necessarily linked to economic status, to intellectual potential, or to educational achievement. Nevertheless, there are overall correlations that tend to hold for total subpopulations that we consider with full awareness of the numerous exceptions.

Templin (1957, p. 147) concluded that children from families in upper socioeconomic levels tend to be more advanced in language development than children from lower socioeconomic families. Templin observed that there are consistent differences in language measures such as articulatory proficiency, phonemic discrimination, word recognition, mean length of utterance, and complexity of syntactical constructions. Insofar as socioeconomic status is positively correlated with factors such as intellectual level of parents, educational level cultural opportunities, and parental attention, as well as attitude to language usage for the young child, the expectations projected by Templin are likely to hold. However, there are economically poor

---

[14] J. Macnamara, ed., "Problems of Bilingualism," *The Journal of Social Issues*, **23** 2 (April 1967). The student interested in, or concerned with, problems of bilingualism should study this monograph. It includes articles by authorities from a variety of disciplines dealing with important aspects and issues of bilingualism.

[15] S. Ervin-Tripp, *Language Acquisition and Communicative Choice* (Stanford, Calif.: Stanford University Press, 1973), 1–91. Also contains significant essays on bilingualism.

homes that are rich in culture, love, and understanding of children, as well as wealthy homes that are impoverished in factors that nourish children intellectually, emotionally, and linguistically.

Bernstein (1961) has attracted considerable attention by his observations and generalizations in regard to the differences between the "quality" of language used by working-class parents in lower socio-economic levels compared with middle- and upper-socioeconomic classes. Bernstein uses the terms *restricted* and *elaborated codes* to indicate the differences between the lower and middle and upper classes in regard to language usage. In effect, if we were to take Bernstein literally and accept his generalizations more seriously than he probably intended, we would conclude that persons of lower economic classes use language as emotional expression rather than for the communication of ideas. The language, as constructed in terms of vocabulary and syntax is essentially noninformative. In contrast, persons in the middle- and upper-economic class are more likely to use language that is informative, more detailed, and at the same time more abstract. For critical comments on this position see Cazden (1972, pp. 132–134) and Labov (1972, pp. 204–240).[16]

Our position is to view both what Bernstein states and his critics' evaluations with considerable reservation. We consider any sweeping generalization as both unscientific and dangerous. On the other hand, we believe that some of the critics, including Labov, protest too strongly and go beyond the intentions of persons they criticize. What is important to the child, what matters in regard to language acquisition and development, is the nature of the particular environment in which the child is reared. Sociopolitics sometimes goes out of hand and influences the interpretation of the findings of sociolinguistics. To deny that some children from one kind of environment may need more help than children from another kind of environment is to deny these children their opportunity for social, intellectual, and educational achievement. On the other hand, to assume that any socioeconomic status is invariably associated with any specific factors is to be perceptually defensive and too busy with prejudices to attend to specific facts and their implications. A true concern for the child should help to put matters in proper perspective in the interest of the child, even where dialects and cultural groups are at issue.

---

[16] Labov, in *Language in the Inner City* (Philadelphia: University of Pennsylvania Press, 1972), takes strong exception to Bernstein's position as well as to the teaching programs that accept the position that lower-class children have poor language and need to be taught Standard English in place of their non-Standard dialects. Labov is particularly concerned with black children and their use of Black English.

STIMULATION TO SPEAK

As indicated earlier, stimulation to speak may come partly from the atmosphere of the home and partly from experiences that provoke linguistic activity. Some social environments provide more stimulation to speak and more good models to imitate than others. When a mother talks to her child frequently and simply and when her own speech is clear and intelligible, the child is likely to speak earlier. If, as the child grows older, he lives with parents who share and enjoy interesting experiences with him, such as going on picnics and talking about books, he tends to speak more fully and with longer sentences than the child who has fewer experiences. Talk cannot thrive in a vacuum; it needs the stimulation of common experiences and adventures. An example of a child who had little stimulation to speak is that of a five-year-old boy who has a seven-year-old sister who is a chatterbox and who almost constantly interprets for him: "He doesn't like his cheese sandwich toasted; he likes it plain." When an adult suggested that he'd like to hear what the little boy thought of toasted sandwiches, the little sister replied, "He's too shy. He doesn't talk much." The poor lad never gets much chance to talk with a loquacious sister at his elbow.

Admittedly, some children may be overstimulated. A seven-year-old boy lived with very verbal and alert parents who were overly interested in bringing up their child with "broad horizons." From the time the child was two, they talked *at* him. As he grew older, they provided him with a wealth of sensory experiences such as listening to classical records and watching the ballet, but he never had time really to enjoy the experiences, for the parents accompanied each one with a barrage of words, most of which were polysyllabic. The overstimulation and the pattern of complex language were too much for the child. The apparent result was that he gave up trying to speak and appeared to be a child with "retarded language development." Though not truly retarded, he had become a reluctant speaker, at least in his home setting.

Problems and Topics for Papers[17]

1. What is meant by the statement: "Speech is a human species-specific function?" Do you agree with this statement? How close do the chimpanzees come to language usage? Do the "talking" chimpanzees meet the criteria?
2. What are the criteria for true speech?

---

[17] Note: Information for many of the problems and topics may be found in the list of References and Suggested Readings.

3. Listen to the free speech of a boy and a girl at each of the following age levels: two, four, and six years. Note differences in articulatory pro- ficiency, vocabulary, and sentence length. Are there any consistent differences between the sexes? Are there differences in syntactic com- plexity?

4. Make the same observations as in No. 3 for a child whom you consider bright and for one you consider to be of average intelligence.

5. Listen to children in the kindergarten and to children in the third grade. What language factors distinguish the two groups?

6. Ask a three-, a four-, and a five-year-old child to repeat the sentence: "Tomorrow Mommy, Daddy, and I will go on a picnic, if it doesn't rain." Note the difference in their elicited imitations.

7. Read and report on two of the references from the list of references and suggested readings that follows.

8. Find a provocative picture in a magazine (one that is likely to induce a story). Ask a five-year-old and an eight-year-old to make up a story based on the picture. Note the differences in use of vocabulary, length, and complexity of each sentence, and in the total length of the story.

9. What are the issues involved in bilingual education? What is your posi- tion?

10. Define bidialectism. Give three or four examples of differences in dialects for names of things. Give examples of three differences in syntactic forms for plurals, tense endings, progressive verbs in Black English, and a standard regional dialect of American English.

References and Suggested Readings

Bernstein, B., "Social Structure, Language and Learning," *Educational Research*, **3**, (1961), 163–176. (This article has produced considerable controversy on the nature and differences between members of social classes and their use of language.)

Bloom, L., *Language Development: Form and Function in Emerging Grammars*, Cambridge: The M.I.T. Press, 1970. (A report on the acquisition of grammar by three children beginning at about 19 months of age. In- terpretations of cognitive functioning are included.)

Braine, M. D. S., "The Ontogeny of English Phrase Structure," *Language*, **39** (January–March 1963), 1–13.

Brown, R., *A First Language: The Early Stages*, Cambridge: Harvard Uni- versity Press, 1973.

——, "The Development of *Wh* questions in Child Speech," *Journal of Verbal Learning and Verbal Behavior*, **7** (1968), 279–290.

——, and U. Bellugi, "Three Processes in the Child's Acquisition of Syntax," *Harvard Educational Review*, **34**, 2 (Spring 1964), 133–151. (An exposition of a study of two children, "Adam" and "Eve," who were selected because they were both very talkative and very intelligible.)

Cazden, C. B., *Child Language and Education*, New York: Holt, Rinehart and Winston, Inc., 1972. (Basically deals with early language acquisition. However, Cazden also includes discussion of dialects and the role of language in cognition. A readable book for nonspecialists.)

Carroll, J. B., "Words, Meanings, and Concepts," *Harvard Educational Review*, **34**, 2 (Spring 1964), 178–202. (An exposition of how word meanings and concepts can be taught effectively by classroom teachers.)

Chomsky, C., *The Acquisition of Syntax in Children from Five to Ten*, Cambridge: The M.I.T. Press, 1969. (Describes the author's investigation of the acquisition of syntactic structures in children between five to ten years of age. Her findings indicate that the grammar of a five-year-old differs in a number of ways from adult grammar "and that the gradual disappearance of these discrepancies can be traced as children exhibit increased knowledge over the next four or five years of their development.")

Dale, P. S., *Language Development: Structure and Function*, New York: Holt, Rinehart and Winston, 1972. (Discusses language acquisition and evaluates language training approaches.)

Darley, F. L., and H. Winitz, "Age of First Words: Review of Research," *Journal of Speech and Hearing Disorders*, **26**, 3 (August 1961), 272–290.

Davis, E. A., *The Development of Linguistic Skills in Twins, Singletons with Siblings and Only Children from Ages Five to Ten Years*, Minneapolis: University of Minnesota Press, 1937. (A classic and basic study of the language development of single and multiple-birth children.)

Dececco, J. P., *The Psychology of Language, Thought and Instruction*, New York: Holt, Rinehart and Winston, Inc., 1967. (A book of readings that includes essays of historical importance as well as some contemporary essays that are provocative and may become important. Present problems of the culturally different who may also be culturally deprived give the readings immediate significance. The editor succeeded in providing a good balance in points of view about the nature and purpose of language as well as current issues and their educational implications.)

Eimas, P. D., E. R. Siqueland, P. Jusczyk, and J. Vigorito, "Speech Perception in Infants," *Science*, **171** (1971), 303–306.

Ervin-Tripp, S., *Language Acquisition and Communicative Choice*, Stanford, Calif.: Stanford University Press, 1973.

———, "Discourse Agreement: How Children Answer Questions," in J. R. Hayes, ed., *Cognition and the Development of Language*, New York: John Wiley & Sons, Inc., 1970. (The *comprehension* of questions develops sequentially from *yes-no* to *what, where, what-do, whose, who, why, wherefrom, how,* and *when.*)

Fry, D. B., "The Development of the Phonological System in the Normal and Deaf Child," in F. M. Smith and G. A. Miller, *The Genesis of Language*, Cambridge: The M.I.T. Press, 1966.

Goldfarb, W., "Effects of Psychological Deprivation in Infancy and Subsequent Stimulation," *American Journal of Psychiatry*, **12** (August 1954), 102–129.

Ingram, D., "Phonological Rules in Young Children," *Journal of Child Language*, **1** (1974), 49–64.

———, and Jon Eisenson, in Jon Eisenson, ed., *Aphasia in Children*, New York: Harper & Row, Publishers, Inc., 1972.

Irwin, O. C., "Speech Development in the Young Child," *Journal of Speech and Hearing Disorders*, **17**, 3 (1952), 269–279.

Jacobs, R. A., and P. S. Rosenbaum, *English Transformational Grammar*, Waltham, Mass.: Blaisdell Publishing Co., 1968.

Jakobson, R., *Child Language, Aphasia and Phonological Universals*, The Hague: Mouton & Company, 1968.

Kimura, D., "Functional Asymmetry of the Brain in Dichotic Listening," *Cortex*, **3** (1967), 163–178. (Dichotic listening, an approach to indicate ear preference, is explained in its relationship to cerebral dominance and language functions.)

Labov, W., *Language in the Inner City*, Philadelphia: University of Pennsylvania Press, 1972.

Lee, L. L., *Developmental Sentence Analysis*, Evanston, Ill.: Northwestern University Press, 1974. (Describes procedures for assessing a child's language status based on a taped language sample.)

———, "Developmental Sentence Types: A Method for Comparing Normal and Deviant Syntactic Development," *Journal of Speech and Hearing Disorders*, **31**, 4 (1966), 311–330. (An approach to the assessment of levels of syntactic development based on comparisons between a normally developing child and one with language delay.)

Lenneberg, E. H., *Biological Foundations of Language*, New York: John Wiley & Sons, Inc., 1967.

———, "Language Disorders in Childhood," *Harvard Educational Review*, **24** (Spring 1964), 152–177. (Devoted to language and learning; highly recommended for teachers and language clinicians.)

Lewis, M. M., *How Children Learn to Speak*, New York: Basic Books, Inc., 1959. (An English author's observations about speech development.)

McCarthy, D., "Language Development in Children," in L. Carmichael, ed., *Manual of Child Psychology*, rev. ed., New York: John Wiley & Sons, Inc., 1954, 492–630. (Deserves reading as a classic report.)

McNeill, D., *The Acquisition of Language*. New York: Harper & Row, Publishers, Inc., 1970. (A fast-moving, technical discussion of language acquisition by children.)

———, "The Development of Language," in Mussen, P. H., ed., *Carmichael's Manual of Child Psychology*, 3rd ed., New York: John Wiley & Sons, Inc., 1970, 1061–1161. (A survey of recent literature on language acquisition emphasizing the relationships among language development, intellect, and maturation in the child.)

Menyuk, P., *Sentences Children Use*, M.I.T. Research Monograph Series, Cambridge, Mass.: 1969.

Piaget, J., and B. Inhelder, *The Psychology of the Child*, New York: Basic Books, Inc., 1969. (Chap. 6 of this book is devoted to an exposition of the development (evolution) of language and thought in the child.)

Prather, E. M., D. L. Hedrick, and A. Kern, "Articulation Development in Children Aged Two to Four Years," *Journal of Speech and Hearing Disorders*, **40** (1975), 179–191.

Sander, E. K., "When Are Speech Sounds Learned?" *Journal of Speech and Hearing Disorders*, **37** (1972), 55–63.

Slobin, D., ed., *A Field Manual for Cross-Culture Study of the Acquisition of Communicative Competence*, Berkeley, Calif.: University of California Press, 1967.

Smith, M. E., "Measurement of the Vocabularies of Young Bilingual Children in Both of the Languages Used," *Journal of Genetic Psychology*, **34** (1949), 305–310.

Templin, M. C., "The Study of Articulation and Language Development During the Early School Years," in F. M. Smith, and G. A. Miller, *The Genesis of Language*, Cambridge: The M.I.T. Press, 1966.

———, *Certain Language Skills in Children: Their Development and Interrelationships*, Minneapolis: University of Minnesota Press, 1957.

Tyack, D., and R. Gottsleben, *Language Sampling; Analysis and Training: A Handbook for Teachers and Clinicians*, Palo Alto, Calif.: Consulting Psychologists Press, 1974.

Van Riper, C., *Speech Correction*, 5th ed., Englewood Cliffs, N.J.: Prentice-Hall, Inc., 1972.

Winitz, H., *Articulatory Acquisition and Behavior*, New York: Appleton-Century-Crofts, 1969, chap. 1. (An excellent review of the research literature on prelingual stages of language development and theories about the onset of speech.)

———, "Sex Differences in Language of Kindergarten Children," *ASHA*, **1** (1959), 86.

8. Stimulating Language Development

As noted in Chapter 7, most children learn to speak well and quickly. Their competence and performance in all aspects of language—phonological, semantic, morphemic, and syntactic—are usually so readily apparent that we take them for granted. The following soliloquy by a kindergartner illustrates performance in language: After considerable, obvious deliberation, she called a Siamese cat a puppy cat. When asked why it was a puppy cat, she responded with: "He's small like a cat... He's on a leash like a dog. ... Walks like a dog. ... Looks half cat, half dog. ... Sounds like a baby." With decided satisfaction and with assurance, she announced, "That's why he's a puppy cat."

For a five-year-old, this child's monologue displayed considerable facility with language. Her phonological system virtually equaled that of an adult with no observable substitutions or omissions of sounds. Although her sentences were mostly simple ones, she did use one with a dependent clause. Her vocabulary was adequate for her explanation. For her age, she displayed an unusual degree of language sophistication through her deductive powers. In her monologue, she used each remark, based on an analogy, as a cue for further extension and expansion of ideas. In this process, she presented a series of concepts. Finally, she arrived at her generalization, "That's why he's a puppy cat."

The next conversation is that of a three-and-one-half-year-old city boy. When *The Big City Book* by A. Ingle (New York: Platt & Munk,

1975) was shown to the child, Joey said, "I wanta read the book. You read the book." Whereupon the book was opened to its fly page, which includes pictures of a taxi, City Hall, a police car, a bus, and a grocery store—all items found in a large city. The adult said, "Joey, tell me about it." The boy enumerated items on the page including a policeman. As there was no policeman in the picture, the adult remarked, "I don't see a policeman." Joey said, "He's inside the car." Then he turned to pages 10 and 11 with buildings and a helicopter. Joey pointed to the helicopter and said *helicopter* very clearly. He responded to "Tell me about it" with "It opens." When this remark was followed by the adult's "Yes?", he added, "It makes a noise. ... It flies." He turned to another page and named the animals such as giraffe [dræf], crocodile, duck, and hippopotamus/hɪpˈɑməˌmɪs/. Then he saw a car on top of a truck of melons and said, "The car is on the flowers." Then he noticed a pileup of cars on one side of the page and announced, "They got in an accident." When prodded with "Tell me about it," he responded with "They did." When he was prodded again with, "Why do you suppose there was an accident?", he responded again with, "They did." Joe's sound production is beginning to approximate that of an adult. Occasionally he uses /t/ and /d/ for /θ/ and /ð/, consistently uses /t/ for /tʃ/ and /d/ for /dʒ/. He did particularly well in naming all of the objects and he spoke grammatically. When Joey was questioned about the policeman, he said that the policeman was in the police car. He used his own experience to call the melons *flowers*, but was accurate in placing the car on top of the flowers. He was not able to tell the "why" of the accident.   Surely at this age, we cannot expect this explanation. This boy, too, is well on his way to using language with proficiency.

All children do not progress as rapidly in the receptive and expressive functions of language as these two children. Probably much of their learning has taken place in their homes with parents helping to motivate their language competence and production. Much of language learning takes place before the child enters school. The school's language arts programs are but extensions of the child's early language training with each individual child organizing his/her own language learning and advancing to another level when ready.

Both the teacher and the clinician are aware of the differences in stages of language development in children. The teacher makes an informal evaluation based on listening to the children's language. The teacher and clinician are equally interested in seeing that the development of language is at the level that is needed for academic achievement. When the level of the children's development appears to be decidedly below the level of their peers, the teacher refers these children to the clinician (or the clinician may have already pinpointed the youngsters in a screening survey). These children's vocabularies may be meager; their phonological and syntactical development, that of a much younger child. In such cases, the speech and language clinician diagnoses the children's language difficulties and plans and carries through strategies designed to develop particular language abilities.

Testing Language Abilities

Thus, the clinician evaluates both linguistic competence and performance. Competence, as noted, refers to the underlying hypothesized rule mastered by the speaker-hearer. Performance refers to how the child strings words together into sentences under, of course, such constraints as memory, attention, motivation, distraction factors, communicative environment—and some physiological and acoustic parameters. That children must comprehend before they produce meaningful utterances is an important concept for clinicians and teachers to appreciate. For instance, Mecham (1971) reports that the children he studied comprehended and responded correctly to adjectives used to designate size and color but that they did not produce these adjectives even after hearing them 24 times.

Language tests assess different verbal behaviors including the broad aspects such as comprehension of language and expression of language, as well as narrower aspects such as syntactical and morphological sophistication and extent of vocabulary and phonological development. Generally, we use tests to find out how children are functioning currently, to discover their strengths and weaknesses, and to compare their performance with others. Although we recognize that children do not perform equally well, we usually compare on the basis of *norms*— what is average for a certain age. This testing provides us with some useful information as to children's performance.

We need to recognize, however, that the tests have been constructed by human beings, each with a hypothesis or theory in mind. Early language assessments relied heavily on the mean language response (average number of words per utterance). In the 1960s, the Illinois Test of Psycholinguistic Abilities (ITPA) (Urbana, Illinois, University of Illinois Press, 1968), based on Osgood's communication model, and The Northwestern Syntax Screening Test (Evanston, Illinois, Northwestern University Press, 1969), based on transformational grammar, were published. Beyond being aware of the rationale of a particular test, we need to realize that individual children vary considerably in their performance during testing. Scharf (1972) found that scores of successive language samples obtained from individual children revealed reversals, sudden change, or no change in performances. He notes that such variations may be more indicative of the child's mood on a given day than of levels of the child's language development.

Language tests provide insights into language behavior although, as noted, clinicians and teachers must be aware that they are accepting the individual test maker's theory and concept of language. For clinicians and teachers, the results of language tests are an essential part of the diagnostic procedure; but, in addition, they must use their own experience with the language behavior of children and their knowledge of language development to diagnose and devise techniques of stimulating language development. At this point, therefore, we examine briefly some of the current language tests. Those tests that are cited are representative of what is available. The selection is by no means complete. Obviously, the perfect language test has not yet been devised.

1. M. J. Mecham, J. L. Jex, and J. D. Jones, *Utah Test of Language Development*, (Communication Research Associates, Salt Lake City, Post Office Box 11012, 1967). This test is designed as a screening device for the early detection of language problems in children between the ages of four and eight. It correlates fairly highly with the ITPA and includes language items from Stanford-Binet, Gesell Developmental Schedules, Vineland Social Maturity Scale, Peabody Picture Vocabulary Test, and the Mecham Verbal Language Development scale.

2. E. Carrow-Woolfolk, *Carrow Elicited Language Inventory* (Learning Concepts, 2501 N. Lamar, Austin, Texas, 1975). This test identifies children aged three through eight with language problems and determines the specific linguistic structures that contribute to these problems. The test consists of a set of plates, each of which contains one or more black and white line drawings; the pictures represent referential categories and contrasts that can be designated by form classes and function words, morphological constructions, grammatical categories, and syntactic structures.

3. C. R. Foster, J. J. Giddan, and J. Stark, *Assessment of Children's Language Comprehension* (Consulting Psychologists Press, 577 College Avenue, Palo Alto, California 94302, 1970.) This test measures the child's ability to understand language without having to produce it. It was designed to help clinicians and teachers define receptive language difficulties in young children and to provide a basis for remedial training appropriate to each child's needs. It uses a core vocabulary of 50 common words, which are combined into two-, three-, and four-element phrases. It delineates (a) a simple receptive vocabulary, (b) the number of critical elements (information words) the child can process, and (c) any pattern in the breakdown of critical element sequences. The

inventory does not include age or developmental norms. It is useful for test-retest purposes.

4. J. Reynell, and R. M. C. Huntley, "New Scales for the Assessment of Language Development in Young Children," *Journal of Learning Disabilities*, **4** (December 1971), 540–557. This test is designed for the assessment of aspects of language development over the age range of one to five years. The scales, based on the normal pattern of development, include (1) Verbal Comprehension A, which requires no speech; (2) Verbal Comprehension B, which requires neither speech nor hand function; and (3) Expressive language, which includes separate sections on language structure, vocabulary, and content.

5. N. B. Fluharty, "The Design and Standardization of a Speech and Language Screening Test for Use with Preschool Children," *Journal of Speech and Hearing Disorders*, **39** (February 1974), 75–86. This test, designed for use with three- to five-year olds, follows the transformation-generative grammar mode. It contains three parts: (1) Identification of 15 common objects, (2) nonverbal responses to sentences incorporating the ten basic syntactic structures, and (3) imitation of ten one-sentence picture descriptions.

6. L. L. Lee, and S. M. Canter, "Developmental Sentence Scoring: A Clinical Procedure for Estimating Syntactic Development in Children's Spontaneous Speech," *Journal of Speech and Hearing Disorders*, **36** (August 1971), 315–340. This procedure evaluates a child's performance in the use of grammatical rules in spontaneous speech and measures the child's grammar against "adult Standard English" (p. 317). Lee and Canter describe a procedure for estimating the status and progress of children enrolled for clinical language-usage training based upon a developmental scale of syntax acquisition. The evaluation is based on 50 complete, different, consecutive, intelligible, nonecholalic sentences elicited from a child in conversation with an adult.

7. L. Luterman, and A. Bar, "The Diagnostic Significance of Sentence Repetition for Language-Impaired Children," *Journal of Speech and Hearing Disorders*, **36** (February 1971), 29–39. This article suggests a diagnostic tool for language-impaired children based on the child's sentence repetitions. Its three conditions are (1) repetition of grammatically incorrect sentences taken from the child's own production, (2) repetition of grammatically correct versions of these sentences, and (3) repetition of the reverse word order of these grammatically correct versions. The evaluation is based on the premise that children will not imitate appropriate features unless they have acquired the rules for the particular parts of the syntax.

8. A. E. Boehm, *Boehm Test of Basic Concepts*, New York, Psychological Corporation, 1971. This test is designed for children in the early

grades who are underachievers. It assesses the mastery of concepts commonly found in preschool and primary grade instructional materials, which are essential to understanding and responding to instruction in the early grades. The concepts belong in four categories: spatial, quantitative, time, and miscellaneous. For example, the concepts in Book I are *top*, *three*, *away from*, *next to*, *inside*, *some*, *not many*, *middle*, *few*, *farthest*, *around*, *over*, *widest*, *most*, *between*, *whole*, *nearest*, *second*, *corner*, *several*, *behind*, *row*, *different*, *after*, *almost*, and *half*.

9. E. D. Critchlow, *Dos Amigos Verbal Language Scales*, Academic Therapy Publications, 1539 Fourth Street, San Rafael, California, 1974. This is an individual test that can be given and scored in ten minutes, which provides information about the dominant language of the child, and about the comparative development of the child's English and Spanish, and yields the functional level of the child's spoken language development.

10. The *Illinois Test of Psycholinguistic Abilities* is described in Chapter 1. The ITPA is widely used both for diagnostic and research purposes. Recent evidence suggests that the ITPA subtests may not measure distinct and separate psycholinguistic abilities (Hare, Hammill, and Bartel 1973; Burns and Watson 1973; Cronkhite and Penner 1975). This is discussed in Chapter 1. It is, of course, a useful test but planning remediation programs based on each of the subtests may not bring about the precision intended in language development programs.

Can Language Development Be Stimulated?

Probably the two language development programs that are most frequently discussed are the "Sesame Street" Television Program and the Peabody Language Kit both of which are linguistically based. Evidence points to the success of both of these programs.

Ball and Bogatz (1971) report on the success of "Sesame Street" with 943 subjects, many of whom have disadvantaged backgrounds. They revealed that:

1. Boys and girls who watched the programs showed greater gains than those who did not.
2. Watching time was positively correlated with learning.
3. Skills that were best learned were those that received the most time and attention on the program.
4. Regular watching by disadvantaged children produced gains

superior to those of middle-class subjects who watched infrequently.

5. Greater gains were made by three-year-olds than by older children.
6. Children who watched the shows and then discussed them with their mothers showed the greatest gains.

Hamre (1972), noting the success of "Sesame Street," recommends that schools plan programs in language stimulation activities in a similar manner. He explains that "Sesame Street" provides a wealth of linguistic experiences some of which might be considered "controlled."

Milligan and Potter (1971) reviewed the studies of the Peabody Kit and concluded that it does accelerate growth in language development with both the advantaged and the disadvantaged. They also concluded that it appears to improve reading.

Strategies in Stimulating Language Development

We believe that language growth and meaningful experiences involving important concepts are intertwined. Young children, to be successful with language, should talk about persons, objects, and ideas with which they are familiar. The teacher or clinician then must take advantage of children's everyday experiences and, in addition, provide them with new, untried exciting ones. Bloom (1971) maintains that therapeutic language programs must give attention to content, for it appears that learning a linguistic code depends upon the child's learning to distinguish, understand, and express certain conceptual relations. Language learning can take place as a result of such experiential activities as trips, science experiments, creative drama, puppetry, and discussions.

In planning strategies for stimulating language development, most of the work should be based on children's experiences with concepts that are well within the intellectual range of the children. In addition, the interaction between the clinician or teacher and the child should be of the kind that will further positive self-images on the part of the child (see Chapter 3). Lastly, the work should be at the level at which the child can achieve success. Just as there is a time for reading readiness, there is a time for readiness for certain language abilities. Language readiness for certain abilities does exist; for example there are significant differences between first and third graders in the discrimination of unfamiliar syntactic constructions (Vasta and Lievert 1973).

Certain guidelines for successful language intervention are essential. Foulke (1974) lists the following that seem applicable in most situations:

1. Allow the child to learn through his best channel.
2. Keep verbalization at a minimum. Explain directions clearly.
3. Plan the environment so that the child can concentrate.
4. Structure the lesson so that the child can succeed. Ask children to "think over" a wrong answer. Do not reinforce wrong answers.
5. Try to begin teaching just below the child's level and lead up as the child is able.
6. Be flexible in your teaching. Back up or change when necessary.
7. Make sure you are familiar with the materials and that they are within the child's ability before teaching a lesson.

Evidence is accumulating that rarely if ever does a child have difficulty with only a single facet of language. The child who has difficulty with syntactic structures may well also have difficulty with the production of sounds (see Menyuk and Looney 1972). Panagos (1974) points out that a misarticulation is but one symptom of a more generalized language disorder, the cause of which may be tied to other deficits of cognitive and linguistic development. Some of the strategies that follow may appear to emphasize one facet of development more than others. Most of the strategies, however, are multifaceted.

Furthermore, while we are suggesting specific language activities, we should like to emphasize again that each activity should possess, if possible, an experiential base and that each activity should not be produced as an isolated exercise but as an integral, meaningful part of the school day's learning. For example, we have used the sentence: Ice cream tastes _____ than oatmeal. Children will not learn the concept of *better* from a repetition of this one sentence. When, however, they talk about: Smelling roses is better than _____; Petting a cat is better than petting a _____; Eating chocolate cake is better than eating _____, they are likely to acquire the meaning and concept of *better*. If, in addition, as they play the roles of two men, one good and one bad, the children talk about Jim's being the better man of the two, another dimension is added to the concept of *better*. With the reminders that meaning is important, that children must feel a need for an activity and find satisfaction in it, we list activities which can serve as examples of many others that stimulate language development.

Strategies for Stimulating Language Development in the Primary Grades

UNDERSTANDING AUDITORY SYMBOLS AND THEIR RELATIONSHIPS

Following simple directions:

Stand up; sit down; put your hand on your head, on your eyes and on your mouth.

Reading nursery rhymes and then answering questions about the content:

Jack and Jill: Who went up the hill?
What happened to Jack?
What happened to Jill?

Little Jack Horner: What was Jack eating?
What did he say when he put his thumb in the pie?

Following more complicated directions:

Individual: Bring me a book and a pencil.
Bring me a book, a pencil, and a piece of paper.
Group: Get up, stand behind your chair; raise your hands.
Clap your hands; jump twice; turn around twice.
Move your paper from one side of your desk to the other side; put your book on top of the paper.

Following directions as given in a book:

H. Rockwell, *I Did It* (New York: Macmillan Publishing Co., Inc., 1974). This book, intended for five- to seven-year-olds, gives simple directions that tell how to do such things as making a paper bag mask, a paper airplane, a secret message, or a mosaic picture.

Reading a story with the children inserting sounds as they are called for:

The Toy Auto
Sounds: key—click, click
dog, —arf, arf
doll—mama

cat—meow, meow
drum—boom, boom
fire engine—r, r, r, r, r, r, r.
toy car—honk, honk—sometimes followed by boohoo.

Every night at six o'clock, Mrs. Brown locked the door of her store (Click, click). The toys all came alive. The stuffed dogs barked (arf, arf); the stuffed cats meowed (meow, meow); the drum went boom, boom (boom, boom); the baby dolls cried (mama, mama); the fire engine wailed (r-r-r-r-r-r). Everyone was having fun except the poor little car. It wasn't very happy (honk, honk—boohoo). Bright, shiny with a horn, a starter, and able to move, it was truly beautiful. But it was very expensive and nobody wanted to buy it. Poor little auto (Boohoo).

One day a little boy came into the toy store. He looked around and saw the dogs (arf, arf), the cats (meow, meow), the drum (boom, boom), the fire engine (r-r-r-r-r), and the little auto(honk, honk—boohoo). But he loved that little red car (honk, honk). But his mother said, "No way. It costs too much." But that night the little boy's mother and father planned a big surprise for the little boy. The next day, the little boy's mother took him back to the store and told him he could have anything in the store he wanted for his birthday present. He went right to the little auto (honk, honk), picked it up, and hugged it. He didn't even look at the dogs (arf, arf), the cats (meow, meow), the drum (boom, boom), the baby dolls (mama, mama), or the fire engine (r-r-r-r-r-r). The little car (honk, honk) snuggled into the arms of the little boy. It was time to close and Mrs. Brown again locked the door of her store (click, click). And the little boy and his new auto (honk, honk) went happily home.

Playing the game, "Simple Simon Says." For example, Simple Simon says, "Jump on one foot." If the leader omits *Simple Simon*, the children do nothing.

Following directions for work at the desk.

On the desk there are red, blue, and green crayons and a dittoed sheet with a wagon, a little boy, and a tree by the road. The teacher's directions might include: Color the little boy's suit blue; color the tree green; color the wagon blue. Put in a big, big sun at the top of the page.

Responding to: Could this happen?

A little boy was eating his desk.
He has fingers on his feet.
She has a thumb on his foot.
She has very dark hair.
With his legs and feet, he can run.

He puts food into his mouth.
She drinks from a plate.
She eats from a glass.
He sometimes has bacon for breakfast.
She sleeps in a bed.
She sits on a chair.

Making changes in wording in some of the following sentences so that they make sense:

The man who paints the house is a plumber.
The man who fixes the electric lights is a carpenter.
The man who drives the limousine for the rich lady is a chauffeur.
The man who cooks the dinner is a cook.
The lady who prescribes medicine for you is a doctor.
The lady who goes to court to try cases is a policeman.
The lady who plans the building of a bridge is an engineer.

Deciding whether the following sentences make sense:

The baby screamed.
The kettle is on top of the burner.
The hot soup is in the refrigerator.
The porch is inside the house.
The rug is on the floor.

Identifying objects inside the room from descriptions:

"I am thinking of something in this room. It is round; it is red. We can eat it. What is it?"

Identifying objects outside the room from descriptions:

"I am thinking of something that goes high into the sky.
The man in it gives us traffic reports in the morning.
It can go from one airport to another. It can land on top of a building or in a field. What is it?

CATEGORIZATION

1. Providing pictures of four green hats and one red hat. The children put those together that belong with each other.
2. Providing pictures of four hats and four caps. The children again sort these into the two proper categories.

3. Providing pictures of cans of fruit, fresh fruit, cans of vegetables, and fresh vegetables. Again the children sort these into the proper categories.
4. Tell me which one in each of the following does not belong:

   cat, tiger, lion, goldfish.
   peaches, pears, squash, apples.
   oaks, elms, daisies, poplars.
   refrigerator, bed, kitchen stove, dishwasher.

MORPHOLOGICAL AND CONCEPT FILL-INS

Here is one pencil. Here are two_____.
Ice cream tastes _____ than oatmeal.
Ice cream with chocolate sauce and nuts tastes _____ of all.
The Empire State Building (or whatever building is the biggest or tallest) is the _____ building in our town.
Today for lunch, I am eating a hot dog. Yesterday for lunch I _____ spaghetti. Tomorrow I _____ hamburgers.

AUDITORY PERCEPTION PROCESSES

Rhyming games:

Which word does goat rhyme with: cat, seek, coat?
"I am thinking of something white that falls from the sky in the winter. It rhymes with *blow*. What is it?

VISUAL PERCEPTION PROCESSES

1. Showing a picture with many boats. The children find all the boats.
2. Drawing on the board a house but leaving off one wall. Ask the child to finish the picture.
3. Cutting several pictures in half. Have the children match the halves accurately.
4. Dividing a series of pictures of people into halves. The children match the halves.
5. Using some of the simple jigsaw puzzles. The children put them together.
6. Using pipe cleaners, make a man but leave one leg off. The child puts the leg on.
7. Using children's literature that shows various shapes clearly and identifies the shapes—

T. Hoban, *Circles, Triangles, and Squares* (New York: Macmillan Publishing Co., Inc., 1974). This book shows shapes common to children's experiences, such as bubbles, signs, playground equipment, eyeglasses, and cookies.

VISUAL MEMORY

1. Making colored chains from paper with the colors in a certain order.
2. Patterning different kinds of beads in the same order.
3. Making up a story about a series of pictures. The children then arrange the pictures in the right order.
4. Making designs from pipe cleaners. Have the children imitate them.
5. Using flannel board patterns. For example, the children arrange a series of pictures depicting a snow storm in the right order: the snow falling, the men shoveling the snow, the snow melting.
6. Cutting various shapes as circle, triangle, and rectangle from different bits of colored paper. Have the children arrange them in the same order as you have. The teacher or clinician will need to use larger shapes for the demonstration—showing them and then removing them.

AUDITORY MEMORY

Dramatic Situations:

A child is sick. After the doctor arrives, the mother must go to the store for aspirin, cold medicine, juices, and ice cream. The mother has to remember all these items and return with them.

Planning on going on a trip. The children are going to Alaska. They pack all their warm clothes: underwear, woolen shirts, socks and sweaters, leather mittens, heavy coats, and boots. They repeat all they are to take, perhaps adding more.

Using stories as a base:

The teacher shows the pictures in such a book as the following: A. Ingle, *The Big City Book* (New York: Platt Munk, 1975). These pictures contain items that belong in schools, television stations, subways, parks, airports, and the like. The teacher enumerates the items, and the children talk about their functions. The children then recall the items in the various spots.

The teacher reads a story with a very definite series of actions. The children then enumerate the actions.

The teacher reads a story with a definite number of persons with different occupations. The children then enumerate the occupations.

Children repeat simple stories such as "The Three Bears."

Finger plays, repitition of.

Nursery rhymes, repitition of.

Children bring their telephone numbers to school and learn the number of two of their classmates. They then pretend to call them on the telephone.

MANUAL AND VERBAL EXPRESSION

Pantomiming Activities:

1. Pantomiming nursery rhymes such as "Humpty Dumpty" and "Little Miss Muffet."
2. Pantomiming such activities as looking for a cat, bouncing a ball, catching a ball, vacuuming the floor, peeling potatoes, beating an egg, eating meat, eating spaghetti, drinking milk, picking flowers, playing a piano or violin.
3. Pantomiming in pairs: looking for a lost ring, rowing in a boat, walking on a very icy street, walking in mud, going through the woods at night when it is very dark, shopping in a store that is very crowded.
4. Pantomiming in groups:

   A fussy old lady, a bashful person, and a big bully being waited on by a brash waiter or waitress in a restaurant.

   After a bomb has gone off at an airport, one relative is looking for two others. They all finally find each other and are very happy.

Adding Verbalization:

1. Pretending to represent certain occupations: cook, bus driver, lawyer, doctor, policeman, policewoman, painter, carpenter, schoolteacher.
2. Dramatizing nursery rhymes as "Mistress Mary" or "Wee Willie Winkie."
3. Dramatizing stories.

4. Making up stories based on some of the children's experiences such as a visit to the supermarket, to the firehouse, or to the post office, or going on a boat ride or a train ride. Or stories may be based on two words such as *ugly* and *beautiful*, or a set of objects.
5. Discussion based on such problems as:
   a. Let us suppose that you saw one of your classmates hide a barometer that you had been using in your science exhibition in his locker. He really loves that barometer. What would you do?
   b. Your cousin, from another town, arrives who is very, very bright and very, very beautiful. She draws attention to her high grades, her ability to write poetry, and her good looks. What would you do in this kind of situation?

Piaget's Contribution to Cognitive Development

Many language arts teachers recently have come to regard the contributions of Piaget as being exceedingly helpful in planning for the cognitive development of children. Piaget is a developmental psychologist who was concerned with changes in cognitive functioning from birth through adolescence. Unlike Skinner, Piaget does not conceptualize behavior in terms of stimuli, responses, and reinforcement. Rather he describes children's behavior by asking them questions, noting their responses, and carefully and in detail observing their verbal behavior at different stages of their lives. Piaget designed his approach to discover the nature and level of development of the concepts that children use and not to produce developmental scales (Wadsworth 1971, p. 5). Because of the influence of his training in biology, Piaget views cognitive behavior as acts of organization and adaptation to the environment.

Piaget believes that the child controls the procuring and organizing of experiences in his own environment. For instance, babies follow with their eyes, explore with their hands, hold crackers and throw them. Such activities provide the base for absorbing and organizing experiences. This process, which Piaget calls *assimilation*, is fundamental to learning throughout life. It is, however, modified by *accommodation*, which steers children into adaptation to the world by resisting some patterns and by bringing in new results, which, in turn, enrich the patterns. A child's learning might be likened to a data-processing operation wherein the child feeds the data that is relevant into the machine and rejects that which is not relevant. The results of this operation represent learning. Piaget's hypothesis is that cognitive development is a coherent process of successive qualitative changes of cognitive structures with each structure and its concomitant changes deriving logically and inevitably from the preceding one (Wadsworth 1973, p. 25).

Piaget's Building Stages

STAGE 1. FIRST TWO YEARS: SENSORIMOTOR PERIOD

The earliest behavior shows no sense of persisting objects or of space or time concepts. But presently, the behavior changes and each month it takes into account more features of the world. At birth, children possess innate reflexes only, but gradually they begin to explore objects in their environment, watching the parts of the mobile move, holding a teddy bear, shaking the rattle. They discover, as a result of their interaction with their environment, that the world is a succession of objects with permanence in its surroundings. They discover tools for eating although they may try to use their rattles for this purpose. They find out that movements in specific directions carried out at specific times lead to the same results; for example, they hold out their arms and they are lifted. They learn to use words as symbols. By two years of age, the child invents new patterns of behavior, using words, actions, and symbolic play with and without words.

STAGE 2. TWO TO FOUR YEARS. PRECONCEPTUAL THOUGHT

At this stage, children really explore their world—walking, touching, pulling, investigating everything they can reach. They climb on top of things, get below them, touch them, manipulate them. They imitate adults—running the vacuum cleaner like Mommy or hitting a nail like big brother. Words begin to symbolize images although a single symbol, in the early part of this stage, may carry many meanings: /bʊ/ for book may mean, "Read to me," "Give it to me." or "Put it away." Slowly words not only accompany actions but represent something. At this stage the child is basically egocentric and he may play by himself putting his dolly to bed and saying, "Put baby to bed." Recently when a ball (on a string) in the form of a music box was pulled down, and "Silent Night, Holy Night" was produced, the three-and-a-half-year-old said, "Christmas," and then "What is it?" (He had begun to classify.) Whereupon he pulled the ball down to hear the music. But the precocious five-and-a-half-year-old said, "It's a music box with a mechanism inside. The pull triggered the music." And then, "Can you get inside it?" This second child belonged in the next stage.

STAGE 3. FOUR TO EIGHT YEARS. INTUITIVE THOUGHT

This boy related the sound heard to the sound in the music box in his own home. He would have liked to get inside it to see how it worked. At this stage, children are busy with what they see around them and what is happening around them. They really put things together— comparing and contrasting. The example given at the beginning of this chapter exemplifies this stage. The child listed a series of analogies until she arrived at "puppy cat." As children begin to categorize, they begin to think. Children at this age should be given opportunities to experiment with a variety of objects and should take part in many happenings such as trips, creative drama, puppet plays, and science experiments such as planting seeds and watching them grow.

STAGE 4. EIGHT TO 11 YEARS. CONCRETE OPERATIONS

At this stage, children increase their logical thought processes. They think in concrete terms and must be given many opportunities to practice this concrete thinking. On reading about a fire in Chicago, they ask and answer, "What started the fire?" They answer the question, "How high is the Trade Center Building?" in terms of the number of stories, which answer is concrete and clear. They may talk about, if they live in Manhattan, "How far away is Times Square?" And then, "How far away is California?" They can understand concepts about lengths, numbers, speed, and sizes. At this stage, teachers give their students many opportunities to reason in concrete terms; *because, although,* and *if* are heard frequently.

STAGE 5. 11 YEARS ON. FORMAL OPERATIONS

This stage is particularly important because here children attain the power of abstract thought. They operate freely with their own imagined possibilities and hypotheses. They can abstract, manipulate ideas about ideas, examine relationships. They set up miniature research studies and carry through their investigations.

From these stages, we can deduce that Piaget does not believe in separating language and cognition. After all, he entitled his book about language, *The Language and Thought of the Child*. We must remember that Piaget did not intend that these stages represent norms; therefore, the ages given are approximate and can vary as much as two years.

Many classroom activities and experiences are available for the various stages. We believe that it is important to introduce children to literature early and consistently. With this bias, we are, therefore, including activities that are largely based on children's literature for the various stages.

Language Arts Activities for the Various Stages

STAGE 3. INTUITIVE THOUGHT (THIS STAGE SHOULD PROVIDE A WEALTH OF EXPERIENCES INVOLVING EVERYDAY HAPPENINGS).

CONCEPT—NUMBERS.

Book—J. J. Reiss, *Numbers*, Scarsdale, N.Y.: Bradbury Press, 1971. This book helps children to count five arms on a starfish, seven segments on a horse chestnut leaf, and 100 legs on a centipede. It can be used to capture an interest in numbers and in counting.

CONCEPT—DIFFERENCES BETWEEN WINTER AND SUMMER

Books: E. Schick, *City in the Winter* (New York: Macmillan Publishing Co. Inc., 1970). E. Schick, *City in the Summer* (New York: Macmillan Publishing Co. Inc., 1960). These books can serve as a basis for a discussion on how the city in the winter differs from the city in the summer. For example, in *City in the Winter*, Jimmy wakes up to find the world is very white. He and his grandmother explore what the snow has caused—bootprints, buried sidewalks, and a closed store. The teacher may then say, "But suppose that Jimmy woke up on a very, very hot day in the summer. What would Jimmy and his grandmother have found then?" Clues can be found in *City in the Summer*. The teacher may go on to explore many differences between winter and summer: play activities, clothes worn, foods eaten, and trips taken.

CONCEPT—ROLES OF MOTHERS

Books: W. Wiesner, *Turnabout* (New York: Seabury Press, 1972). J. Lasher, *Mothers Can Do Anything* (Racine, Wis.: Whitman Publishing Company, 1972). The Wiesner book is a Norwegian tale in which the farmer and his wife change roles for a day. While the wife calmly rakes the hay, the farmer breaks the eggs, lets the cider run out of the keg, spoils the porridge, nearly kills the cow and gets stuck halfway up the chimney.

The Lasher book contains a series of pictures showing mothers on jobs that are fundamentally different from the traditional women's jobs: policewoman, taxi driver, painter, judge, ditch digger, architect, dentist, plumber, cook, archeologist, and astronaut.

These books can serve as the base for a variety of activities: playing the role of mother as the children themselves see the role, playing the roles as suggested in either of the two books; discussing the roles of mothers in their own neighborhood; writing a poem about the roles of mothers.

CONCEPT—THE FIVE SENSES

Books: Aliki, *My Five Senses* (New York: Thomas Y. Crowell Company, 1962). This book points to the functions of the five senses and shows that a combination of senses can be involved in any perception.

P. Showers, *The Listening Walk* (New York: Thomas Y. Crowell Company, 1961). This is the story of a boy who goes walking with his father; they don't talk but just listen to all the sounds around them.

Reading these two books can serve as the initial step in classroom work involving all the senses. From this vantage point, children can talk about the sounds they normally hear: the screeching of tires, the banging of doors, and the wind whistling. Or they may talk about kitchen sounds: the kettle whistling, the coffee pot going "ploppety plop, plop," the toaster going "zing," the dishes clattering, the pans banging, the bell going "brrrrr." Next they may consider smells: smells in the winter, in the summer, in the spring, what smells warn of danger; what smell is the best of all smells; what smell is the worst of all smells. And they can then attack the other senses. This work makes children aware of the world around them and, incidentally, increases their vocabulary. They may well learn new words such as *prickly, sticky, tangy*, or for some the difference between *hard* and *soft*.

CONCEPT—SIBLING RIVALRY

Stegmaier (1974) in an article "Teaching Interpersonal Communication Through Children's Literature" shows how children's literature can provide a vehicle for teaching about conflict between siblings. She suggests two books for this purpose: Ezra Jack Keats's *Peter's Chair* (New York: Harper & Row, Publishers, Inc., 1967) and Russell Hoban's *A Baby Sister for Frances* (New York: Harper & Row, Publishers, Inc., 1964). Another more recent book is Eloise Greenfield's *She Came Bringing That Little Baby Girl* (Philadelphia: J. B. Lippincott Co., 1974). In this book Kevin wanted a baby brother but "she came bringing me that little girl wrapped all up in a pink blanket." Kevin is disappointed and annoyed as he sees relatives and neighbors fussing over a wee, wrinkled baby with tiny hands and feet. From a discussion of the concepts in these books, children recognize that natural rivalries do exist in such situations.

STAGE 4. CONCRETE OPERATIONS (THIS STAGE SHOULD INVOLVE MANY CONCRETE PROBLEM-SOLVING ACTIVITIES.)

Problem: Inability to cope with a new school environment with such problems as making new friends.

> Genevieve Gray, *Sore Loser* (Boston: Houghton Mifflin Company, 1974). (This book tells about Loren who cannot seem to do anything right in his new sixth-grade class. He has trouble adjusting to the school and in making friends. The plot is revealed through letters written by Loren and by his mother, notes to the school principal from his teacher, school bulletins, and essays by students.)
> A number of ways can be used to help solve this problem:
> 1. Playing the story as it is written and then replaying it as it could have been written, adding scenes and changing scenes.
> 2. Discussing Loren's problem and possible solutions to it.
> 3. Asking a counselor in the school to come in to give his viewpoints on the problem.

CONCEPT—NUMBERS

> Book: S. Shapman, *Numbers, How Many? How Much?* (Chicago: Follett Publishing Company, 1972).
> This book contains 14 amusing arithmetic problems involving addition, subtraction, multiplication, and division. Objects in the problems include squishy grasshoppers, mud pies, basketballs, crocodiles, and kissing relatives.
> This book can be used as reinforcement of many of the mathematical concepts and, at the same time, sections of it can be the basis for amusing creative drama.

STAGE 5. PROPOSITIONAL OR FORMAL LOGIC. (AT THIS STAGE TEACHERS SHOULD BE ENCOURAGING ABSTRACTIONS, RESEARCH ABILITIES, AND PROBLEMS THAT INVOLVE EITHER INDUCTION OR DEDUCTION.)

Two examples are given for this stage. The first involved a study of the Erie Canal undertaken by 13- and 14-year-olds. The second, involving a study of literature having to do with *pride*, was undertaken by 15- and 16-year-olds in a drama class in Jamaica High School, Jamaica, New York.

Teachers at both the elementary and high school levels frequently plan their work with their students. As the work of the unit progresses, many speech activities take place. Children give talks, report, discuss, debate, interview, read aloud, and dramatize.

For example, children in an eighth grade were studying the early history of New York State. While studying this era, one 12-year-old, reporting on his trip across New York State on the Thruway, compared the Thruway to the Erie Canal. The report of this trip motivated members of the class to study the building of the canal. The writer of their social studies text explained the reasons for the building of the canal and its values to the country, but the children wanted more information than their text contained. They discussed what more they would like to know about the Erie Canal. Specifically they wanted answers to the following:

- What were the factors that made a canal seem advisable?
- Who decided a canal was necessary?
- Why was Van Buren opposed to it?
- Why did Clinton approve the building of the canal?
- What were the times like in the early 1800s?
- What kind of clothes did people wear then?
- What did they do for entertainment?
- How did they live?
- What did they do for a living?
- How was the building of the canal planned?
- What was the route of the canal?
- What were some of the difficulties encountered in building the canal?
- Who built the canal?
- What was its opening like?
- What were the effects of its opening?

After they had listed these questions on the blackboard, they broke up into groups to decide how to do their research and how to report on their findings. The project demanded oral communication in its planning and in its execution.

Throughout this activity, groups frequently gave progress reports. As the children read, they found other items that they thought should be included. Finally, individuals and groups of individuals reported on what they had read. One boy gave an account of the way people talked in the 1800s. This item was not included originally, but he and the members of his group felt it added to their understanding of the period. "Oh, go sandpaper your nose" became one of the favorite expressions of the group. Another panel of students gave a very interesting discussion of the songs sung during this era. Through such activities children learn to participate in discussion.

The teacher helped these children in a number of ways to prepare and give reports. He reminded them of the necessity of gaining and holding the interest of their listeners. He suggested ways and means of collecting material and of organizing it. He stressed their having a thorough knowledge of their topic, a real interest in it themselves, and a desire to communicate this interest to their listeners.

The teacher also taught them to be more successful participants in a discussion group. He taught them how to state a problem, analyze it, and examine its solutions. The children learned that they must have a basis for the choice of a particular solution. Although these children had already learned to be fairly effective members of a discussion group, the teacher reinforced their learning. Frequently he stressed that they must have knowledge and background before speaking. Because the discussion sometimes went off on a tangent, he emphasized that they must keep it relevant. He helped the students to consider all points of view, participate well, and listen carefully. He encouraged each boy and girl to be a responsible member of the group.

In this work on the Erie Canal the students found it necessary to read aloud from various sources. One boy read the speech made by DeWitt Clinton at the opening of the canal. The teacher helped him to prepare this speech for reading aloud by making sure he understood the material both intellectually and emotionally. As the boy mentioned bringing together the waters of the Hudson River and Lake Erie, his classmates felt pride in his voice. Because he knew the background so well, he needed almost no help in preparing his material to read aloud.

Finally, as a culminating activity, the class wrote and produced a play that depicted the struggle to build the canal. The play included a chorus of singers who sang about the Erie Canal and a choral-speaking group who, dressed in overalls, carrying shovels, and pushing wheelbarrows, spoke, "We are digging the ditch through the mire." The play, quite elaborately staged and executed, ran for three nights.

A drama class taught by Mrs. Kirchman, formerly of Jamaica High School, Queens, studied the various concepts of *pride* as portrayed in a variety of plays. The following is the first page of a booklet that was the end result of the study.

Dear Students,

The word *pride* has been bandied about and used so loosely that we may have forgotten what we mean by it. I thought you would enjoy thinking about the layers of meaning covering the bare bones of the word. After discussing the connotations of the word, via dictionaries, quotations, and illustrations from drama, we were asked to dissect *pride* in a brief composition, poem, or sketch.

We selected fragments from your written work in an effort to explore the anatomy of *pride*. You may like having a copy of this class assignment, written by your classmates.

With proud shades of Antigone, Dr. Stockman, Masha, Kurt Muller, Annie Sullivan, Cyrano, St. Joan, and all the other people we've touched through plays,

> Yours,
> Rose Kirchman

> People are isolated
> By walls of their own making.
> They cannot help each other
> Or tell their problems honestly.
> Shame and false pride
> Lock the doors to understanding.
> While trying to help a friend
> They judge him, but say nothing;
> Their opinions are shadowed in silence.
> Guilt and fear combine and mix.
> They will never remove their facades.
> Being disapproved of is a large enough threat;
> Crying comes later,
> Behind a closed door.
>
> Patricia Truscelli

I sold out to the enemy at Berlin
I begged to go home in a box
But the punishment redeemed me—I died clear-conscienced and with pride
As I plunged head first to the rocks.

I no longer worry about the Proud
Who nurture the cancer in their mind.
I owe Pride nothing—I already gave.
I died for the false star,
My Pride.

Les Cohen

The study of the Erie Canal involved many opportunities for reasoning. For example, the boys and girls talked about the evidence used to prove the feasibility of the canal. They discussed how leaders can put across even unpopular ideas. They were also able to look at progress over several decades—first, the stagecoach; then, the canal; then, the railroads; and finally, airplanes. They projected into the future. What could possibly be available in another 20 years—space ships? They analyzed the attitudes of reactionaries in Clinton's day and made analogies with the attitudes of today's reactionaries.

The high school drama group explored the concepts that can be attached to the word *pride*. They enlarged their horizons both from a cognitive and affective standpoint. They assumed a mental set for the abstractions of what pride can be. They shifted from one concept to another all within the rubric of *pride*. They grasped a variety of concepts having to do with *pride* and put these abstractions into writing.

Following the general philosophy of Piaget, we believe that the classroom teacher helps the child to develop thought processes and appropriate language for logical thinking. This development means that children use language to meet cognitive demands, to compare, to contrast, to draw inferences, to see cause and effect relationships, to take things apart and put them together, to talk about things and events that are present or absent. When the classroom teacher promotes such activities, boys and girls will continue in their language development through high school.

Reading and Speaking

We believe that children must learn to speak and to listen before they learn to read; reading depends upon these two linguistic activities. Involved in these linguistic activities are all four aspects of language: semantic, phonological, morphological, and syntactical.

Most writers today note that many reading skills are present in the oral language of young children; and, as they read, they draw on their previous linguistic knowledge. The children must recognize printed words and their various forms as ones they already know. They must be able to understand how words are strung together to make sentences. They, therefore, need to know the rules of the spoken language before they begin to read. Reading is a language-oriented skill, deliberately taught and learned, which is dependent upon the child's linguistic abilities both as a speaker and listener (see Anastaslow 1971; Wilkinson 1971; Ruddell 1970; and Mattingly 1972).

Investigators who have done research on children with reading disabilities point to the co-occurrence of language difficulties—usually in the areas of oral expression and listening comprehension. For example, Bruininks, Lockes, and Gropper (1970) in comparing the psycholinguistic abilities of good and poor readers found that the poor readers were inferior to good readers on ITPA subtests that required listening and oral expression. Incidentally, there were no differences on those subtests requiring skills involving visual and motor channels of expression. Kirby, Lyle, and Ambie (1972) found that problem readers did not do well on the auditory subtests of the ITPA. Wakefield (1973) found that normal readers did better than clinic readers on the digit span section of the WISC and the auditory sequential memory test of the ITPA. Flynn and Byrne (1970) reported that advanced readers did better on auditory discrimination tests and on two blending tests than did normal readers. Semel and Wiig (1975) discovered that elementary school learning-disabled children showed reductions in both the comprehension and expression of syntactic structures. These studies point to inabilities in competence and in the production of language in reading-disabled children.

Content is as important in teaching reading as it is in stimulating language development. Children in the first grade want to hear of the world around them and what goes on in their street, school, and home. Consequently for teachers of first graders to consider teaching to read through language experiences makes sense (see Stauffer, 1970). That teaching through language experiences also takes into account the level of language development of the children involved is noteworthy. Second and third graders become interested in fairy stories and in funny animals that talk. Those in the middle grades like factual material; later, enthusiasm develops for adventure, travel, biography, and invention. All children enjoy material that is graphic, dramatic, and active. Furthermore, they like to read of human experiences with which they are at least partially familiar.

Having indicated that we believe reading is language based but a somewhat different activity from speaking and that content plays an important role in motivation to learn to read, we now examine some of the relationships of reading and speaking as pointed out by Gibson (1972) and Mattingly (1972):

Relationship Between Speaking and Reading

Gibson (1972) points to the similarities between hearing-speaking and reading-writing. She notes that there exist similarities in the phonological system of hearing-speaking and the graphological system of reading-writing, in the semantic systems of both, and in the syntactic rule structure of both. Further relationships probably exist in the two areas in independence, transfer, and mapping rules.

Gibson draws a parallel between the phonological system and the graphological system: She notes that productive speech begins with babbling (although disagreement does exist as to the role of babbling in speech acquisition) and that graphic production begins with scribbling. In both instances, feedback (one auditory, one visual) provides an opportunity to learn by self-regulation. She quotes Lavine's Cornell University doctoral dissertation (1972) to the effect that the categorical features of writing—a set of distinctive features, recombination of elements, and repetitive regularity—are learned quite early as shown by the child's ability to distinguish samples of writing from other marks on the paper. Gibson also points out that as hearing-speaking has a phonological rule system, so has reading-writing an orthographic system. But she does emphasize that although there may be transfer of learning, the letter is not mapped by the sound and that the nature of the relationship is not simple but complex.

Discussing the semantic relationship, Gibson stresses that spoken words are symbols for real events, things, and ideas, and that written words are but symbols for spoken words. However, she stresses that reading for meaning does not always come easily.

Gibson believes that the syntactic aspects are easier to compare— that rules of grammar are the same for spoken and for written language. A knowledge of syntactic structure in both instances must be picked up to process units that communicate meaning. She notes that how the child does this for reading is not known and that the clues to syntax in both instances are comparable but not identical.

Mattingly (1972) in comparing reading and listening notes that the usual view is that the processes are parallel and summarizes this viewpoint: "... written text is input by eye and speech by ear, but at as early a stage as possible, consistent with this difference in modality, the two inputs have a common internal representation. From this stage onward, the two processes are identical." Mattingly further notes that even with the recent view of speech perception with a different model of linguistic processing wherein the process is active and similar to production, the assumption of a parallel between reading and listening remains.

Mattingly then points out differences between listening and reading: (1) Listening is a more natural way of perceiving language. Listening is easy, and reading is hard although listening is not a more efficient process in all respects. (2) Listening is slower. (3) The manner in which information is presented is basically different in reading and listening. The listener is processing a flow of complex acoustic signals and while listening has to separate the cues from irrelevant detail. Cues are not discrete events but tend to blend into one another. On the other hand, the reader is processing a series of symbols that are quite simply related to the physical medium that conveys them. Readers can see the letters if they want to, for, in writing, a string of separate symbols are connected for practical convenience. Speech signals cannot be viewed in this way.

Mattingly concludes that reading is a language-based skill, that it is parasitic on language. Reading in the visual mode is not a parallel activity to speech perception in the auditory mode; differences cannot be explained by differences of modality. Reading is rather a deliberately acquired language-based skill that is dependent upon the speaker-hearer's awareness of certain aspects of primary linguistic activity.

That more research needs to be done to ascertain how speaking, listening, and reading are related is clear. In the meantime, we develop strategies for both language competence and performance for both the speech communication specialist and the reading specialist.

Stark (1975) summarizes the role of the speech and language clinician in this area:

> ...we believe that there is a significant amount of evidence to indicate that speech and language pathologists can make a very important contribution to the prevention and treatment of reading problems. Assisting parents, teachers, and other specialists by providing information about the nature of language acquisition and training children in linguistic processing may produce highly desirable results. At the least, speech and hearing clinicians may be able to modify currently used teaching techniques and materials so that teachers can more effectively understand the role that language development plays in reading
>
> (Stark 1975, p. 834).

In summary, we subscribe to the theory that normal language acquisition involves a set of skills that develop in a more or less parallel fashion with each skill being possibly related to another, and possibly to some still undesignated language ability that increases with maturity. Sometimes a particular skill may be slow to develop but is still within normal range. In other cases, some of the skills do not develop, and these underdeveloped skills may well interfere with many of the other skills. The clinician intervenes to help the child develop particular language skills, whereas teachers plan to develop all the skills. As language develops, thinking and the ability to attack more complex, cognitive problems develop. Reading is a language-based activity and, consequently, as language skills are built so is a basis for reading. There is a time for language readiness as well as for reading readiness.

Problems

1. Visit a classroom in an elementary school or in a high school. List the activities that went on in the classroom that would stimulate language development. Describe each activity in one sentence.

2. Find five pieces of children's literature and indicate (a) how a clinician would use each piece for language intervention—that is, developing strategies for accelerating specific language abilities; (b) and how a classroom teacher would use each piece of literature for stimulating language development.
3. Visit a nursery school and a third-grade class. Indicate, in general, the differences in vocabulary, sytax, and articulation.
4. Watch "Sesame Street" or "The Electric Company" programs. Indicate the language abilities being stimulated and the strategies used to stimulate them.
5. Try any of the exercises listed for developing language abilities with two kindergarten children. Report on your progress.
6. List and describe one or two language activities for Piaget's stages 3, 4, and 5. Justify your choice.
7. Read and report on one of the following: Aram and Nation 1975; Beving and Eblen 1973; Calder and Angan 1970; Carter 1974; Doyle 1971; Meyer and Shane 1973; Pertz 1971: Semel and Wiig 1975.

References and Suggested Readings

Anastaslow, N., *Oral Language: Expression of Thought*, Newark, Del.: International Reading Association, 1971.

Aram, D. M., and J. E. Nation, "Patterns of Language Behavior in Children with Developmental Language Disorders," *Journal of Speech and Hearing Research*, **18** (June 1975), 229–240. (Classifies children with similar patterns of language based on their ability to comprehend, formulate, and repeat specified phonologic, syntactic, and semantic aspects of language.)

Ball, S., and G. A. Bogatz, "The First Year of Sesame Street: An Evaluation," *Today's Education* (National Education Association Journal), **60** (March 1971), 72.

Baratz, J. C., "A Bi-Dialectal Task for Determining Language Proficiency in Economically Disadvantaged Negro Children," *Child Development*, **40** (September 1969), 889–901. (Compares the language behavior of standard and nonstandard speakers when repeating standard or nonstandard sentences. Concludes that the major difficulty for black children is one of "code-switching" rather than language deficiency.)

——, "Language and Cognitive Assessment of Negro Children: Assumptions and Research Needs, *ASHA*, **11** (March 1969), 87–91.

——, and R. W. Shuy, *Teaching Black Children to Read*, Washington, D.C.: Center for Applied Linguistics, 1969. (Supports the concept that grammatical differences between a black child's dialect and standard English interfere with the child's learning to read.)

Betts, E. A., "Reading: Linguistic Guide Lines," *Elementary English*, **51** (September 1974), 829–831.

Beving, B., and R. E. Eblen, "'Same' and 'Different' Concepts and Children's Performance on Speech Sound Discrimination," *Journal of Speech and Hearing Research*, **16** (September 1973), 513–517.

Blumberg, H. M., *A Program of Sequential Language Development*, Springfield, Ill.: Charles C Thomas, Publisher, 1975.

Bloom, L., "Why Not Pivot Grammar?" *Journal of Speech and Hearing Disorders*, **36** (February 1971), 40–50.

Bright, H. M., "Boehm Test of Basic Concepts—A New Tool for Assessing Language Development," *Language Speech and Hearing Services in the Schools*, **4** (July 1973), 140–141.

Bruininks, R. H., W. G. Lockes, and R. L. Gropper, "Psycholinguistic Abilities of Good and Poor Reading Disadvantaged First-Graders," *The Elementary School Journal*, **70** (April 1970), 378–388.

Burns, G. W., and B. L. Watson, "Factor Analysis of the Revised ITPA with Underachieving Children," *Journal of Learning Disabilities*, **6** (June–July 1973), 36–41.

Bush, W. C., and M. T. Giles, *Aids to Psycholinguistic Teaching*, Columbus, Ohio: Charles E. Merrill Publishing Co., 1969.

Calder, C. R., Jr., and E. M. Angan, *Techniques and Activities to Stimulate Verbal Learning*, New York: Macmillan Publishing Co., Inc., 1970.

Carlson, R. K., "Raising Self-Concepts of Disadvantaged Children Through Puppetry," *Elementary English*, **47** (March 1970), 349–355. (Discusses the use of puppetry as a means of enhancing the children's learning experiences. Lists the kinds of puppetry used.)

Carroll, J. B., *Language and Thought*, Englewood Cliffs, N.J.: Prentice-Hall Inc., 1964.

Carrow, E., "A Test Using Elicited Imitations in Assessing Grammatical Structure in Children," *Journal of Speech and Hearing Disorders*, **39** (November 1974), 437–444. (Describes a test of grammatical categories: articles, adjectives, nouns, pronouns, demonstratives, conjunctions, verbs, negatives, contractions, prepositions, and adverbs.)

Carter, T., "Creative Dramatics for Learning-Disabled Children," *Academic Therapy*, **9** (Summer 1974), 411–417.

Cazden, C., "The Neglected Situation in Child Language and Education," in F. Williams, ed., *Language and Poverty*, Chicago: Markham Publishing Co., 1970. (Lists the aspects of speech situations that affect test scores.)

Chapman, R.S., and J. F. Miller, "Word Order in Early Two and Three Word Utterances. Does Production Precede Comprehension?" *Journal of Speech and Hearing Research*, **18** (June 1975), 355–371. (Supports the view that children's use of word-order information as a cue to subject and object status is limited and acquired late, in contrast to the observance of subject-object word order in their speech.)

Chappell, G. E., "Language Disabilities and the Language Clinician," *Journal of Learning Disabilities*, **5** (December 1972), 611–619. (Indicates where the language performance may break down.)

Chomsky, C., *The Acquisition of Syntax in Children from Five to Ten*, Cambridge, Mass.: The M.I.T. Press, 1969. (Ascertains children's competence in four grammatical structures.)

Cicirelli, V. G., "A Note on the Factor Analysis of Disadvantaged Children: Illinois Test of Psycholinguistic Abilities and Achievement Test Scores," *Journal of Experimental Education*, **41** (Fall 1972), 5–8.

———, B. Granger et al., "Performance of Disadvantaged Children in Revised ITPA," *Psychology in Schools*, **8** (July 1971), 240–246.

Clark, C. M., and B. E. Dodd, "Auditory Factors in Visual Motor Testing and Training," *Journal of Learning Disabilities*, **4** (1971), 582.

Cohen, S. A., and G. S. Kornfield, "Oral Vocabulary and Beginning Reading in Disadvantaged Black Children," *Reading Teacher*, **24** (October 1970), 33–38.

Critchlow, D. E., *Dos Amigos Verbal Language Scales*, San Rafael, Calif.: Academic Therapy Publications, 1974. (Measures the bilingual child's comparative English-speaking language development. Designed to measure the child's level to function in both English and Spanish in such areas as likenesses, differences, and analogies.)

Cronkhite, G., and K. Penner, "A Reconceptualization and Revised Scoring Procedures for the ITPA Based on Multivariate Analysis of the Original Normative Data," *Journal of Speech and Hearing Research*, **18** (September 1975), 506–520.

Doyle, M., "A Review of Three Significant Compensatory Education Language Programs for the Culturally Disadvantaged," *Elementary English*, **48** (February 1971), 193–197. (Shows how programs attempted to give children the verbal sophistication necessary to meet the requirements of the school.)

Duke, C., "Creative Dramatics and English Teaching," Urbana, Ill.: National Council of Teachers of English, 1974.

Dunn, L. M., and J. O. Smith, *Peabody Language Development Kits*, Circle Pines, Minn.: American Guidance Service.

Engler, L. F., E. P. Hannah, and T. M. Longhurst, "Linguistic Analysis of Speech Samples," *Journal of Speech and Hearing Disorders*, **38** (May 1973), 192–204. (Shows the way to contrast a child's speech with that of an adult or other children his own age or development. Tells how to elicit and record the sample.)

Fennimore, F., "Choral Reading as a Spontaneous Experience," *Elementary English*, **48** (November 1971), 870–885. (Describes an informal approach to choral speaking based on the children's own language.)

Fluharty, N. B., "The Design and Standardization of a Speech and Language Screening Test for Use with Preschool Children," *Journal of Speech and Hearing Disorders*, **39** (February 1974), 75–86.

Flynn, P. T., and M. C. Byrne, "Relationship Between Reading and Selected Auditory Abilities of Third-Grade Children," *Journal of Speech and Hearing Research*, **13** (December 1970), 731–740. (Tests for significant differences between advanced and retarded readers on auditory tasks.)

Follman, J. A., and A. J. Lowe, "Empirical Examination of Critical Reading and Critical Thinking: Overview," *Journal of Reading Behavior*, **5** (Summer 1972–1973), 304–316. (Summarizes the results of a research program of two parallel series of fifth and twelfth grade analyses of critical reading, critical thinking, and reading and scholastic achievement scores.)

Foster, C. R., J. J. Giddan, and J. Stark, *Assessment of Children's Language Comprehension*, Palo Alto, Calif.: Consulting Psychologists Press, 1969.

Frentz, T., "Children's Comprehension of Standard and Negro Nonstandard English Sentences," *Speech Monographs*, **38** (March 1971), 10–16.

Foulke, P. N., "How Early Should Language Development and Pre-Reading Experience be Started?" *Elementary English*, **51** (1974), 310–315.

Gibson, E. J., "Reading for Some Purpose," in J. J. Kavanagh and I. G. Mattingly, *Language by Ear and by Eye*, Cambridge, Mass.: The M.I.T. Press, 1972, 3–17.

Goldizer, B. F., *Primer for Perception. How to Help Children Learn to Learn*, Johnston, Pa.: Mafey Associates, 1971.

Goodman, K. S., "Effective Teachers of Reading Know Language and Children," *Elementary English*, **51** (September 1974), 823–831.

Gruenewald, L. J., and S. A. Pollak, "The Speech Clinician's Role in Auditory Learning: Reading Readiness," *Language Speech and Hearing Services in Schools*, **4** (July 1973), 120–126. (Lists auditory activities associated with reading. Shows how the speech clinician is involved with the auditory-vocal language of children.)

Hammill, D. E., and S. C. Larsen, "The Relationship of Selected Auditory Perceptual Skills and Reading Ability," *Journal of Learning Disabilities*, **7** (August–September 1974), 429–435.

Hamre, C. E., "The Sesame Street Challenge," *Journal of Learning Disabilities*, **3** (April 1972), 207–209.

Hare, B. A., D. D. Hammill, and N. R. Bartel, "Construct Validity of Selected Subtests of the ITPA," *Exceptional Children*, **40** (September 1973), 13–20.

Herman, D., and S. Ratliffe, *Speech Activities in the Elementary School*, Skokie, Ill., National Textbook Company, 1972.

———, *Speech and Drama in the Intermediate Schools: MSA Curriculum Guide* 2. Skokie, Ill.: National Textbook Company, 1972.

Herron, R., and B. Sutton-Smith, *Child's Play*, New York: John Wiley & Sons, Inc., 1971.

Higginbotham, D. C., "Psycholinguistic Research and Language Learning," *Elementary English*, **49** (October 1972), 811–817. (Reviews language acquisition theory as it has relevance for educational practice.)

Huizinga, R. J., "The Relationship of the ITPA to the Stanford-Binet Form L-M and the WISC," *Journal of Learning Disabilities*, **6** (August–September 1973), 451–456. (Reports on the relationship between the ITPA and two measures of intelligence.)

Irwin, R. B., "Effectiveness of Speech Therapy for Second-Grade Children with Misarticulations: Predictive Factors," *Exceptional Child*, **32** (March 1966), 471–479.

Isaacs, N., *A Brief Introduction to Piaget*, New York: Schocken Books, Inc., 1972.

Kaliski, L., R. Tankersley, and R. Iogha, *Structured Dramatics for Children with Learning Disabilities*, San Rafael, Calif., Academic Therapy Publishing Company, 1971.

Karnes, M. B., *Helping Young Children Develop Language Skills: A Book of Activities*, Washington, D.C.: Council for Exceptional Children, 1968. (Covers a wide range of language abilities.)

Kirby, E. A., W. Lyle, and B. Ambie, "Reading and Psycholinguistic Processes of Innate Problem Readers," *Journal of Learning Disabilities*, **5** (May 1972), 295–298.

Kirk, S. S., J. J. McCarthy, and K. A. Kirk, *Illinois Test of Psycholinguistic Abilities*, rev. ed., Urbana, Ill.: Institute for Research on Exceptional Children, 1969.

Levenstein, P. "Cognitive Growth in Pre-Schoolers Through Verbal Interaction with Mothers," *American Journal of Orthopsychiatry*, **40** (April 1970), 426–432.

Lee, L. L., and S. M. Canter, "Developmental Sentence Scoring: A Clinical Procedure for Estimating Syntactic Development in Children's Spontaneous Speech," *Journal of Speech and Hearing Disorders*, **36** (August 1971), 315–340.

Leonard, L. B., "A Preliminary View of Generalization in Language Training," *Journal of Speech and Hearing Disorders*, **39** (November 1974), 429–436.

————, "What Is Deviant Language?" *Journal of Speech and Hearing Disorders*, **37** (November 1972), 427–446. (Suggests the way to determine clinically significant aspects of syntactical deviations and to distinguish between the slow language developer and the deviant language developer.)

Lodge, D. M., and E. A. Leach, "Children's Acquisition of Idioms in the English Language," *Journal of Speech and Hearing Research*, **18** (September 1975), 521–529. (Shows strong preference for literal meaning in younger children.)

Longhurst, T. M., and T. A. M. Schrandt, "Linguistic Analysis of Children's Speech: A Comparison of Four Procedures," *Journal of Speech and Hearing Disorders*, **38** (May 1973), 240–249.

Luterman, L., and A. Bar, "The Diagnostic Significance of Sentence Repetition for Language Impaired Children," *Journal of Speech and Hearing Disorders*, **36** (February 1971), 29–39.

MacDonald, J. D., and J. P. Blatt, "Environmental Language Intervention: The Rationale for Diagnostic and Training Strategy Through Rules, Context, and Generalization," *Journal of Speech and Hearing Disorders*, **39** (August 1974), 244–256.

Mattingly, I. G., "Reading for Linguistic Process and Linguistic Awareness," in J. J. Kavanagh and I. G. Mattingly, eds., *Language by Ear and by Eye*, Cambridge, Mass.: The M.I.T. Press, 1972, 133–147.

Mecham, M. J., "Enhancing Environments for Children with Cultural-Linguistic Differences," *Language, Speech, and Hearing Services in the Schools*,

6 (July 1975), 156–160. (Proposes the thesis that attitudinal tensions affect relationships between different socioeconomic classes and that such differences may be recognized in dialectal or linguistic characteristics.)

———, "Measurement of Verbal Listening Accuracy in Children," *Journal of Learning Disabilities*, **4** (May 1971), 257–272.

———, J. D. Jones, and J. L. Jex, "Use of the Utah Test of Language Development for Screening Language Disabilities," *Journal of Learning Disabilities*, **6** (October 1973), 524–527.

Menyuk, P., and P. L. Looney, "Relationships among Components of the Grammar," *Journal of Speech and Hearing Research*, **15** (June 1972), 395–406. (Examines the relationship between the accuracy of repetition of syntactic structures and phonological sequences by language-disordered children and the effect of meaning on the phonological sequence repetition accuracy of a group of language-disordered and normal speaking children.)

Meyer, W. J., and J. Shane, "The Form and Function of Children's Questions," *Journal of Genetic Psychology*, **123** (December 1973), 285–296. (Compares the question-asking behavior between two groups of children separated by a span of some three years. In general, the data support Piaget's conceptualizations concerning question-asking behavior.)

Milligan, J. L., and R. E. Potter, "The Peabody Language Development Kit and Its Function in a Language Development and Pre-Reading Program," *Reading World*, **2** (December 1971), 130–136. (Reviews the studies of the values of the Peabody Kit.)

Muma, J. P., "The Communication Game: Dump and Play," *Journal of Speech and Hearing Disorders*, **40** (August 1975), 296–309. (Explains the dump and play operations and the social enterprise of the speaker-listener situation. Dump operations refer to mental processes in preparing and giving a message. Play operations refer to adapting the message (such as changes in semantic or syntactic structure) so that the listener is able to respond to the message.)

———, "Language Assessment: Some Underlying Assumptions," *ASHA*, **15** (July 1973), 331–337. (Contains an excellent bibliography.)

Nolan, P. S., "Reading Nonstandard Dialect Materials: A Study at Grades Two and Four," *Child Development*, **45** (1972), 270–289.

Panagos, J. M., "Persistence of the Open Syllable Reinterpreted as a Symptom of Language Disorder," *Journal of Speech and Hearing Disorders*, **39** (February 1974), 23–31.

Pertz, D. L., "Urban Youth, Nonstandard English and Economic Mobility," *Elementary English*, **48** (December 1971), 1012–1017. (Attacks the problem of whether to teach Standard English to urban youth.)

Piaget, J., (trans. by M. Gabain), *The Language and Thought of the Child*, New York: New American Library, Meridian, 1974.

———, (trans. by Helen Weaver), *Psychology of the Child*, New York: Basic Books, Inc., 1969.

Ramsey, I., "Comparison of First Grade Negro Dialect Speaker's Comprehension of Standard English and Negro Dialect," *Elementary English*, **49** (May 1972), 688–696.

Rees, N. S., "Auditory Processing Factors in Language Disorders: The View from Procrustes' Bed," *Journal of Speech and Hearing Disorders*, **38** (August 1973), 304–315. (Cites the evidence and the lack of it for an auditory perceptual factor in language learning and disorders.)

————, "Bases of Decision in Language Training," *Journal of Speech and Hearing Disorders*, **37** (August 1972), 283–304. (Discusses six theoretical bases for selecting grammatical structures in training language-disordered children. These are viewed as points of reference that suggest possible answers to the language clinician's choice of strategies for training.)

————, "Imitative and Language Development Issues and Clinical Implications," *Journal of Speech and Hearing Disorders*, **40** (August 1975), 339–350.

————, "The Speech Pathologist and the Reading Process," *ASHA*, **16** (May 1974), 255–257. (Talks about the contribution that the speech pathologist can make to the process of reading acquisition both in normal and learning-disabled children.)

Reynell, J., and R. M. C. Huntley, "New Scales for the Assessment of Language Development in Young Children," *Journal of Learning Disabilities*, **4** (October 1971), 549–557.

Rice, J. A., and E. B. Doughtie, "I.Q. and the ITPA: Classification versus Diagnosis," *Journal of Learning Disabilities*, **3** (1970), 471–474.

Robinson, H. A., "Psycholinguistics, Sociolinguistics, Reading, and the Classroom Teacher," *International Reading Association Conference Papers*, **17** (1972).

Rodnick, R., and B. Wood, "The Communication Strategies of Children," *The Speech Teacher*, **22** (March 1973), 114–124. (Researches the use by children of language as a tool—based on three referents—eating, sleeping, and playing.)

Ruddell, R. B., *Reading Language Instruction: Innovative Practices*. Englewood Cliffs, Prentice-Hall, Inc., 1974.

Ruddell, R., "Psycholinguistic Implications for a System of a Communication Model," in H. Singer, and R. Ruddell, eds., *Theoretical Models and Processes of Reading*, Newark, Del.: International Reading Association, 1970, pp. 239–258.

Schiach, G. M., *Teach Them to Speak: A Language Development Programme in 200 Lessons*, London: Ward Lock Educational, 1972.

Schiefelbusch, R. L., and L. L. Lloyds, eds., *Language Perspectives: Acquisition, Retardation, and Intervention*. Baltimore: University Park Press, 1973.

Semel, E. M., and E. H. Wiig, "Comprehension of Syntactic Structures and Critical Verbal Elements by Children with Learning Disabilities," *Journal of Learning Disabilities*, **8** (January 1975), 46–53.

Sharf, D. J., "Some Relationships between Measures of Early Language Development," *Journal of Speech and Hearing Disorders*, **37** (February 1972), 64–74.

Shewan, C. M., "The Language Disordered Child in Relation to Muma's

Communication Game," *Journal of Speech and Hearing Disorders,* **40** (August 1975), 310–314. (Indicates that the concept of communicative competence is clinically relevant and important.)

Shields, M. M., and E. Steiner, "The Language of Three- to-Five-Year-Olds in Preschool Education," *The Journal of Educational Research,* **15** (February 1973), 97–105.

Shriner, T. H., "A Review of Mean Length of Response as a Measure of Expressive Language Development in Children," *Journal of Speech and Hearing Disorders,* **34** (February 1969), 61–67. (Reviews and discusses the studies dealing with mean length of response as a measure of children's language development.)

Siegel, G. M., "The Use of Language Tests," *Language, Speech and Hearing Services in the Schools,* **6** (October 1975), 211–216. (Talks about today's emphasis on helping develop the language of the schoolchild. Emphasizes the role of the clinician in evaluation of language performance.)

Simon, C. S., "Talk Time! Language Development in Readiness Classes," *Language, Speech and Hearing Services in the Schools,* **6** (July 1975), 161–168. (Describes a program entitled "Talk Time," which furthered communication among the members of the team of the language underdeveloped in terms of auditory and language skills.)

Smith, E. B., K. S. Goodman, and R. Meredith, *Language and Thinking in the Elementary School,* New York: Holt, Rinehart and Winston, Inc., 1970.

Sperry, V., *A Language Approach to Learning Disabilities,* Palo Alto, Calif.: Counseling Psychologist Press, 1972.

Stark, J., "Reading Failure: A Language Based Problem," *ASHA,* **17** (December 1975), 832–834.

————, R. L. Rosenbaum, D. Schwartz, and A. Wisan, "The Nonverbal Child: Some Clinical Guidelines," *Journal of Speech and Hearing Disorders,* **38** (February 1973), 59–72. (Describes principles and procedures related to language training for nonverbal children.)

Stauffer, R. G., *The Language-Experience Approach to the Teaching of Reading,* New York: Harper & Row Publishers, Inc., 1970.

Stegmaier, N. K., "Teaching Interpersonal Communication Through Children's Literature," *Elementary English,* **51** (October 1974), 927–932. (Explains how children's literature can be a vehicle for communicative activities that further honest, wholesome, and sound interpersonal relationships.)

Stern, C., and W. Tupta, "Ethnic Responding of Disadvantaged Preschool Children as a Function of Type of Speech Modeled," *Journal of School Psychology,* **8** (1970), 24–27.

Stewig, J. W., *Spontaneous Drama: A Language Art,* Columbus, Ohio: Charles E. Merrill Publishing Co., 1973. (Demonstrates how creative drama can build verbal and nonverbal language skills.)

Uhl, N. P., T. Fillmer, and J. E. Yano, "Receptive and Expressive Vocabularies of Upper-Middle and Low SEL Children," *Elementary English,* **49** (May 1972), 725–734.

Vasta, R., and R. M. Lievert, "Auditory Discrimination—Syntactic Structure," *Developmental Psychology*, **9** (1973), 79–82.

Wadsworth, B. J., *Piaget's Theory of Cognitive Development*, New York: David McKay Co., Inc., 1973.

Wakefield, M. W., "Sequential Memory Responses of Normal and Clinic Readers," *Elementary English*, **50** (September 1973), 930–939.

———, and N. J. Silvaroli, "A Study of Oral Language Patterns of Low Socioeconomic Groups," *The Reading Teacher*, **22** (April 1969), 622–624. (Attempts to discover whether differences in speech patterns were influenced more by the ethnic or socioeconomic background of the children. Results indicated that economic background was a stronger influence on language than ethnic background.)

Way, B., *Development Through Drama*, London: Longmans, Green and Company, Ltd., 1967. (Includes chapters on imagination, movement, and the use of sound, speaking, sensitivity and characterization, improvisation, play making and play building, and social drama.)

Wepman, J. N., "Relationships of Auditory Discrimination to Speech and Reading," *ASHA*, **1** (1969), 96.

Wilkinson, A., *The Foundations of Language*, New York: Oxford University Press, 1971.

Woolfolk, E. C., *Carrow Elicited Language Inventory*, Austin, Tex.: Learning Concepts, 1975.

9. Delayed or Retarded Language Acquisition and Development

Delayed Development

Until recently, a child who was severely delayed in language development was not likely to be found in the "normal" classroom. Even if the severe delay was not associated with mental retardation, the child's admission to graded classes may have been postponed. In some instances a child with moderate language retardation was enrolled in a class for exceptional or educationally handicapped children. With a contemporary move to "mainstream" as many exceptional children as possible, even the severely delayed-in-language child may now be enrolled in "regular" classrooms. Occasionally we may find one in a class with normal children of a younger age group. For the most part, however, the "regular" classroom teacher is more likely to have children with mild language delay, children whose history may include slower onset of speech and somewhat slower development in articulatory, vocabulary, and syntactic (grammatical) proficiency.

The term *delayed language development* may be applied among school-age children to a range of problems, from cases in which there is a complete failure to use oral language[1] to those where the vocabulary

---

[1] Complete failure to develop language in children with hearing, is likely only for those who are in the low-grade idiot range of intelligence.

and sentence control seem adequate, but speech is not readily intelligible. However, as we consider later, children who persevere in infantilisms are also likely to be retarded in their syntactic development. There are however, exceptions of all kinds to this general statement. Some late starters catch up quickly once they get going, and by school age, are on a par with their age peers. Some children, whose speech is faulty for one or two sounds, and who may lisp or lall, are nevertheless completely intelligible with good or better than average vocabularies and with comparable syntactical proficiency. At the other extreme we find some children who employ gestures as substitutes for oral language as well as those who use single words or phrases accompanied by gestures at age four or five. A few, after making a slow start with a vocabulary of a dozen or so single-word utterances, may give up the effort and withdraw to become almost silent children by age four or five.

Many children who enter school with delayed language development are likely to present articulatory problems by the time they reach the second or third grade. These children do not suddenly develop their articulatory difficulties. For the most part, their articulatory proficiency was delayed as one aspect of their language development. By the time the children begin to manage language, the articulatory aspect of their overall development becomes more apparent.

Menyuk (1964) compared 10 children diagnosed as using infantile speech with 10 matched children, ages 3.0 years to 5.10 years. The I.Q.s of the two groups were approximately 126, based on the Ammons Full-Range Picture Vocabulary Test. Menyuk concluded from her data that the term *infantile*, in regard to articulation, appears to be an incorrect designation because "at no age level did the grammatical production of a child with deviant speech match or closely match the grammatical production of a child with normal speech from two years on." Our own observations support those of Menyuk, with even greater differences found for children who are within the normal or below-average range of intelligence.

Children with serious delay in language (oral words) per se are not likely to progress normally in the primary grades. There are, of course, occasional and important exceptions. We sometimes find children with severe oral linguistic impairments who nevertheless learn to read and to write and so evidence their educational achievement. More often, however, children with serious delays in language development also have difficulties in learning to read and to write and are generally retarded in educational achievement.

For the most part, the classroom teacher of the nonexceptional child may have one or two children who have the residuals of delayed language. These children often need the help of the speech clinician to improve their articulatory proficiency. They are likely also to need help with other aspects of language development.

MENTAL RETARDATION

Despite recent criticism of intelligence tests as instruments for assessing mental capacity and intellectual potential, the relationship between functional mental retardation and language delay continues to be evident. We are still able to observe that the chief cause of prolonged language (speech) delay is mental retardation. This is so for the onset of speech as well as for the development of speech after onset. There is, however, considerable recent evidence that with direct teaching and training, many mentally retarded children are able to learn to speak even though they could not acquire speech by a "normal" amount of exposure in an essentially normal language environment.[2]

With due reservation for and about intelligence testing and testers of intelligence, we present some studies that indicate the relationship between mental retardation and language delay. However, we again emphasize that *findings are reversible and are, often,* happily, influenced by therapy.[3]

Lillywhite and Bradley (1969, p. 11) report that in a survey of communication impairment among the educably mentally retarded in the Portland, Oregon, public schools, 12 per cent were found to have speech and/or language defects, as compared with 4.5 per cent among the nonretarded. Generally, in their survey, Lillywhite and Bradley observed that the most severely retarded, those with I.Q.s ranging from 40 to 70, presented a variety of defects, including articulatory, functional, and organic voice quality disturbances such as excessive nasality, huskiness, and language delay. "All of the children showed speech and language functioning in one way or another significantly

---

[2] In an experiment at the Institute for Childhood Aphasia at San Francisco State University, a group of severely retarded children (I.Q.s below 50) who had no functional speech were directly taught language in a program regularly used for aphasic children. Most of the children acquired considerable functional language after a five-month, four-hour-per-week, training period. Emphasis was on vocabulary building, language concepts, and syntax. Most of the children reached the level equivalent of a two-to three-word mean length of utterance. This is comparable to the normal acquisition of children between 15 to 18 months of age. All of the children learned some socially useful language.

[3] P. W. Drash in "Habilitation of the Retarded Child: A Remedial Program," *The Journal of Special Education*, **6** (1972) reports on a delayed language child who tested at age four in the mid-50 to mid-60 I.Q. range on standardized tests of intelligence. After two years of speech and language training, the child tested well within the normal range of intelligence. Academic achievement in two years of elementary school was also well within the average range.

inferior to expectation based upon mental age." They were, of course considerably more inferior based upon actual age expectations. Contributing causes of speech defects are hearing losses, found in greater incidence among retardates than among nonretardates, as well as sluggish control of palatal and pharyngeal structures.

Luchsinger and Arnold (1967, pp. 513–544) report that 52 per cent (69 of 134 cases) diagnosed as having delayed language development in a large New York City clinic tested on intake as having Intelligence Quotients below 75. Another 16 tested at the borderline level (I.Q. 80). As in the Lillywhite and Bradley survey, contributing or associated causes were also present. These included mongolism, childhood schizophrenia, and endocrine disturbances.

Let us accept the notion of mental retardation as representing present capacity related to past experience and innate but not necessarily realized potential. On this basis we will find correlations between mental retardation and language proficiency along the following lines. The most severely mentally retarded may never acquire functional speech. Moderately retarded children usually do acquire speech, but often with numerous defects in articulation, impoverished vocabularies, and very limited syntax. Mildly retarded children acquire speech, but are likely to have limited vocabularies and use relatively simple sentence constructions. In general, moderate and mildly retarded children parallel and "shadow" normal children in all aspects of language development. Naremore and Dever (1975) studied the language performance of educable mentally retarded and normal children in the six to ten years age range. They found that the retarded children tended to use simpler grammatical constructions than the normal children. Specifically in regard to ten-year-olds, the investigators observed that the retarded children used few subordinate clauses and more "and" or "and then" constructions to relate parts of sentences. However, "The development . . . appears to be in the same direction as that of the normal child, although the same levels are not attained."

We sometimes find children with moderate mental retardation who seem to have as many words as their age peers. A discerning listener may be able to note, however, that these children use the words less meaningfully and that the words lack depth and richness of concept. It is our observation that some mentally retarded children who are well trained and well taught are able to acquire appropriate words on a low level of meaning for many situations and events.

Some mentally retarded children who "know the words but not too many of the meanings" may manage to get through the primary grades without too much trouble. These children, by virtue of the "halo effect" of their apparent linguistic ability, may not seem to be

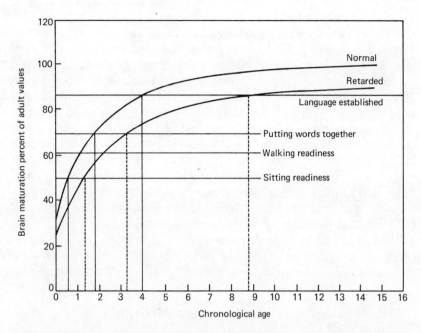

Figure 10. On the ordinate, Lenneberg combined all the parameters of brain maturation into a single factor. "Retarded children presumably attain the maturational values later in life than normal children. Attainment of brain maturation is correlated with behavioral achievements shown here as 'horizons.' A comparison of the growth curves of normal and retarded children explains why the relative distances among the various milestones become greater with advancing age. Normally, a child begins to join words together about 15 months after he is ready to sit up; in a retarded child it may take 24 months to achieve this. It takes about two years to acquire the general basis for language establishment once a normal child has begun to put words together. In a retarded child it may take five years or more to acquire the same facility in language."*

mentally retarded until they reach a level in school where the teacher begins to note their difficulty in dealing with concepts or ideas that cannot readily be objectified.

It is also important to recognize that there are some children whose difficulty with oral language makes them appear to be mentally retarded when they are not. Some children who are suspected of being mentally retarded because of their delayed development may, upon examination with nonlanguage tests of intelligence, turn out to be normal, or even above average, in intelligence. Other causes, such as

---

* From E. H. Lenneberg, *Biological Foundations of Language*, (New York: John Wiley & Sons, Inc., 1967), p. 169

slow general physiologic development, emotional disturbances, or hearing loss, may account for the language delay. The possibility of error in arriving at a causal diagnosis of mental retardation for language delay points to the need for a competent clinical psychologist or school psychologist to examine the suspected child and make an evaluation. If this cannot be done, the language clinician as well as classroom teacher may entertain hypotheses about the concerned child, but judgments should be withheld until justified. They should be especially careful to reserve judgment about possible mental retardation for the child with uneven school achievement. If the child does average or better work when oral language is not required, but does poorly in areas that require speech competency, we should seek the cause for the disparity rather than conclude that we are dealing with a "nontypical" but nevertheless mentally retarded child.

Figure 10, taken from Lenneberg (1967, p. 109) presents a graphic comparison of the language development of retardates and normal children in relationship to milestones for sitting and walking.

THERAPEUTIC APPROACHES: THE MENTALLY RETARDED

Treatment for the mentally retarded, whether we are dealing with "biological types" or with those who may be functionally delayed, should take the form of education and training geared to the capacities of the individual child. Our emphasis would be on vocabulary building, language concepts, and syntax (grammar) with intelligible communication as the goal. For low level retardates, socially functional language may be both the immediate and ultimate goal. However, an effort for more advanced language should be tried, even for children regarded as among the most severely mentally retarded.

Stimulation and improvement of the home environment, if this is possible, should help to bring the retardate to a level where potential for language usage and articulatory proficiency become highly and positively correlated. Specific training for the correction of specific articulatory and vocal defects is indicated for the higher grade retardates. Such children may be members of slow progress or "special" classes. For most children, a reasonable achievement objective is to strive for the proficiency level of a normal child whose chronological age is equal to that of the mental age of the retardate. In the absence of sensory, motor, or personality involvements, this level of achievement may be reached for most higher level retardates. Little progress, however, may be expected beyond age 14 (Goda and Griffith 1962 and Lenneberg 1967, pp. 154–155).

Although voice and articulatory defects occur in a higher incidence in retardates than in children of normal intelligence, the chief factor in the mentally retarded child's communicative difficulties are to be found in limited and inadequate language. This, as Wood (1964, p. 39) points out, may have either organic or nonorganic associated causes.

What in language do we teach (stimulate and motivate) retarded children who are slow in language development? By slow we imply even slower than we may have a right to expect based upon their degree of retardation. Miller and Yoder (1972) provide an answer. Based upon a review of the literature completed in 1970, they concluded that mentally retarded children who do have language develop their language code in a manner similar to that of normal children *but at a slower rate*. The implication of this finding is that what we know about normal language acquisition provides a basis for the language training of retarded children. The sample syntactic structures presented in our chapter on the Development of Language constitute a body of information based upon normal language acquisition. Beyond this, we can endorse Miller and Yoder's (1974, pp. 507–508) principles and criteria for the individual retarded child. With some modification to reflect our own position, we have incorporated the Miller and Yoder criteria as follows.[4]

1. A language training program should begin with regard to where each child is linguistically (stage or level of development as ascertained by standardized testing or the analysis of a representative language sample). The program should project increments as to where the child should be helped to advance.
2. A program should be based on a realistic set of goals or behaviors in regard to language, both for the communication of ideas and the expression of feelings. The latter, admittedly, may come more easily and spontaneously as acquisitions by exposure to older speakers in the environment. A program should include intermediate and tentative terminal behaviors. These should be related and relevant to the child's home, social, and educational environment as well as to individual development capacities.
3. A program should be founded on what we now know about normal language acquisition.
4. A program should anticipate the variety of circumstances and

---

[4] Although these criteria are presented as specific to retarded children, we believe that they pertain to all children who are retarded in language development.

situations that involve children and older speakers in their environments.

5. Overall communicative competence, both verbal and nonverbal, should be aspects of the social goals.

6. A program should have a systematic approach to help the child achieve appropriate and proficient language. The systematic approach may employ operant procedures and techniques, or other approaches compatible with the teacher-clinician and the child. Seldom does inspiration of the moment suffice. However, a sensitive teacher-clinician will follow a child's lead if unexpected circumstances or unexpected language behaviors are presented.

HEARING LOSS: THE DEAF[5]

Deaf children have insufficient hearing, at the time when speech normally is learned, to enable them to acquire oral language ability through the sense of hearing. Children with a hearing loss that is severe enough for them to be diagnosed as deaf do not learn to speak orally unless they are specially trained to do so through the use of devices and techniques that are not necessary for children with normal hearing. Virtually all children with severe hearing loss are likely to have significant defects of articulation, voice, and almost always of language development (vocabulary and syntax). However, as we observed in our discussion of the prelingual stages in language development, up to six months of age the vocalizations of deaf children are not ordinarily different from those of hearing children. Between six and eight months of age, deficiencies in vocalizations and utterances between the deaf and the hearing tend to be quantitative rather than qualitative (Lenneberg 1964, p. 153). The deaf infant has a reduced inventory of sounds and spends less time in sound play than does the hearing child. This observation has an important therapeutic implication. If the child is recognized early as one with a severe hearing loss every effort should be made by the parents to encourage vocalization and sound play. The parents should, for example, make certain that the child sees the parent who is talking, especially in direct parent-child interchange. Simple repeated statements should be directed to the child. A mirror, strategically placed above the child, may stimulate talking to the mirror image. Such activities will encourage the deaf child not to become a silent child. The child may be responsive to the

---

[5] The problems of the deaf and hard-of-hearing children are considered in some detail in Chapter 14.

low-pitched vocalization of the adult, that is, to the voice per se, and then learn to look and see, and perhaps begin to face-read some of the speech of the adult. Appropriate gestures accompanying the speech of the adult may well enhance the deaf child's understanding of the adult's speech.

The problems of the deaf child for language learning are sometimes complicated by some degree of associated mental retardation or by slower mental maturation. However, Lenneberg (1964, p. 156), after reviewing the literature on cognitive, nonverbal investigations of deaf children, observes: "On strictly cognitive tasks it has been experimentally shown that even pre-school and thus 'pre-language' deaf children perform no worse than hearing children."

The extent of delay in language development for many, if not for most, deaf children may be appreciated when we realize that the normal hearing child at primary school age has a *speaking* vocabulary of 2,000 or more words—and several times that number for comprehension. In sharp contrast, the deaf child who enters a school for the deaf at age five may have no working vocabulary at all. The deaf child who has not acquired either an oral or a gesture (sign) system that can be used with at least one other person to communicate and express thoughts and feelings is without functional language.

This is the basis of the position taken by Furth (1966, pp. 226–228) on the need to establish an early visual language (gesture) system for congenitally deaf children. Learning to talk, and so to think, without recourse to oral language enhances the deaf child's cognitive and intellectual development. Waiting to establish an oral language system may impair such development. So, Furth argues, "as a direct result of linguistic incompetence, the deaf fail or are poor in all tasks which are specifically verbal or on a few non-verbal tasks in which linguistic habits afford a direct advantage." As an indirect result, the deaf lack information and exhibit a minimal amount of intellectual curiosity. Moreover, "they have less opportunity and training to think." Based on these observations, Furth proposes that the deficiencies associated with the linguistic incompetence of the deaf "would be avoidable if non-verbal methods of instruction and communication were encouraged both at home in the earliest years and in formal school education." He suggests that at home "parents must have recourse to distinguishable signs and use these together with speech. Practically all deaf children, instead of the present 10 per cent, could then be expected to reach a basic competence in English, just as all hearing children in any society learn the language to which they are exposed."

Furth may be overoptimistic in his projection of the training of deaf children through nonverbal (we believe he means nonoral) means.

However, we accept his position that the intellectual potentials of most deaf children, as well as their linguistic limitations, could be improved if the implications of his suggestions were followed.

There are some exceptions among deaf children in regard to language development. Most of the exceptions are found among bright deaf children, especially among those whose parents were aware of the hearing impairment and initiated early training along the lines suggested. Other exceptions may be found among deaf children with sufficient residual hearing who are able to make use of their limited hearing, those who have learned to attend to speakers and to read their faces and their articulatory and accompanying manual gestures. Some children, though deaf, may have their residual hearing enhanced by a properly fitted hearing aid and so learn considerably more about speech and speakers than if they relied on vision alone. Still other exceptions are found among children who became deaf (adventitious deafness) after they had acquired speech. In general, however, the incidence of speech defects and of language retardation is almost universal among preschool deaf children.

Most deaf children of school age have a slower rate of academic achievement than do their hearing peers. However, unless mental retardation is an associated problem, most deaf children learn to read and to write, and to progress in other school subjects.

Silverman (1971, p. 411), sums up his position as well as a consensus of the literature as follows:

> The deaf child does not learn at the same rate as the hearing child. With the need to master new vocabulary and language, it takes about two or more years to achieve second grade school level and an additional one and a half to two years to complete the third grade.

Silverman, in common with other authorities on the deaf, believes that most deaf children do not achieve academically up to their intellectual potential. "The gap between mental ability and academic achievement can be reduced but is seldom eliminated." Improved instructional methods may, we hope, reduce the gap for some children and eliminate it for the most fortunate of the deaf.

DEAF-APHASIC CHILDREN

Before leaving the subject of the deaf, we briefly discuss a small subgroup of congenitally (developmentally) aphasic-deaf.[6] Such child-

---

[6] For a survey of the literature of the evolving concept of developmental aphasia and the auditory and perceptual impairments of aphasic children, see H. Myklebust, in L. E. Travis, ed., *Handbook of Speech Pathology and Audiology* (New York: Appleton-Century-Crofts (Prentice-Hall, Inc.), 1972), chaps. 46–47.

We present our own view of the aphasic child in Chapter 16.

ren, who are also referred to as having central deafness, are not able to perceive and assign meanings even to sounds which, when reinforced by amplification, are physically received. We assume that such children, in addition to peripheral hearing loss, also have incurred damage or have severe maturational delay of an area, or areas, of the cerebral cortex that normally serves for the analysis of speech sounds. A child who is both peripherally and centrally deaf (aphasic), is likely to ignore and reject even very loud speech, and may be disturbed by and refuse to use hearing aids. The child is probably wise in doing so. If the youngster is unable to make sense out of any received human speech sounds, confusion and frustration may result from mere reception without perception. Such a child may be trained initially through a straight visual approach, with gesture and finger spelling and later through graphic media alone for reading and writing. We need to emphasize, however, that the deaf-aphasic child constitutes a very small subgroup of the deaf. Nondeaf congenitally aphasic children, also a small group, are considered in Chapter 16.

THE HARD-OF-HEARING

Language retardation and voice and articulation defects are prevalent in children who have sufficient hearing to learn to speak through the auditory modality, but whose hearing is sufficiently impaired to create problems in the easy and comfortable reception of speech signals. O'Neill (1964, p. 4) considers the term *hard-of-hearing* to designate "a person who experiences difficulty in auditory reception but not complete loss of auditory reception (as exists in the deaf). Auditory reception can be improved by amplification or training."

With important exceptions, the incidence of speech (voice and articulation) and language defects are positively related to the severity of hearing loss and to the time in the child's life at which the loss began. The child who develops a hearing loss at age three or four, when his speech is well established, is likely to have much less impairment for language, and possibly also for voice and articulation, than is the congenitally hard-of-hearing child, or one whose hearing loss was acquired before he spoke in sentences. Some children whose pure-tone audiometric results might lead us to expect severe speech difficulties may do better than those whose hearing impairment might be considered relatively mild judging by their audiograms. "Just as there are gradations in the usefulness of hearing, so there are gradations in the quality and intelligibility of the speech of the hard-of-hearing. Many hard-of-hearing children speak so well that the lay observer notices no abnormality, whereas the severely impaired may be almost unintelligible to those who are not accustomed to this type of speech" (Silverman 1972, p. 431).

We need to appreciate that both the quality and the quantity of the language of the hard-of-hearing child depend on many individual factors. These include the intelligence of the child, the early recognition of the hearing loss, and the motivation of both parents and child toward speech learning. A bright child who is well motivated and who has well-informed parents may achieve normal speech through combining lip (speech) reading and the maximum use of hearing. Amplified sound and the use of a hearing aid, if possible and appropriate, may be of considerable help.

SPEECH DEFECTS ASSOCIATED WITH HEARING LOSS

Almost all children who are more than mildly hard of hearing have some degree of difficulty in articulation and appropriate vocalization. Depending in part on the type and degree of hearing loss, distortions and omissions of consonants, and especially fricative sounds, are common. There is also likely to be some difficulty in distinguishing between voiced and voiceless cognates such as *b* and *p*, *d* and *t*, *v* and *f*, and the *th* sounds. Vowels and diphthongs may be distorted.

The improvement of the speech of the child with a recognized and appreciable hearing loss is the task of the professional speech clinician rather than the classroom teacher who specializes in "normal" children. The nonspecialist classroom teacher has an important auxiliary role in cooperating with the speech clinician and special educator. In this instance, the special educator is one whose responsibilities are specific to children who have significant hearing impairment.

INTERMITTENT OR OCCASIONAL HEARING DIFFICULTY

Many teachers have had children who on occasion seem to have some difficulty in hearing. It is possible that some of these children have relatively slight though chronic difficulty with hearing, but are usually able to make up for the loss by good attentive effort. However, if such a child has a head cold, or suffers from enlarged adenoids because of a temporary inflammation, the hearing problem may be temporarily increased. Fatigue or ill-health may produce comparable results. There are, of course, other children who, for reasons related to their emotional problems in or out of the classroom, on occasion seem not to be able to hear. Perhaps these children block out human speech sounds because of difficulties that arise when they hear, understand, and respond to speech. If the teacher suspects the latter to be the case, an understanding of what may be the basis for the nonhearing rather than a scolding is in order.

Whenever hearing loss is suspected, an audiological evaluation, which should include speech perception, is recommended. If hearing loss is found, its cause and possible treatment should be determined by a physician. Fortunately, in some instances, medical treatment can minimize or entirely clear up temporary difficulty in hearing, resulting from pathology.

THE HARD-OF-HEARING CHILD IN THE CLASSROOM[7]

The teacher can be of appreciable help in the classroom for a child believed to have a hearing loss. Among the things that can be done to be of direct help to the particular child are

1. Make certain that the teacher is constantly in direct view of the child during instructional periods.
2. Permit changing of seats to keep the teacher's face in direct view of the child.
3. Speak louder and somewhat more slowly when an activity is anticipated that will involve a specific response from the child suspected of having a hearing loss.

EMOTIONAL PROBLEMS

The history of many children with language delay includes an item indicating that they began to speak at an age within normal limits but then seemed to give up speaking. On questioning, one or both parents may reveal that the cessation of speaking seemed to be associated with an unhappy familial situation. In some instances, it becomes apparent that the parents were disturbed about their own relationship, and frequently spoke harshly to each other in the presence of the young child. Occasionally, an admission is obtained that when the parents spoke to each other at all, it was in emotional outbursts. The young child apparently became afraid of the consequences of speech and retired into the relative safety and security of not speaking at least to the parents at home. Such a child may continue to be apprehensive about the consequences of speaking in other situations, including in school where the teacher may be perceived as a parent away from home. If the child meets any penalty resulting from speech behavior during the early school experiences, his/her apprehensions are confirmed. This kind of child may prefer to be ignorant or "dumb" or accept a scolding for apparent inattention or negativism rather than risk the greater penalty

---

[7] See Chapter, 1 and 4 for a more detailed discussion of the teacher's role.

of saying the wrong thing. The child may decide that it is safer to be the "quiet one" than the one who becomes involved in difficulties for speaking thoughts or feelings.

Another situation associated with regression or cessation of speech and occurring frequently enough to be worthy of note is the birth of a new child. The two- or three-year-old may look upon the crying, non-speaking infant as a usurper of attention and affection. With what seems fair logic, the older sibling may decide that the only way to compete with the usurper is to imitate the newcomer's behavior. So speech, at least for a while, may regress to prelingual stages or come to a halt.

There are other children, more severely involved in their emotional relationships and human identifications, whose early history also begins with comparatively normal onset and development of speech. These children appear to be normal, at least as far as speech is concerned, until they are about two years of age. Then they regress or cease to talk or become fixed at the one-word labeling stage. These children also show other withdrawal behavior of sufficient degree as to be identified as childhood schizophrenics. Goldfarb (1961) presents a psychiatrist's view of the nature and treatment of children with childhood schizophrenia. Other psychiatric, psychological, and psycholinguistic viewpoints are included in the writings of Pronovost and Wakstein (1966), Rimland (1964), Rutter (1971), and Wing (1966). A behavior modification approach that is realistic both as to objectives and achievements is presented by Lovaas, Schreibman, and Koegel (1974).

PARENTAL EXPECTATIONS AND DELAYED SPEECH

In the chapter on the Development of Language we presented four basic assumptions relative to the parents and the home environment that were considered conducive to a child's normal acquisition of speech (see p. 160). Some parents, perhaps in their effort to provide normal stimulation and have a normal speaking child, become anxious in their expectations. Perhaps they fail to understand that child speech is not adult speech in miniature form. A child speaks as a child, not only in thoughts but in phonology, vocabulary, pronunciation, and syntax. Perhaps it is well for us to remember that "When I was a child, I spoke as a child . . . When I became a man, I put away childish things" (*Corinthians*, 13, 11).

Chess and Rosenberg (1974) report on referrals made to them in a clinical psychiatric practice limited to children. Children with speech problems, they observe, are brought in earlier (peak ages four to five) than are children without speech problems (peak ages eight to nine).

Out of a population of 563 children, 139 (24 per cent) had some type of language difficulty at the time of referral. Of this group, 81 had delayed onset of speech (fewer than 15 words by two years of age) and 51 immature speech (speech usage significantly below age expectation).

Chess and Rosenberg make two important clinical observations. "In the cognitively normal child with speech usage below age there may be a tendency to inhibit speech in situations where rebuff or misunderstanding are anticipated." The second observation is related to the higher incidence of boys to girls (three boys to one girl) in the clinical population. "Whether this is a function of the high language expectations of middle-class parents has not been determined." The findings of Wood (1946) and Peckarsky (1952) suggest that unrealistic parental expectations are in fact related to speech delay in children.

Other findings reveal that the parents of delayed-speech children are often inclined to be rigid and restrictive in their demands upon their children, as well as upon one another. Possibly as a result of the frustration experienced by the parents, there is an air of excessive tension in the conduct of the home. Many of the parents admit to being "perfectionists" but use the term with pride rather than insight. It is possible that children brought up in such homes unconciously feel rejected. It is possible also that the parents, consciously or unconsciously, are rejecting their children. Certainly these parents are rejecting the efforts and accomplishments of their children, and the children respond to this attitude as if they were being entirely rejected. A child whose early speech attempts are ignored as being unworthy of notice, or who is criticized for not being readily understandable, may well hesitate to talk in order to avoid any unfavorable parental response.

Some of the feeling of apprehension continues to characterize the behavior of children who were delayed in speech. The classroom teacher in the first or second grade would do well to be permissive in attitude and to avoid correcting the articulation or pronunciation of children who have a delayed-speech history. These children need the security of acceptance of themselves as they are so that their speech efforts will not be conducive to disapproval or fear. Remedial speech work of specific speech faults may well wait until the third or fourth grade for these children. Of course, indirect efforts at correction take place whenever the child is exposed to a kind and permissive environment that stimulates good but not unrealistically perfectionistic speech. An attitude of permissiveness, incidentally, should be consistent and should not vary from day to day according to the whims of the adult.

Kleffner (1973, pp. 11–12), on the basis of rich clinical experience, observes that three factors are common in parental reactions to young children who have disorders of speech. Kleffner's observations are particularly relevant to the child who appears to be delayed in speech development.

1. Parental anxiety tends to produce "an insidious and pervasive pressure for the child to talk. Paradoxically, this pressure can co-exist ... with a reduction in the parent's efforts to engage in functional communicative interactions with the child."
2. Parents tend to intensify their efforts to evoke what little language their children have acquired rather than to help them to acquire new language or to broaden their concepts about language. Parents encourage labeling by asking children to name pictures or objects (What's this?) rather than presenting situation and themselves talking about the picture, for example, "The bird's wings are spread open when it flies."
3. Parents seem to have difficulty in determining the level of language usage and language stimulation that will result in an optimum verbal interchange. "Sometimes they talk far above the child's head; at other times reverting to rudimentary or even nonverbal communication well below the child's ability levels."

FAULTY MOTIVATION

Human beings, we have emphasized, are expected to speak. The drive to speak is so strong in almost all children that we need to do little more than provide a decent environment for a child to have one who will speak. However, the quantity of the child's speech and, to some degree, the quality of speech may well be modified by an unfavorable environment. In the preceding pages we considered the possible effects of parental anxiety and unrealistic and perfectionistic expectations. Now we turn our attention to what may well be the other side of the coin, the overprotected child.

The child who suffers—and suffers is really the word—from overprotection is a comparatively rare child. The overprotected child does start to talk and most likely will continue to acquire speech that is at least normal in syntax unless the child is completely overwhelmed by parents. But for the rare child who has adequate intellectual, sensory, and motor equipment, who does make a start but does not seem motivated to continue in language acquisiticn, what is presented in the next few paragraphs is relevant.

Children are not likely to develop many new skills, language acquisition included, unless such skills provide them with a sense of satisfaction and accomplishment that they cannot otherwise obtain. Though almost every child is born to speak, and will have a normal age for onset of speech, the members of the family may either nurture or retard later speech development. Children whose wants are regularly anticipated may be denied the opportunity for expressing their wants, thereby frustrating their need to do so. The magic of speech is the right of each child who is capable of exercising such potency. Parents who are over-protective, because of past or present injuries or illnesses of their children, and who hover over them when they first attempt to stand alone or to walk, do nothing to encourage standing or walking. Parents who cannot wait until their child completes a gesture without over-whelming the youngster with a number of things the gesture might signify produce a state of "what's the use" and confusion in the child. Children have the need and right to speak for themselves *just as soon as they are able.* Some overprotected children may be fortunate in having other less anxiety ridden and overprotective adults or older siblings with whom they can identify. Speech may then be selectively produced. But the less fortunate of the overprotected children may begin to speak at the expected age but not make the expected acquisitions after onset. Among the immediate improvements and modifications sought for these children are the following:

1. An understanding on the part of parents, and any other over-anxious, overzealous members of the child's environment, that the child is deserving of the right to entertain a want or a need, even if it is necessary to cry about it.
2. When an attempt at speech is made, the attempt is to be heard out before the adults jump to do something about it.

For children who have not begun to speak, or who have not gone beyond "mama" and "dada" in their early naming, the following suggestions are in order:

1. A repeated vocalization, especially if it accompanies a repeated gesture in association with a given situation, may be the beginning of word usage. The adult should imitate the vocalization in the recurring situation before responding to the act of gesture-vocalization. In this way, attention is directed to the oral activity rather than to the pantomine.
2. Once repeated vocalization is established, the parent should take the initatitive and give a simple monosyllabic name to a toy or object frequently used and desired by the child. This name should include sounds the child has successfully made and repeated in his sound-play activity. For example, if "da" is frequently uttered by the child, the name "da" can be given to a doll or some other plaything enjoyed by the child. The

sound should be spoken by the parent each time the object is given to the child, and each time the adult, when present, observes the child reaching for the object. After one or two days of this practice, the object should be withheld, but not with a look of apprehension or threat, until the child makes some attempt to utter the sound-name for it. If the child is reasonably successful in making a sound that closely resembles, if not directly reproduces the sound-name, quick approval for the effort is in order. This, however, does not mean that the child is to be rewarded by another toy or overwhelmed with a flow of words too numerous and too rapid for assimilation or understanding. Easy is the mode for early parent-child interchanges. The longer this mode is maintained, the better are the interchanges.

BILINGUAL INFLUENCES

In Chapter 7 on Language Development, we discussed bilingualism and bidialectlism. These subjects, however related, should not be confused. Neither should we fail to be aware of the sociopolitics involved in considerations of bilingualism. It is beyond the scope of this book to become involved in the questions and issues of bilingual or bidialectal education. (For an objective review of these matters, the reader is referred to Cazden (1972, pp. 143–181). Our concern in this chapter is to consider the influence of bilingualism relative to the acquisition and development of speech in children who have no choice as to whether they might prefer a bilingual or monolingual environment or which of two languages they are to be exposed to first.

As suggested in the chapter on Language Development, children who come from a bilingual environment include a higher proportion of ones with delayed language development than do children exposed to a single language from birth. The research data, unfortunately, are sparse as to the specific effects of bilingualism on onset of speech, lexical, phonological, and syntactic acquisitions. Even more rare are studies on the effect of conceptualization and verbal meaning for bilingual children. The bilingual children we see in a clinical setting are found frequently to have been delayed in onset of speech and even more delayed in their language acquisitions after onset. But this is a selected population of children referred for diagnosis or treatment because of their evident difficulties. We know very little about bilingual children who have no difficulties. An exception is a study by Smith (1949) who investigated the effect of bilingualism (Chinese and English) among children in the Hawaiian Islands. Smith found that even when the vocabularies of the two languages were combined, only two fifths of the children exceeded the expected norms for monolingual children. On the strength of her data Smith concluded that "only the superior bilingual child is capable of attaining the vocabulary norms of monoglots . . . "

A significantly different conclusion was reached by Lambert, Just, and Segalowitz (1970, p. 233). However, these investigators—sociolinguists—were involved with the results of teaching a second language (French) to children brought up in monolingual (English) homes. The teaching was carried on in Montreal schools in the kindergarten. The authors consider that this age and school level is critical to the results. The teachers were French speaking and described as highly skilled. Moreover, in addition to vocabulary building and listening comprehension, the children were taught art and music and played games in French. So, learning French became both fun and status achievement. Lambert et al. say that the children in this ideal school situation "demonstrate a very high level of skill in both receptive and productive aspects of French, the major language of instruction; a generally excellent command of all aspects of English, the home language of the children; and a high level of skill in a nonlanguage subject matter, mathematics, taught through the foreign language only."

On the basis of these two references of studies made over a considerable distance and difference in social cultures and time, we are not ready to come to any conclusions. However, for children who are simultaneously exposed to two languages, and who do present indications of delayed or disordered speech, we can suggest the following:

On the whole, it would seem much safer for a child to have one language well established before being exposed to a second. If multiple language exposure cannot be avoided, as is the case in many homes and many cultures, the use of a given language should be identified consistently with a person or a situation. Some children seem to find it necessary to fit themselves and the speaking situation into a linguistic "groove" and to maintain that groove in a consistent manner. For example, if the parents spoke only English, and the grandparents, nurse, or housekeeper spoke a second language, the child would learn to associate a language pattern—a way of speaking—with a person or persons and so have less conflict than if the parents spoke English on some occasions and a second language on others. When the other times are unpredictable, or when the other times are reserved for admonishments, difficulty with the second language may intensify. So, also, unfortunately, may the child's attitude toward language behavior in general.

The observations we have made in regard to bilingual exposure hold true also for children who appear to have difficulty in language development. Many children present no such difficulty. Such children are often found in middle- and upper-socioeconomic-class homes. Penfield (1959, pp. 221–255) recommends that children who live in bilingual environments, as, for instance, in Montreal, Canada, should intentionally be taught two languages by the direct method—that is, by having the children exposed to both languages in their home, but each in a systematic way—during the early preschool years. The argument for this natural and direct approach is that the child's brain before school age has a maximum plasticity and capacity for acquiring more than one language. A young child may respond "reflexively" to whatever language is spoken. The children will not, of course, realize that they may be speaking French on one occasion and to one person, and English to another person or on different occasions.

If, however, a child who has been exposed to more than one language appears to have difficulty in learning to speak, we strongly recommend that the parents decide which language is to be essential for the child and that the youngster be exposed to only one language until the child's speech behavior has become established. This frequently calls for control and modification of the home environment as well as of aspects of the environment outside of the home. Although such control and modification may not always be easy to achieve, it is important that it be done.

Bilingualism may present a variety of problems relative to language proficiency as well as to psychological and social development. These problems are discussed in a monograph edited by Macnamara (1967).

BIDIALECTISM: BLACK ENGLISH

We have already indicated the need to distinguish between delayed and defective speech and the use of a dialect in which there are differences in phonology, vocabulary, and syntax with another dialect of the same language. Thus, children who speak Black English, or any other dialect of English for that matter, should be evaluated for how well they are doing in the particular dialect before decisions are made as to whether their speech is delayed or defective.

The matter of whether a child's dialect should be changed involves educational and sociolinguistic considerations. We earnestly hope that it is not solely a political consideration. If the decision is made to encourage the child to change from Black English to another dialect of English that is more representative of a majority of speakers in the country or area in which the child lives, then necessary procedures can be undertaken. Another decision may be to establish bidialectism. In any event, it is essential that the clinician or teacher who is responsible for motivating and bringing about changes, *or teaching* a "standard" dialect, understands the child's first dialect.

Because the issues of bidialectism are so involved, we can make no definitive statements. We do suggest, as educators as well as clinicians, that if one dialect interferes with a second because of numerous over-lapping features, a choice will need to be made as to whether a minority or majority dialect should be taught. Again we hope that the interests of the child rather than sociopolitical influences will determine the choice.

Before closing this necessarily brief consideration of bidialectism and its implications for children whose first English dialect is Black English, an observation of caution is in order. We previously advised to keep separate dialectical differences and delayed language develop-ment or defective speech. It is equally important that we do not attri-bute to a dialect actual delay in language development or indications of defective speech. In fairness to the children involved, we should keep in mind that developmental problems may be expected for any group within a culture that for reasons of its own or because of imposed causes has children who are "at high risk." By "high risk" we refer to children who are prematurely born, whose mothers were not well nourished or who are themselves malnourished in their early years. The incidence of such children who are delayed in language and often in intellectual and cognitive development, as well, is higher than in the general population. *The Language of Poverty*, a term used for Black English, should not be confused with the effects of impoverishment on some of the children brought up in poverty.[8] The effects of poverty are by no means limited to blacks.

MULTIPLE BIRTHS

To what extent may we accept the observation that twins are double trouble? And if we double the potentialities for trouble with twins, is there a progressive likelihood of difficulty as the number of children per birth increases? Although most of our data are on twins, the answer in general is "Yes." With awareness that as individual children, children born as twins range in their intelligence, motor development, language

---

[8] We strongly recommend the book *Language and Poverty*, edited by F. Williams (Chicago: Markham Publishing Co., 1970), for an excellent series of essays on dialects and their implica-tions for attitudes on social change and education. We also recommend *Black English: Its History and Usage in the United States* by J. L. Dillard (New York: Random House, Inc. 1972). Dillard claims that 80 per cent of American blacks speak Black English as one of their dialects of American English.

development, and the like from retarded to precocious, we nevertheless find more delay and more problems in speech among twins than among single-born children. When the twins are identical, the liabilities, and happily some of the assets, are also likely to be amazingly similar.

After reviewing the literature on twins, Lenneberg (1967, p. 253) concludes:

> The developmental history of identical twins tends to be much more synchronous than that of fraternal twins. Among the former, motor milestones, menarche, change of voice, and growth rate are more likely to occur at the same time than among the latter. The same is reflected in the onset of speech (that is, the age at which the first few words appear, words are joined into phrases, and grammatical mistakes become minimal). It is only among the fraternal twins that difference in onset occurs, whereas identical twins seem to progress simultaneously. It is the general consensus of the investigators that these divergences cannot be simply explained on the grounds of imitation or differential treatment by parents.

Lenneberg (p. 252) summarizes the findings on delayed language and twins with the observation that 65 per cent of identical twins were delayed in onset of speech compared with 60 per cent of fraternal twins. Identical twins showed considerably more similarity in the features of their delay than did fraternal twins.

Onset of speech is delayed in twins, and twins are retarded in language acquisition up to about age four. The evidence suggests that most twins do catch up with single-born children by the time they enter the elementary school grades. Early language retardation among twins may be attributed both to organic causes and to an atypical social environment—the influence of each twin upon the other.

According to Nelson (1959, p. 305), most twins are prematurely born. Prematurity of birth is associated in many instances with vascular defects and with brain damage. Even when there is no clear evidence of damage to the brain, there is considerable evidence of a lag in overall physical maturation, which continues at least until the time the child is of age to enter school. Lags in psychological and social development parallel those for physical development. These disadvantages, we should emphasize, are associated with the combination of twinning and premature birth. Though there is evidence that some prematurely born children "may never catch up" (Silvern 1961), we are more inclined to accept the point of view of the geneticist Newman (1940), who maintains that if twins survive the hazards of being born and the consequences of prematurity, by the time they are well along in school they are as capable as their single-born peers.

Twins provide an atypical environment for one another. As they grow up they seem to be satisfied with their mutual social situation and so are less demanding of the attentions of older persons. Even if attention is demanded, it must be divided. Unfortunately, twins are not well qualified as language stimulators. The result is that they are exposed less to adults than are single children, and more to poor language stimulation. An interesting linguistic phenomenon among twins is their development of a special code for expression and communication—an idioglossia—which seems to serve the twins adequately but baffles all other members of the family. Because of the evident satisfaction twins derive from their idioglossia, they may not be motivated to learn the language of their homes or their more extended environment.

Evidence that most twins tend to catch up with single-born children comes from a study by Mittler (1970) on a middle-class population of twins in England. Mittler compared a population of 200 four-year-old twins with 100 singletons of the same age. All the children had just entered nursery school. The Illinois Test of Psycholinguistic Abilities—ITPA—(Kirk and McCarthy 1968) was used as the assessment measure. Mittler found that the twins' scores on all of the ITPA subtests paralleled those of the singleton children. Mittler concludes "thus, twins do not appear to show any characteristic pattern of linguistic organization, and their performance can best be described as a more or less uniform retardation or immaturity." The retardation in this study amounted to approximately six months.

Another finding that is worthy of note is that coming from a middle-class home was not as strongly a favorable factor for twins as for single children. Mittler speculates that by virtue of being a twin, each child is less receptive to the usual positive language values that are attributed to being a member of a middle socioeconomic family. ". . . It might be argued that the middle class twin remains a 'restricted' code user by virtue of the 'twin situation' which renders him less receptive to the 'elaborated' linguistic code used by his parents, whereas working class twins, who are mainly exposed to restricted codes in any case, are relatively less handicapped" (p. 755).

Though most twins do catch up by school age, there is a higher incidence of those who are retarded in language than in the population at large. A school-age population may not include many children who cannot be accepted or who are not accepted in schools by virtue of their language and associated retardations.

If twins arrive at school age still using their special language, they should, if at all possible, be put in separate classes. If this is not possible they should be put in separate groups so that they may associate with children using more conventional language.

THE ROLE OF THE CLASSROOM TEACHER WITH DELAYED-LANGUAGE CHILDREN[9]

As indicated earlier, regular classroom teachers are not likely to have many children with seriously retarded language development among their pupils. By the time children of normal intellect, who began by being delayed in language, reach school age, they are likely to be speaking well enough to be accepted in the regular class. However, some of the residuals of the problem may remain. Some of the children who were formerly delayed in speech may still be apprehensive about speaking and show anxiety when responsibility for communication is fixed upon them. These children are likely to be freer when responding as members of a group than when they are required to recite alone or to speak with, rather than in front of, their classmates. Others may have limited vocabularies or more than a normal number of speech faults. If teachers can determine which of the causes of retarded language development were present for any of the children, they can be of great help in controlling or preventing the pressure associated with the original cause for language retardation. These children need to learn that speech is enjoyable before they become aware that with the acquisition of speech there is an assumption of communicative responsibility. When pleasure replaces apprehension, goals for increased speech proficiency can be set. The children should be directed gently toward these goals and not goaded toward their attainment. Incidentally, we strongly urge that children who have just started their school careers be given no cause to become self-conscious about their lack of speech proficiency. Teachers must provide motivation, stimulation, and good and attainable models, as well as reinforcement for improvement. However, teachers should avoid any negative indications that might lead children to hold back on talking, or worse still, cause self-

---

[9] The current practice for "mainstreaming" to include as many children as possible in regular classes at least for part of their academic day may alter the situation in regard to serious language-delay problems. Regular classroom teachers may have to add another specialty to their broad array of general practice" specialties." We hope that at a minimum regular classroom teachers will have the assistance of language clinicians in their work with children who are seriously delayed in their language development.

interruptions of what they, however improficiently, might be trying to say.

Problems and Topics for Papers

1. What are the chief causes of delayed speech? What is *the* chief cause?
2. What is the relationship between emotional upheavals in the family and possible speech delay? Can you recall such a case?
3. Check with the parents of five children as to the ages when their children began to speak. Average the ages for the boys and for the girls. Which group had an older average age?
4. Twins have been found to begin to speak at a later age than single children. How do you account for this?
5. Read two of the references mentioned on childhood schizophrenia and childhood autism. Compare the early clinical histories of these two "types" of children with emotional problems. Are all autistic children schizophrenic? Are all schizophrenic children autistic?
6. Read the article by J. Stark, J. J. Giddan, and J. Meisel, "Increasing Verbal Behavior in an Autistic Child," *Journal of Speech and Hearing Disorders*, **33** (1968), 42–47. What methods were used to get the child to speak? Did the child generate any new utterances based on the vocabulary and syntax he was taught?
7. Compare the approaches in the Stark *et al.* article with those described by E. G. Wolf and B. A. Ruttenberg, "A Communication Therapy for the Autistic Child," *Journal of Speech and Hearing Disorders*, **32** (1967), 331–36, and those in Lovaas et al., referred to in this chapter.
8. There is considerable evidence that children who have difficulty in learning to read include more than a "normal" number of children with delayed-speech onset. Can you account for this?
9. Compare a three-year-old child's motor and speech development with the motor and language milestones of the table adapted from Lenneberg. (See Chapter 7 on language development.) Make the same comparisons for a three- or four-year-old who has been designated as being delayed in speech. Where are the greater disparities?
10. In the light of the present move to "mainstream" as many children as possible in regular classes in the public schools, are there any additional responsibilities and roles the classroom teacher has that were not suggested in this chapter?

References and Recommended Readings

Berry, M. F., *Language Disorders for Children*, New York: Appleton-Century-Crofts, 1969. (A broad treatment of the major causes of language disorders in children. A highlight of the book is the detailed clinical and treatment histories of some children with serious language delay.)

Cazden, C., *Child Language and Education*, New York: Holt, Rinehart and Winston, Inc., 1972. (A down-to-earth treatment of language development in the child. Reviews theories, facts, and their educational implications.)

Chess, S., and M. Rosenberg, " Clinical Differentiation Among Children with Initial Language Complaints," *Journal of Autism and Childhood Schizophrenia*, **4** (1974), 99–109.

Day, E. J., "The Development of Language in Twins, *Child Development*, **3** (1932), 179–199. (A classical study.)

Dillard, J. L., *Black English: Its History and Usage in the United States*, New York: Random House, Inc., 1972. (As the title indicates, the book reviews the history of the origins of Black English in the United States. A readable and authoritative book.)

Drash, P. W., "Habilitation of the Retarded Child: A Remedial Program," *The Journal of Special Education*, **6** (1972), 149–159.

Furth, H. G., *Thinking Without Language*, New York: The Free Press, 1966. (An important book that emphasizes the need to teach deaf children cognition even before they begin to learn a language system.)

Giradeau, F. L., and J. E. Spradlin, eds., *A Functional Analysis Approach to Speech and Language*, ASHA Monograph No. 14, Washington, D. C.: American Speech and Hearing Association, 1970.

Goda, S., and B. G. Griffith, "Spoken Language of Adolescent Retardates and Its Relation to Intelligence, Age, and Anxiety," *Child Development*, **32** (September 1962), 489–498.

Goldfarb, W., *Childhood Schizophrenia*, Cambridge: Harvard University Press, 1961.

Keaster, J., "Impaired Hearing," in W. Johnson et al., *Speech-Handicapped School Children*, New York: Harper & Row, Publishers, Inc., 1967, chap. 8.

Kirk, S., and J. McCarthy, *The Illinois Test of Psycholinguistic Abilities*, Urbana: University of Illinois Press, 1968.

Kleffner, F. R., *Language Disorders in Children*, New York: The Bobbs-Merrill Co., Inc., 1973. (A brief and highly personal, clinical exposition of the nature of language disorders in young children.)

Lambert, W. E., M. Just, and N. Segalowitz, "Some Cognitive Consequences of Following the Curricula of the Early School Grades in a Foreign Language," in J. E. Alatis, ed., *Twenty-first Round Table Bilingualism and Language Contact*, Washington, D.C.: George University Press, 1970.

Lenneberg, E. H., "Language Disorders in Childhood," *Harvard Educational Review*, **34**, 4 (Spring 1964), 152–177. (A review of causes, prognoses, and therapeutic procedures for children with moderate and severe language disorders.)

———, *Biological Foundations of Language*, New York: John Wiley & Sons, Inc., 1967.

Lillywhite, H. S., and D. P. Bradley, *Communication Problems in Mental Retardation*, New York: Harper & Row, Publishers, Inc., 1969. (Includes discussions of background, causes, and management of communication problems of mentally retarded children.)

Lovaas, O. I., L. Schreibman, and R. L. Koegel, "A Behavior Modification Approach to the Treatment of Autistic Children," *Journal of Autism and Childhood Schrizophrenia*, **4** (1974), 111-129.

Luchsinger, R., and G. E. Arnold, *Voice-Speech-Language*, Belmont, Calif.: Wadsworth Publishing Company, 1967.

Macnamara, J., ed., "Problems of Bilingualism," *The Journal of Social Issues*, **23**, 2 (April 1967).

McReynolds, L. V., ed., *Developing Systematic Procedures for Training Children's Language*, ASHA Monograph No. 18. Washington, D.C.: 1974.

Menyuk, P., "Comparison of Grammar of Children with Functionally Deviant Articulation," *Journal of Speech and Hearing Research*, **7**, 2 (June 1964), 109–121.

Miller, J. F., and D. E. Yoder, "An Ontogenetic Language Teaching Strategy for Retarded Children," in R. L. Schiefelbusch, and L. L. Lloyd, eds., *Language Perspectives-Acquisition, Retardation, and Intervention*, Baltimore: University Park Press, 1974, pp. 505–528.

————. "On Developing a Content for a Language Teaching Program," *Mental Retardation* (April 1972), 9–11.

Mittler, P., "Biological and Social Aspects of Language Development in Twins," *Developmental Medicine and Child Neurology*, **12** (1970), 741–757.

Myklebust, H., in L. E. Travis, ed., *Handbook of Speech Pathology and Audiology*, New York: Appleton-Century-Crofts (Prentice-Hall), 1972, chaps. 46–47.

Naremore, R. C., and R. B. Dever, "Language Performance of Educable Mentally Retarded and Normal Children at Five Age Levels," *Journal of Speech and Hearing Research*, **18** (March 1975), 89-95.

Nelson, W. E., *Textbook of Pediatrics*, 7th ed., Philadelphia: W. B. Saunders Company, 1959.

Newman, H. H., *Multiple Human Births*, New York: Doubleday & Co., Inc., 1940.

O'Neill, J. J., *The Hard of Hearing*, Englewood Cliffs, N.J.: Prentice-Hall, Inc., 1964.

Peckarasky, A., *Maternal Attitudes Toward Children with Psychogenically Delayed Speech*. Doctoral dissertation (unpublished), New York University, School of Education, 1952.

Penfield, W., and L. Roberts, *Speech and Brain Mechanisms*, Princeton, N.J.: Princeton University Press, 1959, pp. 251–255.

Pronovost, W., and M. P. Wakstein, "A Longitudinal Study of the Speech Behavior and Language Comprehension of Fourteen Children Diagnosed Atypical or Autistic," *Exceptional Children*, **33** (1966), 19–26.

Rimland, B., *Infantile Autism*, New York: Appleton-Century-Crofts, 1964. (An extensive report on theories as to the cause of autism in children. Excellent research on information available up to the date of the publication of the book.)

Rutter, M., ed., *Infantile Autism: Concepts, Characteristics and Treatment*, London: Churchill, 1971. (A multi-authored book that includes pertinent essays on childhood autism, cognition and language.)

Silverman, S. R., in L. E. Travis, ed., *Handbook of Speech Pathology and Audiology*, New York: Appleton-Century-Crofts (Prentice-Hall), 1972, 398–430.

Silvern, W. A., *Dunham's Premature Infants*, 3rd ed. New York: Paul B. Hoeber, 1961, pp. 76–83.

Smith, M. E., "Measurement of Vocabularies of Young Bilingual Children in Both of the Languages Used," *Journal of Genetic Psychology*, **74**, (June 1949), 305–310.

Van Riper, C., *Speech Correction*, 5th ed., Englewood Cliffs, N. J.: Prentice-Hall Inc., 1972, chap. 4. (The chapter surveys the causes and treatment of delayed speech and contains suggestions for stimulating language in reluctant speakers.)

Williams, F. ed., *Language and Poverty*, Chicago: Markham Publishing Co., 1970. (A series of essays on dialects, especially of persons who are economically disadvantaged. Attitudes of dialect speakers and the educational and social implications of "substandard" dialect speakers are considered.)

Williams, F., and R. Naremore, "Social Class Differences in Children's Syntactic Performances," *Journal of Speech and Hearing Research*, **12** (1969), 777–793.

Wing, J. K., ed., *Early Childhood Autism*, Oxford, England: Pergamon Press, 1966.

Wood, K. S., "Parental Maladjustment and Functional Articulatory Defects in Children," *Journal of Speech Disorders*, **11** (December 1946), 255–275.

Wood, N. E., *Delayed Speech and Language Development*, Englewood Cliffs, N. J.: Prentice-Hall, Inc., 1964. (A concise monograph on language development, causes of delayed speech, and therapeutic procedures; includes many pertinent annotated references on delayed speech.)

10. Defects of Articulation (I) Theory

Of all speech disorders, public school personnel encounter articulatory defects most frequently. Neal (1976) indicates that his study of public school speech clinics shows that 65.5 per cent of the cases handled by the speech clinicians involve articulation disorders. The National Institute of Neurological Diseases and Stroke (1969) cites that 3.0 per cent of the population within the ages from five to 21 have functional articulatory defects. This percentage is higher than for all the other speech difficulties combined; in fact, in this population, about three fifths of all speech defects are of an articulatory nature.

Definition of Articulatory Defects

Articulatory defects fall, in general, into three categories: (1) the substitution of one sound for another; (2) the omission of sounds; and (3) the distortion of sounds.

This categorization is based on the way the listener perceives the sounds. Since clinicians today generally diagnose articulatory defects in this way, the categorization based on listener perception is used. On the other hand, we might have looked at the problem of articulatory difficulties from the viewpoint of the child-speaker who may be applying a deviant but consistent set of phonological rules.

233

SUBSTITUTION OF ONE SOUND FOR ANOTHER

The substitution of one sound for another is the type of articulatory error that children in the primary grades make most frequently. In a detailed study, Snow (1963) reports on the sounds most frequently substituted for other sounds. She found these substitutions most frequent: /ʃ/, /ts/, and /s/ for /tʃ/; /θ/ and /f/ for /s/; /f/, /s/, /t/ for /θ/; /s/ and /tʃ/ for /ʃ/; /d/ and /v/ for /ð/; /dz/ and /tʃ/ for /dʒ/; /dz/ and /s/ for /z/; /z/, /dʒ/, /dz/ for /ʒ/; /w/ for /r/; /w/ for /l/; /w/ for /ʍ/, and /l/ for /j/. An examination of these data reveals that the substitutions have many of the same phonetic features as does the incorrect sound. For example, in comparing /θ/ and /s/, both are fricatives and both are unvoiced; the difference lies in the parts of the articulatory mechanism involved. /θ/ involves the tip of the tongue and the cutting edges of the teeth, whereas, /s/ involves the tip of the tongue and the alveolar ridge or the ridge behind the lower teeth. In comparing the sounds in the substitution /w/ for /r/, both are glides and both are voiced. The difference again lies in the involvement of particular articulatory agents. In comparing /d/ for /ð/, both are voiced but the manner of articulation is different, for /d/ is a stop whereas /ð/ is a fricative. Furthermore, the articulatory agents involved are different, for /d/ is made with the tip of the tongue on the teeth ridge and /ð/ is made with the tip of the tongue against the cutting edges of the teeth. All in all, the phonetic features of the substitutions and the correct sounds share many characteristics; despite their differences, there are many basic similarities.

The following are substitutions made by a seven-year-old boy and by a six-year-old girl. Indicate the substitutions, as /s/ for /θ/, and, according to the system just described, identify the changes as:

	/s/	/θ/
Place of Articulation	Tip of tongue and alveolar ridge.	Tip of tongue on cutting edges of teeth.

Then, using the system of distinctive features as noted in Chapter 6, list the changes in features as:

	/s/	/θ/
	/+ strident/	/- strident/

Substitutions made by Mary, a six-year-old girl in a large school system:

[sʌm]	for *thumb*
[tusbrʌʃ]	for *toothbrush*
[tæt]	for *cat*
[stos]	for *stove*
[naɪs]	for *knife*
[tɪkɪ]	for *chicken*

Substitutions made by Jimmy, a seven-year-old boy:

[stɝ·ɔl]	for *squirrel*
[prʌʃ]	for *brush*
[trʌm]	for *drum*
[lɛlo]	for *yellow*
[fɛdɚ]	for *feather*

Most children seemingly are not consistent in their substitutions. They may substitute /f/ for /θ/ in one word and not in another. They may substitute /f/ for /θ/ but also substitute /θ/ for /s/. Consistent patterns of substitution may seem to occur infrequently. But when the substitutions are analyzed carefully, a pattern usually emerges (see Oller 1973). The child devises a set of rules that translates the usual sounds heard in adult speech into a different but particular phonetic form. Usually, as noted later, the substitutions maintain many of the features of the target sound and are easier to produce. In general, children are more likely to make substitutions when the sound occurs in the middle or at the end of a word than when it occurs at the beginning of a word.

THE ROLE OF DISTINCTIVE FEATURES IN SUBSTITUTIONS

Research by Menyuk (1968) points to the importance of the distinctive features of consonants. She studied the mastery of consonantal sounds in terms of gravity and diffuseness (aspects of place of articulation); stridency, nasality, and continuancy (aspects of manner of articulation); and the vocal component (presence or absence of voice) for two groups: (a) children with normal speech development for whom data were obtained by transcribing phonetically the substitutions made as the children were spontaneously generating sentences, and (b) children with articulatory difficulties, for whom data were obtained by giving the Templin-Darley Articulation Test and analyzing the results.

The data for the group with normal speech development were analyzed by determining the percentage of sounds containing a feature that was used correctly at various ages in the developmental period of two and a half to five years of age. The rank order of use of features in correctly uttered phonemes was (1) nasal, (2) grave, (3) voice, (4) diffuse, (5) continuant, (6) strident. In other words, the feature first mastered in terms of percentage of correct usage was nasality (the presence of nasal resonance as in /m/ and /n/); the second, grave (being produced at the periphery of the speech mechanism as /p/, /b/, /k/, and /g/); the third, the voicing or unvoicing feature; the fourth, the diffuse feature (involved in anterior sounds such as /t/, /d/, and /θ/; the fifth, the continuant feature; and the sixth, the strident feature, where interference is high as in the /tʃ/ and /s/.

Prather, Hedrick, and Kern (1975) in a study of 147 children found a somewhat similar progression in learning. The order they discovered was (1) nasal, (2) grave, (3) diffuse, (4) voice, (5) continuant, and (6) strident—reversing Menyuk's study in categories three and four and five and six. As Menyuk analyzed phonological developmental data, she found the rank order for Japanese children to be identical with that for American children. From this, one can hypothesize that the ability of children to perceive and then to produce distinctive linguistic features of sounds is universal. The features dominating the acquisition of phonemes in the early stages of morphemic structure are two aspects of manner of production—use of nasality and use of voice—and one aspect of place of articulation, grave—placement in periphery of the mechanism.

In her analysis of distinctive features of phonology of children with articulatory defects, Menyuk makes the point that children in learning to utter a phoneme must perceive several features. She notes that distinction between sounds that differ in the feature of place of articulation causes the greatest difficulty. In *tate* for *cake*, /t/ and /d/ are alike except that /t/ is an alveolar sound and /k/ is a palatal sound. The other feature she mentions is continuancy in manner of production, as *tink* for *think*. She observes that when two features are disturbed, as *date* for *cake*, where the substitution involves both the place of articulation and voicing, the speech becomes less intelligible.

It is obvious that considerable phonetic likenesses exist between the substituted sound and the target sound. Usually the change involves no more than two features and often only one. Much of the change seems to be related to ease of production. For example, in the substitutions of /f/ for /θ/ and /w/ for /l/, the only distinctive feature change is from /+coronal/ to /-coronal/ (a feature involving the front of the tongue). When we think in terms of articulatory phonetics, the only change is in the manner of production in both substitutions (see Cairns and Williams 1972; and McReynolds, Engmann, and Dimmitt 1974). Winitz (1972) notes that the phonetic similarity of the sound to be learned and the sound that is substituted may be an important variable governing phonetic acquisition.

Leonard (1973) found that the feature errors of the children in the Cairns and Williams (1972) study were precisely those used most frequently by children he studied who were receiving therapy in a public school setting. Both groups of children used errors that were characterized by distinctive feature sets that required only the addition of one or two features to achieve the target sound. He notes that children who exhibit such errors as substituting /w/ for /r/, /d/ for /ð/, and /f/ for /θ/ eventually will develop standard articulation. Maturity will help these children to reach adult articulatory proficiency.

Leonard points out, however, that another group of children acquire articulation in a deviant manner. He bases this conclusion partly on the Menyuk study just cited. He notes that children who follow the Menyuk schedule but who are acquiring sounds later than their peers are simply using a less mature phonological system. Other children, however, are following a deviant pattern wherein the features /+ strident/, /- anterior/, and /+ continuant/ are seldom maintained in their substitutions. Leonard found that out of 200 children with articulatory difficulties not caused by known organic or intellectual factors, 70 per cent showed deviant errors.

Some writers point out that the existing distinctive feature systems are not always practical for the speech clinician. They believe that a particular distinctive feature may be overgeneralized and may encompass too great a phonetic space. Walsh (1974) contrasts the Jakobsonian theory of distinctive features with one of language-specific articulation features, which he believes helps the clinician to see the sort of articulatory problems involved in certain cases. He illustrates with the use of the substitution of /j/ for /l/, noting that this would be described in (Jakobsonian) theory as a change in such features as vocalic, consonantal, and coronal, all of which are used to differentiate large classes of sounds. Walsh describes his preference as follows:

	/l/	/r/
Lower articulator	+ tongue tip	- tongue tip
	- tongue blade	+ tongue blade

Upper articulator	+ tooth ridge	- tooth ridge
	- prepalate	+ prepalate

Walsh notes that when the substitution is described in this way, the misarticulation can be seen either as a retracted articulation rendering a lateral release impossible or as a motor failure requiring compensatory articulation in a retracted position.

Such lack of precision in the distinctive feature analysis of phonetic events, as illustrated, leads to questions concerning the theory's potential as a model of speech production. For example, Gallagher and Shriner (1975) found that /s/ and /z/ were more likely to be produced correctly when followed by /t/ and /d/ than when followed by other sounds. Distinctive feature theory would classify /s/ and /z/ as having more features in common with /θ/ and /ð/ than with /t/ and /d/. Gallagher and Shriner explain that their results may be influenced by the similarity between /θ/ and /ð/ and their children's incorrect productions of /s/ and /z/. In this area, the need for more research and phonological analysis is evident.

OMISSION OF SOUNDS

A sound may be omitted. The following are examples of omissions of sounds by David, a ten-year-old boy:

[bɛd]	for *bread*
[dɛs]	for *dress*
[taɪ]	for *try*
[ten]	for *train*

Most youngsters will not be as consistent as this child in omitting sounds. Their omissions may be more like those of Susie, a five-year-old, whose examples follow:

Air you dowin? [er jʊ doɪn]	for *Where are you going?*
Me ante o too. [mi ɑntə o tu]	for *I want to go too.*
I or? [aɪ or]	for *Why for?*

Omissions occur much more frequently in the young child's speech than they do in the older child's speech. Children omit final consonants more often than the initial or medial consonant. They commonly omit one of the sounds in clusters of two consonants, such as *tr*[tr], *pr*[pr], *st*[st], or *sl*[sl]. But as children grow older, their *pide* becomes *pride*. Omissions then are not particularly common and tend to decrease after the age of three.

The clinician needs to be aware that some omissions of sounds are indexes of lack of syntactical rather than articulatory development. For instance, the child who says *ask* for *asked* or *five pencil* for *five pencils* may not have as much of an articulatory problem as a syntactical one.

DISTORTION OF SOUNDS

A sound may be distorted. The listener recognizes the sound for what it is, but is distracted by it. The way the sound is made calls attention to it. Laymen, in describing a distorted *s*, make such remarks as: "Her *s* whistles" or "Her *s* has a slushy *sh* sound." In the whistling *s*, too much air is escaping, and in the slushy *s*, air is escaping over the sides of the tongue.

Winitz (1975, p. 2) defines *distortion* as a substitution of an uncommon English sound for the target sound. He describes a lateral lisp as a sound that is voiceless, made with more frication than the normal /s/, and lateralized. He uses the symbol /ɬ/ for the lateral lisp. The /l/ indicates the lateral quality (both sides of the tongue are lowered); the /-/ indicates the dark quality of the /l/; and /o/ indicates the voiceless quality.

Degree and Severity of Articulatory Difficulty

The severity of an articulatory difficulty depends on how greatly it reduces the intelligibility of the speech and the concern it gives the producer. The degree of intelligibility is related to the number of sounds omitted, substituted, and distorted; the distortion of sounds is least important in intelligibility. When the child omits many sounds and substitutes many sounds for others, speech becomes almost unintelligible. The simplest way for a classroom teacher to evaluate the severity of a defect is to count the number of sounds that are omitted, substituted, and distorted. Many quite complex systems of evaluation of degree of severity have been devised. Most of these still need refinement and are used mainly by speech clinicians.

Children may either accept and acknowledge their difficulties, reject them, and/or insist they do not exist, or be overly concerned with them.

A teacher is of inestimable worth in fostering the attitude of acceptance and in motivating students to do what they can to correct the difficulty. Both the teacher and the clinician may have to help the children see that their speech needs to, and should be, corrected. The teacher and clinician must assist the children in perceiving their errors in articulation and in isolating them. In some cases, parents insulate the child against therapy because they believe that a particular articulatory error is attractive. On the other hand, overperfectionist, nagging parents may cause the child to be unduly anxious about the difficulty. In one instance, the deviation or difference is approved; in the other it is penalized. The teacher must be aware of how the child perceives his/her own difficulty.

Concomitant Difficulties

Other speech problems may be associated with articulatory difficulties. For example, the child with a denasal voice has three defective sounds: m[m], n[n], and ng[ŋ]. The child with the muffled voice keeps his/her mouth almost clenched shut; the quality is in part the result of the lack of clear-cut articulation of sounds. These two difficulties are labeled voice disorders. The term *retarded speech development* includes many articulatory defects—omissions, substitutions, and distortions; in fact, some writers include their discussion of the articulatory defects of the primary-grade children under retarded speech development. Retarded speech development, however, does connote, in addition to articulatory difficulties, meager vocabulary, overly simple structure, and, in general, retarded language development. Cleft-palate speech and defective speech caused by impaired hearing are also characterized by articulatory difficulties. Even in cluttering, because of its rapid rate, the child noticeably slurs over and distorts the consonantal sounds. Thus, defective articulation may be a single problem to a child or it may be a symptom of a more complex syndrome.

Articulatory Disorders and Maturation

Because some parents show undue concern about their young children's ability to articulate, teachers must be particularly aware of the need for recognition of the maturing factor in diagnosing articulatory defects. One mother of a five-year-old boy in kindergarten came to a school to demand speech help for him. The only error he made with any consistency was to substitute [t] and [d] for the two *th's*[θ], [ð]. But at times even these sounds were correct. Occasionally he said a [w] for [l]. The mother insisted his speech was not "normal," explaining that his sister had spoken better at the same age, that his cousins of the same age spoke very well, and that the neighborhood youngsters who were even younger spoke more clearly. The little boy was a verbal child who expressed himself unusually well with very few articulatory errors. The teacher explained the part maturity plays in the development of articulation. Because the mother remained unconvinced, the teacher called in the clinician to reassure her. The teacher also suggested that the mother remain in the kindergarten room to listen to how other kindergartners spoke. In such a situation, referring to norms of the acquisition of sounds is sometimes helpful. A table of norms for articulatory acquisition follows.

NORMS FOR THE ACQUISITION OF SOUNDS

Schedules for the acquisition of sounds are listed on pages 151–153. A schedule, which is school grade oriented, is included here. This schedule (Sax 1972) is based on the criterion that 93 per cent of the children produce the sound accurately.

Grade	Males	Females
Beginning kindergarten	/p/, /b/, /m/, /w/, /j/, /h/, /t/, /d/, /n/, /k/, /g/, /ŋ/.	/p/, /b/, /m/, /w/, /j/, /h/, /t/, /d/, /n/, /k/, /g/, /ŋ/, /f/
Beginning first grade	/f/	—
End of first grade	/v/	/v/, /ð/
End of second grade	/ð/	/θ/, /l/
End of third grade	/θ/	/r/
End of fourth grade	/ʃ/, /ʒ/, /tʃ/, /dʒ/.	/ʃ/, /ʒ/, /tʃ/, /dʒ/
End of fifth grade	/l/	—

PROGNOSIS FOR IMPROVEMENT THROUGH MATURATION

Maturation alone takes care of some of the articulatory difficulties in the primary grades. For some children, the impact of the regular kindergarten curriculum and maturation will bring about satisfactory phonological development. The amount and kind of language stimulation provided in the kindergarten may make a considerable difference in the child's development. Other children, however, even with time do not develop phonologically. Therefore, the clinician needs to be able to predict which of the children will need speech help. Almost all of the studies point to stimulability scores as one index of whether a child will develop a normal phonological system. Therefore, to find out whether children can imitate the clinician's utterance of the target sound in a nonsense syllable and in words seems to be one index of subsequent improvement (Carter and Buck 1958; and Farquhar 1961).

A more precise way of predicting is through the Van Riper and Erickson *Predictive Screening Test of Articulation*, 3rd ed. (1973) (Western Michigan University Continuing Education Office, Kalamazoo, Michigan). This test identifies those primary-age school children with functional misarticulations who are not likely to acquire normal, mature articulation by the time they reach third-grade level. As the results of a study of the predictive capability of this test, Barrett and Welsh (1975) conclude that it is a valuable instrument in the speech adequacy screening of the first-grade population. They note that the test can identify first-grade children whose articulation problems are not likely to disappear without therapy by the third grade. The clinician can, therefore, efficiently select those children who need clinical help.

More generalized predictive factors were reported by Irwin (1966). In a study to identify factors or measures predicting improvement in speech, language, and auditory skills, she found that improvement in articulation can be predicted by mental age, scores in articulation, and stimulability. The more severe the articulatory defect, the more improvement appears to occur. Good stimulability scores at the beginning of therapy will predict probable success.

Testing for Errors

Various screening devices are used to locate children in a school population who may need articulation therapy. This initial screening is usually planned by the clinician and is often administered by the classroom teacher. It includes such items as the following:

1. Giving name and address.
2. Naming of objects in pictures that contain the sibilant sounds /s/, /z/, /ʃ/, /ʒ/, /tʃ/, /dʒ/; the two *th* sounds /θ/ and /ð/; /l/, /r/, and /j/ as in *yellow*.
3. Counting to ten or naming the days of the week.
4. Holding conversations often based on children's books that will hold the interest of young children. These books should contain pictures

that will evoke conversation that will include the sounds most likely to be inaccurate. Two such books are:

Gunella Walde, *Tommy and Sarah Dress Up* (Boston: Houghton Mifflin Company, 1972). Tommy and Sarah find a trunk in Sarah's attic with many old clothes. The two children proceed to "dress up."

E. Rice, *Oh, Lewis* (New York: Macmillan Publishing Co., Inc., 1974). Lewis and his mother and sister go shopping. Lewis has to have help buckling his boots, zippering his jacket, finding his mittens, and getting his coat hood on right. He has just as much trouble getting his outer clothes off.

Screening test results, whether administered by the clinician or by the teacher, are influenced by many factors. Regardless of training, examiners often differ in their estimates of a child's articulatory ability. Even when they administer the same test to the same child, differences in test results may exist. Such factors as the following influence the results: (1) The rapport the child feels with the examiner may make considerable difference; psychological studies note that reinforcement with nothing but an appreciatively uttered "m-m-m-m" makes a difference in psychological scores. (2) One examiner's perception of sounds uttered by a child may be different from another's. For instance one may hear an /s/, which seemingly approximates a /θ/, whereas another may hear the same /s/ as within a normal range. (3) The distractions within the environment play a role. To test a child in a teacher's room with teachers constantly entering and leaving is bound to modify the child's performance. (4) Obviously examiners may use different instruments some of which may be more successful than others in locating articulatory deviations.

An example of differences in judgment is provided by Irwin's study (1970), which investigated the consistency of the clinician in making judgments of articulatory production and the effect of instruction, experience, and varying intervals of time on the judgments. Undergraduates in speech pathology were relatively consistent in the way they responded to the evaluation of articulation production. Inconsistencies were higher when misarticulations were being evaluated than when correct productions were being considered. There was more inconsistency when the testing occurred by means of trios (as *that, goat, cake*) than in words or phrases. As students advanced in training in speech pathology, more inconsistencies appeared. Their standards for correct production may have been uncertain; or perhaps there existed some inadequate perceptual abilities.

Testing is done either through imitation (Say after me), spontaneously (Look at this picture. What is this?), or in a combination of the two. Studies seem to indicate that the spontaneous method elicits more errors than the imitative one. The same results hold for children of ages six through 11, kindergartners, first graders, and even four-year-olds [see Lencione and Trent (1965), Smith and Ainsworth (1967), and Krescheck and Socolofsky (1972)].

Tests that were especially devised to evaluate phonological behavior are most often administered by speech clinicians. Sounds are usually tested in three positions: initial, where the sound begins the word; medial, where it is in the middle of the word; and final, where it ends the word.[1]

Criteria on which clinicians base their choice of articulation tests include the following:

1. The rationale behind the test (order of development of sounds, distinctive features, frequency of occurrence of sounds, coarticulation of sounds that can indicate the influence of one sound on another, connected speech, single words, or phrases).
2. Administrative facility (time to administer and to score, and ease of administration and scoring).
3. Population to be tested. For example, Drumwright, Van Natta, Camp, Frankenburg, and Drexler (1973) describe the development of an articulation screening test for economically disadvantaged children.
4. Diagnostic purposes.

The following tests are representative of many in the field that test the accuracy of each of the American English phonemes both singly and in blends. The errors are usually recorded as substitutions, omissions, or distortions.

Goldman and Fristoe's Test of Articulation (American Guidance Service, Circle Pines, Minnesota), based on a filmstrip, evaluates all necessary phonemes and obtains an adequate and accurate sample of

---

[1]Authorities debate whether the medial position should be legitimately included, because a sound in a medial position usually begins or ends a syllable. If one considers position in relation to syllables, only initial or final sounds would be included. Curtis and Hardy note that Stetson's analysis of articulatory dynamics, supported by considerable experimental data, appears to indicate that a consonant's function as either an initiating or terminating element of a syllable may be more significant than its position in a word (J. F. Curtis and J. G. Hardy, "A Phonetic Study of Misarticulation of /r/," *Journal of Speech and Hearing Disorders*, 2 (September 1959), 244–257). They note that classifying a sound as medial denotes the possible difference in functions, since a consonant in the medial position may be either initiating or terminating with respect to the syllable. Hence they use the classification as to whether the sound occurs before a vowel (prevocalic) or after a vowel (postvocalic) within a syllable. J. S. Keenan, "What Is Medial Position?" *Journal of Speech and Hearing Disorders*, 26 (May 1961), 171–177, also suggests that the medial concept be discarded and that the classification be based, as Curtis recommends, on whether the consonant begins a syllable and precedes a vowel, whether it ends a syllable and follows the vowel, or whether it is part of a cluster (as the *l* in *pl*). Certain writers also express concern about the effect of neighboring sounds on the sound to be tested. Most current tests take these factors into consideration.

a child's behavior. Children are asked to respond to pictures by naming familiar objects or by answering questions about the pictures.

The Arizona Articulation Proficiency Scale (Western Psychological Services, Los Angeles, California) includes each phoneme of American English and /l/, /r/, and /s/ clusters with the norm age of the acquisition of each sound. It is based on the rationale that the more frequently a misarticulated sound is heard in speech, the greater is the weight of the articulatory problem.

These two tests are used largely to assess the adequacy of the child's articulatory performance. They are used to determine which children need to be in attendance at the school speech clinical facility. A second type of test, much more detailed, determines the ability of the child to use sounds in various phonetic contexts. In consequence, it provides the clinician with information on the child's ability to produce sounds not only in various positions but also in different phonetic contexts. In addition, it can be used to compare therapy, to evaluate progress, to select case loads, to determine consistency of misarticulations, and to identify factors related to misarticulations such as distinctive features. Brief descriptions of two such tests follow:

The Templin-Darley Test of Articulation, 2nd ed. (Bureau of Educational Research and Service, The University of Iowa, Iowa City, Iowa) is a revision and expansion of the original edition of the Templin-Darley Screening and Diagnostic Test of Articulation. The 141-item Diagnostic Test is subdivided into nine overlapping subtests including a screening test and the Iowa Pressure Articulation Test. A cutoff score is available for each age.

Another diagnostic test is McDonald's Deep Test of Articulation: Picture and Sentence Forms (Stanwix House, Pittsburgh, Pennsylvania). This test offers a different approach to the assessment and treatment of functional articulatory problems, for it is based on constructs derived from motor and acoustic phonetics, control theory, developmental psychology, and linguistics. It disavows the traditional concept of initial, medial, and final consonants, and assesses instead simple and abutting consonants in a representative sampling of phonetic contexts.

Factors Associated with Articulatory Difficulties

LANGUAGE DEFICITS

Many authorities believe that most children with deficiencies in articulatory development also have deficiencies in other aspects of language development. Ferrier's (1966) study, reported in some detail in Chapter 1, indicates that children with articulatory difficulties do not do as well in language as measured by all nine tests of the Illinois Test of Psycholinguistic Abilities (1st ed.) as do children with normal speech. For the children with articulatory defects, the scores on four tests were substantially lower, indicating that these children do not do as well as normal-speaking children in expressing ideas verbally, using grammatical structures automatically, recalling a series of digits presented to them orally, and recalling a series of geometric forms presented to them visually. Smith (1967) reports a correlated finding on a digit recall test.

Marquardt and Saxman (1972), in a study of language comprehension and auditory discrimination in articulatory-deficient kindergarten children, found that those children with normal articulatory ability performed significantly better than those with poor articulatory ability on Carrow's Test of Auditory Language Comprehension. They noted that the level of linguistic knowledge is less for the poor articulation group than for the high articulation group, and that the children who made the greater number of articulatory errors also tended to make the greater number of auditory comprehension errors.

Other studies point to the ability of normal-speaking children to use more sophisticated syntactical structures than do children with functional articulatory abilities. Menyuk (1964) reports that in comparing children with infantile speech[2] with children with normal speech (ages 3–5.10), the normal-speaking children used significantly more transformations than the defective-speech group, and the group with infantile speech used more restricted forms and used them much more frequently than the normal-speaking group. The child with normal speech rapidly acquired structures that required increasingly complex rules for their generation over the two- to three-year period, and exceeded in acquisition of structures even the oldest infantile-speech child. There was no significant difference in the mean number of sentences used.

The results seem to indicate that the most meaningful factor is the difference in the two groups' ability to determine the complete set of rules used to generate and differentiate structures at any level of grammar. Examples of transformation types are

---

[2] This category would seem to be comprised of the more severe articulatory cases. According to Menyuk (1964, p. 119) the most frequent sound errors were omissions and substitutions. Furthermore, 50 per cent of the infantile-speech children omitted initial /s/ and final /t/, and more than 50 per cent of the children used these substitutions: /w/ for /r/ and /l/, /t/ for /k/ and / θ/, /d/ for /g/ and / ð/.

Negation—*He isn't a good boy.*[3]
Question—*Are you nice?*
Contraction—*He'll be good.*
Auxiliary *be* placement—*He is not going.*
Relative clause—*I don't know what he is doing.*
Iteration—*You have to drink milk to be strong.*

Examples of restricted forms are:

Verb phrase omission—*This green.*
Noun phrase redundancy—*I want it the paint.*
Preposition substitution—*He took me at the circus.*
Pronoun subject substitution—*Me like that.*

Similarly, Vandemark and Mann (1965) found that the significant difference between a group of 50 normal-speaking children and 50 children with defective articulation was in the syntactical complexity, which involved grammatical completeness and complexity of response. According to this study, children with defective articulation are not inhibited in terms of amount of verbal output but are deficient in areas of grammatical completeness and complexity of response.

Shriner, Holloway, and Daniloff (1969), in a study of 30 children with normal articulation and 30 with defective articulation, found that the mean number of words per response was significantly lower for the speech-defective group than for the normal-speaking group. They agree with Vandermark and Mann that the children with defective articulation do not use as developed a syntactical structure as the normal-speaking children. This study used a method of evaluating the complexity of sentences that differed from the Vandermark and Mann study in that these researchers counted the number of noun phrases and verb phrases.

Lee (1966) compared the syntactical development of two boys— one normal, the other deviant in articulatory development. She found marked differences between them. Not only was the speech deviant slower in following a normal pattern of behavior but he failed to produce certain types of syntactic structures.

The lack of syntactical development may be related to the lack of articulatory development. Perhaps a neurological impairment, maturational delay, or a defective auditory and/or proprioceptive feedback that causes the defective articulation may bring about syntactical lags.

---

[3] Transformed from such basic structures as *He is a good boy* and *You are nice.*

Or the child who misarticulates, having been made aware of his inadequacy, may speak infrequently and thus have less of an opportunity to experiment with syntactical forms. More research is needed before the significance of the coexistence of deficits in syntactical and articulatory development can be explained.

LOW INTELLIGENCE

Some studies show a high incidence of articulatory defects among children who are definitely feeble-minded. Undoubtedly, many organic conditions, such as brain injury, contribute to both deficient articulatory and mental abilities.

In a study, representative of others, of the articulatory development of 415 mental retardates, Wilson (1966) found that 53.4 per cent had defective articulation, whereas 46.6 per cent had normal speech. As the mental age increases, the total number of deviant sounds decreases but the articulatory pattern is not orderly. Several sibilant, affricative, and fricative sounds are never produced by 90 per cent of the children through the nine-year mental age level. The articulatory development of the mentally retarded does not parallel the development of normal children even when the mental age of the retardate is matched against the chronological age of the normal child.

When the articulatory defect is typed according to omission, substutution, or distortion, and even to the type of sound substitution, the relationship between intellectual ability and articulatory difficulties is refined. For example, Prins (1962b), in a comparison of speech-handicapped and normal children, found that children with defective articulation errors of the omission type were lower in intelligence as measured by a receptive vocabulary test than were the normal-speaking children. But when the articulatory errors consisted chiefly of interdentalization of /s/ or /z/, or the use of phonemic sound substitutions in which only one articulatory feature is altered, there was no significant difference in intellectual ability as measured by a receptive vocabulary test.

SOCIOECONOMIC STATUS

Prins (1962a) also did correlations between a variety of articulatory variables and socioeconomic status. He found that subjects with a high proportion of interdental lisping (where /s/ is produced with the tongue visible between the teeth) tend to come from high socioeconomic levels, whereas subjects with a high proportion of omission-type errors come from low socioeconomic levels.

Adler (1973) in a study involving articulatory deviances and social class membership lists these results: (1) Lower-class children manifested a greater number of omissions and substitutions in all positions than did middle-class children. (2) There was no great distinction between classes for the omission of final consonants. (3) Middle-class children exhibited a higher incidence figure in distortions on all three sound positions in words. (4) Many /θ/ and /ð/ deviances existed regardless of social class. (5) /r/ was incorrectly produced more often by white children than by black children.

HEARING LOSS

We have already stressed the relationship between adequate hearing and the ability to learn to speak. Although children's hearing may be sufficient for understanding conversation and what goes on around them, it may be insufficient for learning to make all the sounds. Some sounds children may not hear at all. Their own speech, therefore, reflects their inability to hear. Peripherally deaf children almost always have defective articulation, for they are unable to imitate sounds. They cannot compare the sounds they utter with those produced by others. In fact, they cannot hear the sounds of any model. Their abilities to see and to feel cannot make up for their inability to hear. We discuss the problem of the child with a hearing loss more fully in Chapter 14.

STRUCTURAL ABNORMALITIES

Anomalies of the tongue, lips, teeth, and palate have long been associated with articulatory difficulties. Recently, however, attitudes have changed on the responsibility of organic deviations of the articulatory mechanism for articulatory defects. For instance, the literature in the field of speech therapy presents opposing viewpoints on the responsibility of dental abnormalities for defective articulation. Undoubtedly, for some children, malocclusion of the teeth or an abnormally large tongue contribute to the child's lack of articulatory development. But some children with similar organic difficulties do not misarticulate the same sounds whereas other children with a normal mechanism do misarticulate them. Poor structures may, however, be a contributing factor in explaining poor articulation.

TEETH AND GUM RIDGE

The teeth and/or gum ridge are involved in the sounds [f], [v], [θ], [ð], [s], [z], [ʃ], [ʒ], [tʃ], and [dʒ]. In [f] and [v] the upper teeth touch the lower lip. In [θ] and [ð] the tongue tip is placed against the biting edge of the upper teeth or between the two rows of teeth. In the sibilant sounds, the air is directed against the teeth in a variety of ways. In some cases the teeth have difficulty reaching the lower lip, the biting edge is badly located, or the teeth are so formed that it is difficult to find a surface of teeth against which to direct the air.

The condition where the upper front teeth protrude abnormally beyond the lower teeth is called an overbite. When the upper lip meets the lower one with difficulty, [p], [b], and [m] may be defective. The tongue lies forward in the mouth, sometimes over the lower teeth. The lower teeth are so far back that they cannot provide the necessary friction to make a good [s] or [z]. With this condition the lower jaw usually recedes.

In other cases the lower jaw protrudes and the lower front teeth project over the upper front teeth. This condition is called an underbite and is usually associated with an undershot jaw.

In still other cases, a space occurs between the upper and lower teeth when they are brought together. This condition is called an open bite. Normally the upper incisor overlaps its counterpart on the lower jaw so that about one third of the surface of the visible lower incisor is covered by the upper incisor. In an open bite [s] and [z] are most frequently defective since the narrow stream of air cannot be directed against the cutting edge of the teeth. Sometimes [ʃ], [ʒ], [θ], and [ð] are distorted. If the lips cannot be brought together [p], [b], and [m] may be defective. When the lower lip cannot touch the teeth easily, [f] and [v] may be inaccurate.

Finally, a space may occur between the central incisors or the canine teeth may be irregularly placed. In both these instances [s] may be defective. When the space occurs, too much air is allowed to escape. Where the teeth are irregularly placed, they may interfere with the tongue so that the air is allowed to escape over one or both of its sides. Frequently, however, individuals themselves, finding compensatory movements, speak well in spite of having teeth that are very irregular.

It should be noted that many children with missing or abnormal teeth do make sounds correctly and some children with normal teeth do not make sounds correctly. Teachers and clinicians should also remember that missing teeth usually do not permanently influence the speech production of children.

TONGUE

The term *tongue-tied* is applied when the frenum of the tongue (the little web of tissue underneath the front part of the tongue) is abnormally short so that the tip of the tongue cannot move to points such as the ridge behind the upper teeth. This condition, where it severely disturbs articulation, is comparatively rare in children.

Other conditions may involve the tongue. The sounds that may be disturbed because of the tongue are [k], [g], [ŋ], [θ], [ð], [l], [r], [s], [z], [ʃ], and [ʒ]. In some few cases the tongue is so large or sluggish that it cannot make the small, precise, and quick movements that are necessary for certain sounds. Sometimes the tongue may be paralyzed or weak. At other times, there may be poor muscular coordination. Occasionally a thyroid deficiency causes sluggishness and poor control of the tongue, the result of generally poor motor coordination.

In [l] and [r], the tongue tip points to the teeth ridge. In [s] and [z], the tongue is grooved to direct a small stream of air against the teeth. In [n], [t], and [d], the tongue touches the teeth ridge. In [ʃ] and [ʒ], the tongue directs a broader channel of air against the teeth. In the sibilant sounds, the tip of the tongue may reach toward the upper gum. In teaching the sibilants, however, clinicians sometimes find it better not to have the child try to reach toward the upper gum but to have him or her reach toward the gum behind the lower teeth. The tongue is obviously an important articulatory agent.

TONGUE THRUST

Some dentists refer children to the speech clinician for a neuromuscular syndrome commonly called "tongue thrust." Some clinicians attempt to differentiate between tongue thrusting as a temporary developmental phase and as a permanent practice and attempt to retrain. Swallowing, however, is a complex reflex action that is difficult to retrain permanently. At this point more research is needed to establish clearly the role of the speech therapist in tongue thrusts. Because of the uncertain status of myofunctional therapy (teaching of proper tongue posturing and movements), the American Speech and Hearing Association in cooperation with a committee from the American Association of Dental Schools (1975) drafted the following position paper:

A growing concern with the creation of clinical programs of myofunctional therapy and the involvement of some speech pathologists in these programs led the American Speech and Hearing Association to seek an assessment of the current status of these clinical management procedures from the Joint Committee on Dentistry and Speech Pathology-Audiology. The Committee is composed of representatives of the ASHA and the American Association of Dental Schools (AADS). Based on a comprehensive study of relevant literature and a thorough evaluation of current clinical methodologies used to manage patients with an allegedly deviant pattern of deglutition frequently called tongue thrust swallow, the Committee developed the following statement

STATEMENT

Review of data from studies published to date has convinced the Committee that neither the validity of the diagnostic label tongue thrust nor
the contention that myofunctional therapy produces significant consistent
changes in oral form or function has been documented adequately. There
is insufficient scientific evidence to permit differentiation between normal
and abnormal or deviant patterns of deglutition, particularly as such
patterns might relate to occlusion and speech. There is unsatisfactory
evidence to support the belief that any patterns of movements defined as
tongue thrust by any criteria suggested to date should be considered
abnormal, detrimental, or representative of a syndrome. The few suitably
controlled studies that have incorporated valid and reliable diagnostic
criteria and appropriate quantitative assessments of therapy have demonstrated no effects on patterns of deglutition or oral structure. Thus,
research is needed to establish the validity of tongue thrust as a clinical
entity.

In view of the above considerations and despite our recognition that
some dentists call upon speech pathologists to provide myofunctional
therapy, at this time, there is no acceptable evidence to support claims of
significant, stable, long-term changes in the functional patterns of deglutition and significant, consistent alterations in oral form. Consequently, the
Committee urges increased research efforts, but cannot recommend that
speech pathologists engage in clinical management procedures with the
intent of altering functional patterns of deglutition (*ASHA*, 1975, p. 331).

PALATE

In sounds such as [ʃ] and [ʒ], the palate plays a part. When the
palate is abnormally high and narrow, the child's tongue may have
difficulty in making the necessary contacts. When an opening occurs
along the middle line of the palate, the condition is serious. This condition is discussed in a later chapter.

MOTOR ABILITY

Some children are poorly coordinated. Some youngsters run, go up- and
downstairs, and jump much more easily than others. One youngster
will put a jigsaw puzzle together and fit the pieces with little or no
effort; another will struggle with it. This motor ability develops with
maturation. But children of the same age vary widely in this ability.
Sometimes poor coordination is evident around the mouth; the tongue,
jaw, and palate are awkward. Some studies have shown that children
with articulatory defects tend to score significantly lower on tests of
motor ability than do children with normal speech. Such a study is
one undertaken by Jenkins and Lohr (1964) who compared motor

proficiency as measured by the Oseretsky Test of Motor Proficiency given to 38 first-grade children with "severe articulatory defects" and 38 normal-speaking controls matched for age, sex, and I.Q. The results of the study showed that the speech-defective group was significantly lower on the total test score and on each of the subtests administered. The tests involve maintaining bodily balance for a given period without gross movements of limbs or torso, performing coordinated hand activities within a time limit and with accuracy (cutting paper), maintaining balance while performing a given movement of the whole body, as in running or hopping, simultaneous voluntary movements, as in tapping the left and right feet alternately, or performing a given muscular activity without extraneous movements, such as clenching the teeth without wrinkling the forehead.

AUDITORY DISCRIMINATION AND AUDITORY MEMORY

As noted earlier in the discussion of articulatory testing, the examiners, the situation in which the child is being examined, the mood of the child, and the test itself all have impact on the assessment. The assessment is only as effective as are these components. The same attributes apply to the examination of a child's ability to discriminate or to remember sounds. In this testing situation you may find a child who is either consistently negativistic or consistently attempting to please the adult. Or the child may have an off day when nothing is of interest. Lastly, the test may actually test other variables than discrimination. Many discrimination tests present a series of paired comparisons. About the only place the child encounters paired words is in tests or in clinical situations (see Schwarz and Goldman 1974). Elenbogen and Thompson (1972) pose the question as to whether the Wepman Test of Discrimination does not measure a vocabulary factor in addition to auditory discrimination. Their study showed that social class differences in error scores disappeared when a distorted form of the Wepman Test with nonsense words was used.

Whether articulatory production depends on correct identification or whether correct identification depends upon production is not completely clear. Perception may well be somewhat more closely related to articulation than to the acoustic stimuli, and consequently phonemic perception may be a function of motor mediation (Monin and Huntington 1974). For example, Williams and McReynolds (1975) found that articulatory production training was effective in changing both articulation and discrimination, whereas discrimination training was effective only in changing discrimination. Gottesman (1972) notes that the implication of her investigation is that differences in auditory discrimination between children speaking the Negro dialect and those speaking Standard English may be explained by differences in pronunciation; she found no differences between the two groups in auditory discrimination performance on words that could be commonly differentiated in the speech of all the children. Marquardt and Saxman (1972) report that in their study the articulatory proficient group made fewer errors in discrimination than did the poor articulatory group.

Similar questions arise as to auditory memory. Locke and Kutz (1975), emphasizing what may be the effect of motor feedback, make the point that whereas speech learning requires memory, memory also depends on speech. Spontaneous speech and subvocal rehearsal both facilitate memory performance. Locke and Kutz found that children who could distinguish between /w/ and /r/, but who consistently spoke /w/ for /r/, made more /w/-/r/ confusions in recall than did children who produced /w/ and /r/ accurately. They suggest that the differences in the production but not in the perception of /w/ and /r/ of the two groups may be the result of the motor experience, which directly or indirectly provides the salient memory clues.

More research needs to be undertaken to determine the roles of auditory discrimination and memory in articulatory production.

Problems

1. Give an articulatory test to two first graders.
   a. List the substitutions.
      1) By checking with the norms and by using a stimulability test, indicate your conclusions as to whether the substitution will be taken care of with maturation.
      2) By using a feature analysis, compare the substitutions with the target sounds. Find out whether you can detect a pattern.
   b. If a distortion exists, indicate the type of distortion phonetically.
   c. By observation or by use of a language test, note what you think the relationship is between articulatory development and syntactical development.
2. Give a sound discrimination test to two children—one in the primary grades and one in the middle grades. Note any differences that may exist.
3. If a case history of a child with an articulatory defect is available, note the information as to the child's:
   a) intellectual and language maturity.
   b) organs involved.
   c) diagnosis.

4. Give a screening test to two kindergarten children, following the procedures suggested in this chapter.
5. Find three children with missing front teeth. Is there a relationship of this condition to their production of /s/ and /z/?
6. Read and report on any one of the following references:
Faircloth and Faircloth 1970.
Gottesman 1972.
Lawrence and Potter 1970.
Perozzi 1973.
Sommers, Cox, and West 1972.

References and Suggested Readings

Adler, S., "Articulatory Deviance and Social-Class Membership," *Journal of Learning Disabilities*, **6** (December 1973), 650–654.

American Speech and Hearing Association Joint Committee with Dentistry, "Position Statement of Tongue-Thrust," *ASHA*, **17** (May 1975), 331–337.

American Speech and Hearing Association, "Task Force Report on School Hearing and Language Screening," *Language, Speech, and Hearing Services in Schools*, **4** (July 1973), 109–119. (Gives basic principles in screening and suggests methods and materials for screening.)

Barrett, C. M., and H. R. Hoops, "The Relationship Between Self-Concept and the Remission of Articulatory Errors," *Language, Speech, and Hearing Services in Schools*, **5** (April 1974), 67–70. (Studies children who do not spontaneously remit articulation errors in terms of self-concept and discrepancies between self-concept and ideal self-concept.)

Barrett, M. D., and J. W. Welsh, "Predictive Articulation Screening," *Language, Speech, and Hearing Services in Schools*, **6** (April 1975), 91–95. (Gives results of predictive capability of Van Riper Predictive Screening Test.)

Block, E. L., and L. D. Goodstein, "Functional Speech Disorders and Personality: A Decade of Research," *Journal of Speech and Hearing Disorders*, **35** (August 1971), 295–314. (Includes a section on relationship of articulatory defects to (a) personality and adjustment of parents, and (b) personality and adjustment of children themselves.)

Cairns, H. S., and F. Williams, "An Analysis of the Substitution Errors of a Group of Standard English-Speaking Children," *Journal of Speech and Hearing Research*, **15** (December 1972), 811–820.

Carter, E. T., and M. Buck, "Prognostic Testing for Functional Articulation Disorders among Children in the First Grade," *Journal of Speech and Hearing Disorders*, **23** (May 1958), 124–133.

Cohen, J. H., and C. F. Diehl, "Relation of Speech-Sound Discrimination Ability to Articulation-Type Speech Defects," *Journal of Speech and Hearing Disorders*, **28** (May 1963), 187–190.

Cole, R. A., "Perceiving Syllables and Remembering Phonemes," *Journal of Speech and Hearing Research*, **16** (March 1973), 37–47. (Supports the concept that a syllable is a temporal grouping of independently coded phonemes, that children are able to remember an entire syllable as a single perceptual unit in memory.)

Compton, A. J., "Generative Studies of Children's Phonological Disorders," *Journal of Speech and Hearing Disorders*, **35** (November 1970), 315–339. (Contains an analysis of two boys' development of a phonological system.)

Dickson, S., "Differences Between Children Who Spontaneously Outgrow and Children Who Retain Functional Articulation Errors," *Journal of Speech and Hearing Research*, **5** (September 1962), 263–271. (Studies the differences in motor proficiency, auditory discrimination, and emotional characteristics of parents of two groups: (1) those who outgrew functional articulatory errors, and (2) those who did not.)

Drumwright, A., P. Van Natta, B. Camp, W. Frankenburg, and H. Drexler, "The Denver Articulation Screening Examination," *Journal of Speech and Hearing Disorders*, **38** (February 1973), 3–14. (Describes the development of an articulation screening test for economically disadvantaged children.)

Elenbogen, E. M., and G. R. Thompson, "A Comparison of Social Class Effect in Two Tests of Auditory Discrimination," *Journal of Learning Disabilities*, **5** (April 1972), 209–212.

Faircloth, M. A., and S. R. Faircloth, "An Analysis of the Articulatory Behavior of a Speech-Defective Child in Connected Speech and in Isolated Word Responses," *Journal of Speech and Hearing Disorders*, **35** (February 1970), 51–61. (Supports the need for testing in connected speech.)

Farquhar, M., "Prognostic Value of Imitative and Auditory Discrimination Tests," *Journal of Speech and Hearing Disorders*, **26** (November 1961), 342–347.

Ferrier, E. E., "Investigation of ITPA Performance of Children with Functional Defects of Articulation," *Exceptional Child*, **32** (May 1966), 625–629.

Gallagher, T. M., and T. H. Shriner, "Articulatory Inconsistencies in the Speech of Normal Children," *Journal of Speech and Hearing Research*, **15** (March 1975), 168–175. (Shows that inconsistent production of /s/ and /z/ is related to motor sequencing constraints independent of word boundaries.)

———, "Contextual Variables Related to Consistent /s/ and /z/ Production in the Spontaneous Speech of Children," *Journal of Speech and Hearing Research*, **18** (December 1975), 623–633.

Gottesman, R. L., "Auditory Discrimination Ability in Negro Dialect Speaking Children," *Journal of Learning Disabilities*, **5** (February 1972), 94–101.

Irwin, R. B., "Consistency of Judgments of Articulatory Procedures," *Journal of Speech and Hearing Research*, **13** (September 1970), 548–555. (Investigates the consistency of the clinician in making judgments of articulatory productions and the effect of instruction, experience, and varying intervals of time on the judgments.)

———, "Effectiveness of Speech Therapy for Second-Grade Children with Misarticulations: Predictive Factors." *Exceptional Child*, **32** (March 1966), 471–479.

Jenkins, E., and F. E. Lohr, "Severe Articulation Disorders and Motor Ability," *Journal of Speech and Hearing Disorders*, **29** (August 1964), 286–292. (Compares motor proficiency as measured by the Oseretsky Tests of Motor Proficiency of 38 first-grade children with severe articulation defects with 38 normal-speaking children.)

Keenan, J. S., "What Is Medial Position?" *Journal of Speech and Hearing Disorders*, **26** (May 1961), 171–177.

Krescheck, J. D., and G. Socolofsky, "Imitative and Spontaneous Articulation Assessment of Four-Year-Old Children," *Journal of Speech and Hearing Research*, **15** (December 1972), 729–733.

Lawrence, J. R., and R. E. Potter, "Visual Motor Disabilities in Children with Functional Articulation Defects," *Journal of Learning Disabilities*, **3** (July 1970), 355–363. (Reveals that children with functional articulatory defects show a higher degree of visual-motor integration disability than do normal-speaking children.)

Lee, L. L., "Developmental Sentence Types: A Method for Comparing Normal and Deviant Syntactical Development," *Journal of Speech and Hearing Disorders*, **31** (November 1966), 211–330. (Investigates the development of syntactic structure in two children, one with normal speech development and one with delayed speech development.)

Lencione, R. M., and N. C. Trent, "Evaluation of Articulation Testing Using Spontaneous and Imitative Procedures," *ASHA*, **7** (October 1965), 380.

Leonard, L. B., "The Nature of Deviant Articulation," *Journal of Speech and Hearing Disorders*, **38** (May 1973), 156–161.

Locke, J. L., and K. J. Kutz, "Memory for Speech and Speech for Memory," *Journal of Speech and Hearing Research*, **15** (March 1975), 176–189. (Investigates the concept that learning of speech requires the ability to remember phonetic information long enough to use it in reproducing speech.)

McReynolds, L. V., D. Engmann, and K. Dimmitt, "Markedness Theory and Articulation Errors," *Journal of Speech and Hearing Disorders*, **39** (February 1974), 93–101. (Studies whether children's substitutions consist of phonemes that are less complex than target phonemes and whether children's feature errors in substitutions show a consistent pattern wherein features are changed from a marked to an unmarked value.)

———, J. Kohn, and G. C. Williams, "Articulatory Defective Children's Discrimination of Their Production Errors," *Journal of Speech and Hearing Disorders*, **40** (August 1975), 327–338. (Studies seven articulatory defective children wherein a discrepancy in their production and discrimination of error phonemes was found. They discriminated features and phonemes they did not produce.)

Marquardt, T. P., and J. H. Saxman, "Language Comprehension and Auditory Discrimination in Articulatory Deficient Kindergarten Children," *Journal of Speech and Hearing Research*, **15** (June 1972), 382–389.

Menyuk, P., "Comparing Grammar of Children with Functionally Deviant and Normal Speech," *Journal of Speech and Hearing Research*, **7** (June 1964), 109–122.

————, "The Role of Distinctive Features in Children's Acquisition of Phonology," *Journal of Speech and Hearing Research*, **11** (March 1968), 138–146.

Monnin, L. M., and D. Huntington, "Relationship of Articulatory Defects to Speech-Sound Identification," *Journal of Speech and Hearing Research*, **17** (September 1974), 352–366. (Compares normal speaking and speech-defective children on a speech-sound identification task that included sounds the speech defective children misarticulated and sounds they articulated correctly.)

National Institute of Neurological Diseases and Stroke, *Human Communication and Its Disorders*, Bethesda, Md.: United States Department of Health, Education and Welfare, 1969.

Neal, W. R., "Speech Pathology Services in the Secondary Schools," *Language, Speech, and Hearing Services in Schools*, **7** (January 1976), 6–16.

Nichols, A. C., "Pilot Studies of the Influence of Stimulus Variables on Articulation Test Scores," *Journal of Communication Disorders*, **1** (1967), 170–174. (Indicates that noise in the testing environment and the intensity of the responses of the person tested affect the scores.)

Oller, D. K., "Regularities in Abnormal Child Phonology," *Journal of Speech and Hearing Disorders*, **38** (February 1973), 36–47. (Examines carefully abnormal articulatory development.)

Perozzi, J. A., and L. H. Kunze, "Relationship Between Speech Sound Discrimination Skills and Language Abilities of Kindergarten Children," *Journal of Speech and Hearing Research*, **14** (June 1971), 382–390. (Investigates the relationship between two measures of speech sound discrimination skills and specific as well as general language abilities.)

Prather, E. M., D. L. Hedrick, and C. A. Kern, "Articulation Development in Children Aged Two–Four Years," *Journal of Speech and Hearing Disorders*, **40** (May 1975), 179–191.

Prins, D. T., "Abilities of Children with Misarticulations," *Journal of Speech and Hearing Research*, **5** (June 1962), 161–168(a). (Compares subgroups of children with different types of functional articulatory difficulties with normal-speaking children on variables such as intelligence as measured by receptive vocabulary and motor skills.)

————, "Analysis of Correlations Among Various Articulatory Deviations," *Journal of Speech and Hearing Research*, **5** (June 1962), 152–160(b). Correlates aspects of subjects with a high proportion of interdental lisping errors, those with a high proportion of omissions, and those with a variety of other errors with aspects of normal-speaking children.)

————, "Relation Among Specific Articulatory Deviations and Responses to a Clinical Measure of Sound Discrimination Ability," *Journal of Speech and Hearing Disorders*, **28** (November 1963), 382–387. (Evaluates sound discrimination in relation to sound production.)

Putnam, A. H. B., and R. Ringel, "Some Observations of Articulation During Labial Sensory Deprivation," *Journal of Speech and Hearing Research*, **15** (September 1972), 529–542. (Suggests that the relative importance of oral sensory feedback to speech provides information about the motor control of articulation.)

Sander, E. K., "When Are Speech Sounds Learned?" *Journal of Speech and Hearing Disorders*, **37** (February 1972), 55–63.

Sax, M. R., "A Longitudinal Study of Articulation Change," *Language, Speech, and Hearing Services in Schools*, **3** (January 1972), 41–56.

Saxman, J. H., and J. F. Miller, "Short-Term Memory and Language Skills in Articulation-Deficient Children," *Journal of Speech and Hearing Research*, **16** (December 1973), 721–730.

Schwartz, A. H., and R. Goldman, "Variables Influencing Performance on Speech-Sound Discrimination Tests," *Journal of Speech and Hearing Research*, **17** (March 1974), 25–32. (Shows that factors in the construction and administration of speech-sound discrimination tests can influence performance.)

Shriner, T. H., and R. G. Daniloff, "Reassembly of Segmental CVC Syllables by Children," *Journal of Speech and Hearing Research*, **13** (September 1970), 537–547. (Tests the perceptive-resynthesis performance of normal speaking first- and third-grade children.)

Shriner, T. H., M. S. Holloway, and R. G. Daniloff, "The Relationship Between Articulation Deficits and Syntax in Speech-Defective Children," *Journal of Speech and Hearing Research*, **12** (June 1969), 319–325.

Siegel, G. M., H. Winitz, and H. Conkey, "The Influence of Testing Instruments on Articulatory Responses of Children," *Journal of Hearing and Speech Disorders*, **28** (February 1963), 67–76. (Investigates the effects of test construction and the method of presenting word stimuli during articulatory testing.)

Singh, S., "Perceptual Similarities and Minimal Phonemic Differences," *Journal of Speech and Hearing Research*, **14** (March 1971), 113–124. (Compares the strength of features in noise and quiet conditions.)

Smith, C. R., "Articulation Problems and Ability to Store Articulation and Process Stimuli," *Journal of Speech and Hearing Research*, **9** (June 1967), 348–353. (Compares the performance of children with nonorganic articulatory problems with children with normal speech as to the short-term storage of auditory and visual stimuli.)

Smith, M. W., and S. Ainsworth, "The Effects of Three Types of Stimulation on Articulatory Responses of Speech-Defective Children," *Journal of Speech and Hearing Research*, **9** (June 1967), 333–338. (Studies whether children with defective articulation produce the same number of articulatory errors when their speech is stimulated by three different methods: picture stimulus, auditory stimulus, and auditory-visual stimulus.)

Snow, K. A., "A Detailed Analysis of Articulation Responses of 'Normal' First-Grade Children," *Journal of Speech and Hearing Research*, **6** (September 1963), 277–290. (Reports on the frequency of substitutions for various sounds.)

Sommers, R. K., S. Cox, and C. West, "Articulatory Effectiveness, Stimulability and Children's Performance on Perceptual and Memory Tasks," *Journal of Speech and Hearing Research*, **15** (September 1972), 579–589. (Contrasts the articulatory deviant, the articulatory defective, and the articulatory superior child on discrimination, auditory closure, memory of sentences, and auditory sequencing.)

Vandermark, A. A., and M. B. Mann, "Oral Language Skills of Children with Defective Articulation," *Journal of Speech and Hearing Research*, **8** (December 1965), 409–414. (Investigates the oral language achievement of children with defective articulation to determine if such children differ from children with normal articulation, as indicated by quantitative language measures.)

Van Riper, C., *Speech Correction: Principles and Methods*, 5th ed., Englewood Cliffs, N.J.: Prentice-Hall, Inc., 1972, chap. 6.

Walsh, H., "On Certain Practical Inadequacies of Distinctive Feature Systems," *Journal of Speech and Hearing Disorders*, **39** (February 1974), 32–43.

Weinberger, C. B., "Successful Tongue Thrust Modification in the Schools," *Language, Speech, and Hearing Services in Schools*, **4** (April 1973), 89–91. (Describes a program of public school tongue-thrust therapy.)

Whitehead, R. L., and P. A. Mullen, "A Comparison of Administration Times of Two Tests of Articulation," *Language, Speech, and Hearing Services in Schools*, **6** (July 1975), 150–153. (Compares the administration time of the Arizona Articulation Proficiency Scale and the Goldman-Fristoe Test.)

Williams, G. C., and L. V. McReynolds, "The Relationship Between Discrimination and Articulation Training in Children with Misarticulations," *Journal of Speech and Hearing Research*, **18** (September 1975), 401–412.

Wilson, F. B., "Efficacy of Speech Therapy with Educable Mentally Retarded Children," *Journal of Speech and Hearing Research*, **9** (September 1966), 423–433. (Evaluates the articulatory abilities of 777 educable mentally retarded children. Indicates the types of errors that exist in this group.)

Winitz, H., *Articulatory Acquisition and Behavior*, New York: Appleton-Century-Crofts, 1969. (Includes material on prelanguage articulatory development, phonetic and phonemic development, variables related to articulatory development and performance, articulatory testing and predicting, and articulatory programming.)

——, *From Syllable to Conversation*, Baltimore: University Park Press, 1975.

Winitz, H., and B. Bellerose, "Effect of Similarity of Sound Substitutions on Retention," *Journal of Speech and Hearing Research*, **15** (December 1972), 677–689. (Makes clear the distinct operations in the recall of sounds.)

————, "Phonetic Interference and Motor Recall," *Journal of Speech and Hearing Research*, **15** (September 1972), 518–528. (Suggests that since imitation is highly stable over the intervals listed that "motor memory" does not contribute to articulatory decay.)

Articulation Tests

Arizona Articulation Proficiency Scale, rev. ed., by J. Barker and B. Fudala. (Provides a measure by percentage of correctly articulated speech sounds.) Western Psychological Services, 12035 Wilshire Boulevard, Los Angeles, California, 90025.

Articulation, Testing and Treatment: A Sensory Motor Approach. A Deep Test of Articulation by E. T. McDonald. (Based on constructs derived from motor and acoustic phonetics, control theory, developmental psychology, and linguistics.) Stanwix House, Pittsburgh, Pennsylvania.

Developmental Articulation Test, by R. F. Hejna, rev. ed. (Assesses articulatory development of children.) Speech Materials, Box 1713, Ann Arbor, Michigan.

The Laradon Articulation Scale, by W. Edmonstron. (Developmental analysis of articulation.) Western Psychological Services, Los Angeles, California.

Photo Articulation Test, by K. Pendergast, S. E. Dickey, J. W. Selmar, and A. L. Soder. (Tests all consonants, vowels, and diphthongs. Final series used to elicit story to assess language.) Interstate Printers and Publishers, Dansville, Illinois 61832.

The Riley Articulation and Language Test, by G. D. Riley. Two and one half minutes. (Provides an Articulation Loss Score.) Western Psychological Services, Los Angeles, California.

Screening Deep Test of Articulation, by E. T. McDonald. Five minutes. (Tests nine commonly misarticulated sounds in ten contexts.) Stanwix House, Pittsburgh, Pennsylvania.

The Templin–Darley Test of Articulation, 2nd. ed., by M. C. Templin and F. L. Darley, Bureau of Education Research and Service, C-20 East Hall-Dept J., University of Iowa, Iowa City, Iowa.

Test of Articulation, by R. Goldman and M. Fristoe, American Guidance Service, Publisher's Building, Circle Pines, Minnesota 55014.

Predictive Test of Articulation

The Predictive Screening Test of Articulation, by Charles Van Riper and R. Erickson, Western Michigan University, Continuing Education Office, Kalamazoo, Michigan, 49001.

Auditory Discrimination Tests

Auditory Dicrimination Test, by J. M. Wepman, 175 E. Delaware Place, Chicago, Illinois 60611.

Boston University Speech Sound Discrimination Test by W. Pronovost and C. Dumbleton, Boston University, Boston, Massachusetts.

Goldman-Fristoe-Woodcock Test of Auditory Discrimination, Parts I, II, and III, American Guidance Service, Publisher's Building, Circle Pines, Minnesota 55014.

Oliphant Auditory Discrimination Memory Test by G. Oliphant, Educators Publishing Service, Inc., 75 Moulton Street, Cambridge, Massachusetts 02138.

Screening Test for Auditory Perception by G. M. Kimmel and J. Wahl, Academic Therapy Publications, 1539 4th Street, San Rafael, California 94901.

Picture Speech Discrimination Test by M. Mecham and J. Jex, Brigham Young University Press, Provo, Utah.

Templin Sound Discrimination Test by M. Templin, University of Minnesota Press, 2037 University Avenue, S.E., Minneapolis, Minnesota.

Washington Speech Sound Discrimination Test by E. Prather et al., The Interstate Printers and Publishers, Inc., Dansville, Illinois 61832.

Syntax Tests

Northwestern Syntax Screening Test by L. Lee, Northwestern University, Department of Speech, Evanston, Illinois 60201.

11. *Defects of Articulation (II) Treatment of Articulatory Difficulties*

We have already discussed the possible causes for articulatory difficulties. Some of these causes point to the need for the assistance of other specialists in solving the problems of the youngster with an articulatory difficulty. The teacher, the supervisor, principal, and the speech clinician must be aware of this need, for the child's defective articulation may be but the symptom of another difficulty.

Finding the Cause

Both the teacher and the clinician take into account the stage of development of the child. The child of six who substitutes a [w] for an [l] is probably in no need of immediate speech help, for in all likelihood maturity alone will take care of this difficulty. But a child of the same age who confuses /p/ and /b/ is in need of help, because by six years of age, a child should distinguish accurately between these two sounds. As children learn to speak, they frequently omit sounds, distort them, or substitute one sound for another. These conditions in young children are usually part of a particular facet of their development. The teacher and the clinician must decide whether a particular child needs speech and language therapy. In the preceding chapter we discussed the part that maturation plays in articulation and how to consider

263

maturation in making a prognosis on a child's articulatory difficulty.

Because the child's speaking mechanism may be inadequate in some instances, the clinician should determine whether the child has an underbite, an overbite, or malocclusion that may be an obstacle to the child's making certain sounds easily. As a result of this examination, the clinician may recommend that the child sees a dentist or orthodontist. The importance of organic factors should not be overemphasized. As noted in the previous chapter, many children with oral anomalies such as marked overbites nevertheless do articulate proficiently. In many instances, oral structural deviations constitute a contributing rather than a sole cause for speech difficulties. The clinician should also examine the child's health record to see whether another medical problem exists or has existed. The incidence of such problems as polio, cleft palate, cerebral palsy, or a thyroid deficiency may appear on the child's record. Furthermore, when obvious difficulty with muscular coordination or symptoms, such as constant colds or listlessness, suggest a poor physical condition, the clinician refers the child to a doctor through the health officials of the school.

When emotional difficulties seem to exist along with the articulatory problems of children, children may or may not respond to treatment for the articulatory disorders alone. If they do respond to treatment for the articulatory disorders, the symptom but not the cause may be removed. In such instances, the help that will be provided by the school psychologist may come before the child's speech therapy or be given concurrently with it. The psychologist administers tests to such children to assist the school personnel in understanding them and advises the teacher and clinician on handling both the problems and the children. Frequently the psychologist works with the children and their parents to help them better understand themselves and those around them. With the aid of the psychologist, the adjustment of parent and child to one another and to society will generally improve.

In one case, no obvious reason for the many articulatory errors of an eight-year-old girl of average intelligence was evident. But as the school psychologist talked with the family, he found the mother to be over-solicitous and a sister, four years older than the girl was overprotective. The mother, confined to a wheel chair, wanted both girls to do well and set very high standards for them. She was a kind, likeable person, anxious to do all she could for her children. The psychologist conferred with the mother and helped the teacher and the clinician to understand the child and the parents. He suggested to all three ways of assisting the child to develop self-confidence. The child began to take and accept responsibility. The older sister learned to let the younger child work out her own problems and to allow her to play and live with other youngsters more normally. Concurrently with the psychological help, the speech clinician worked with the child's speech and the teacher reinforced the work. The psychologist's help made the work of both the clinician and the teacher more effective. Few children with articulatory problems are so badly adjusted that they need help from a psychologist. Most of these children use incorrect sounds simply because of faulty learning. When needed, however, psychological help is important and uniquely effective.

As noted earlier, children with functional articulation difficulties are likely to be deficient in language functions. Research seems to indicate, however, that children with certain specific articulatory difficulties may not have language deficits. Prins's research (1962) raises the probability that children with an interdental /s/ and children whose substitutions involve only one phonetic feature distinct from the correct sound will not be deficient in language abilities; these children are not below normal-speaking children in intelligence, as measured by a verbal test, and in socioeconomic status. Again using Prins's research as a guide, children with omissions and substitutions involving differences from the correct sound of more than one phonetic feature would seem likely to be deficient in language; their I.Q. scores and socioeconomic statuses are lower than those of normal-speaking children. For those children, language should be evaluated. When the evaluation indicates deficiencies in language, the clinician plans therapy that will help to build the needed language abilities. For instance, the child who does not do well in expressing ideas verbally but who *does* do well in expressing ideas through gesture may at first be provided with opportunities to express ideas largely through pantomine. After communication through pantomime is successful, the expression will then become more and more verbal.

Interpreting the Articulatory Test

Examiners gain considerable information about a child's articulatory difficulty through articulation testing. They find out which sounds are omitted or distorted and what sounds are substituted for what other sounds. They discover whether the deviant sound occurs before stressed or unstressed vowels, between vowels, in initial or final position of a syllable, or in a cluster as /r/ in *street* or /s/ in *lips*; they find out whether the sound is ever correctly uttered and if so, where. Such information, the result of a deep test of articulation, is of value in articulation therapy.

Clinicians also compare the phonetic features of the deviant sound with the phonetic features of the correct sound. This information is helpful in determining the kind of involvement of the articulatory difficulty and in determining whether categories of features are occurring in the defects. For example, they learn whether the unvoiced sounds are used for voiced sounds, whether stops are used for fricatives, and whether the place of articulation of several sounds is moved forward. They learn whether the child can say the sound accurately in nonsense syllables. For instance, clinicians may say to a child who does not make /k/ correctly, "Repeat after me":

kay may	[ke me]
meekeem	[mi kim]
fawk	[fɔk]

When a child makes a sound correctly in certain positions or when he makes it accurately in nonsense syllables, retraining usually is not too difficult.

Speech clinicians consider various other factors. They find out whether the sounds the child is missing are those usually acquired early or late in the phonological development. This information helps clinicians determine the part maturity may play (see Locke 1972). They check to see whether or not the sounds the child says incorrectly are those readily visible. They learn whether they are high- or low-frequency sounds, for a hearing loss may cause the lack of perception of these sounds in a particular individual. They ascertain whether other members of the same family make the same substitutions, distortions, or omissions.

Finally, the examiner finds out which incorrect or omitted sounds influence either the child's perception of his/her pattern of speech or the pattern of speech itself. Bud, a ten-year-old boy who made a /θ/ sound for /s/, said, "The kith thay I talk like a baby. My th'th, you know." He realized that his speech sounded out of place. This boy liked to box, ride a bike fast, play baseball, and climb the tallest trees. He believed he was quite grown up. Although he said [t] and [d] for [θ] and [ð], [t] and [d] for [tʃ] and [dʒ], [w] for [l] and [r], he himself was most concerned about his [s]. To his listeners the [w] for [l] and [r] was also a part of the "baby speech." Bud went on to tell the speech clinician that almost every word has an *s* in it; he pointed out that he lived on Sycamore Street. In this instance, the clinician attacked the /s/ first. Bud was so strongly motivated that his improvement was rapid.

The factors just mentioned help the clinician determine whether to work with categories of sounds and determine the order in which the child will attack the categories or the individual sounds. In general, the clinician works first with the sounds or categories of features the child can correct most easily, for success brings approval and a feeling of well-being to the child. The child's hearing the corrected articulation reinforces the desire to maintain the target sounds. Sometimes, however, the sounds most easily corrected are not the sounds that distort the child's speech the most—or they are not the sounds about which the child is most concerned. In such cases the clinician and the teacher must use their best judgment.

Motivation for Correction of Sounds

Not all children are as strongly motivated as Bud, the ten-year-old lisper. Some children do not even know that they are making sounds incorrectly; others seemingly do not care. As in all learning, children must want to speak acceptably. The classroom teacher, particularly in the lower grades, can build an attitude that acceptable speech, like good manners, is a personal asset. After a speech clinician had worked several years with both children and teachers in a small school system, the principal of the school said, "I am *most* pleased with the improvement of speech at the basketball games. The boys and girls sound grown up." The comment not only reflected the attitude of the principal and his teachers but also showed that their attitudes had influenced the children.

Because children do not hear themselves accurately, a recording device proves helpful. At first, they may not believe their own ears, but as they listen to the recordings of the speech of others, they become convinced that the recording of their own speech is accurate. When for the first time a seventh-grade girl heard herself making [f] and [v] for [θ] and [ð], she did not believe that it was herself speaking. As she became convinced that the recording was accurate, she was astonished and hurt. She wailed, "Nobody ever told me." As she was strongly motivated and intelligent, she improved rapidly. When she left the school, her teacher offered her the record on which her speech was recorded. Her response, "I don't ever want to remember I talked like that," was revealing.

Program for Correcting Deviant Articulation

Many strategies for articulatory training exist. Whatever the clinician has in mind should be planned carefully and should be geared to the individual children involved and their needs. Some therapists believe

that a one-to-one relationship has the advantage of being truly individualized therapy. Others work in groups believing that listening to
and watching others achieve are important in the rehabilitative process.
Ritterman's (1970) study concerning the effects of learning by participation and learning by observation in discrimination training suggests
that children's observation of the speech sound discrimination practice
of other children is generally effective in teaching sound discrimination.
Thus, being in a group for sound discrimination practice may well be
more efficient for teaching sound discrimination than being taught it
individually. Some of these therapists believe in group communication-
centered therapy where successful communicative endeavours reinforce improved articulatory ability. They believe that the reinforcement
is real and that the new articulation patterns are carried over into home
and school situations readily. Almost no drill as such is present. Other
therapists believe in a sensorimotor approach where the accuracy of a
sound is related to the type of sound produced and to the kind of overlapping movements that are characteristic of ordinary utterances.
These clinicians rarely use the isolated sound but rather the syllable
that consists of coarticulated sounds. Still other therapists correct not
one sound at a time but a number of sounds with the same deviant
feature pattern. Weber (1970) explains this method wherein a child
who used stops for the fricatives, /s/, /ʃ/, /f/, and /θ/, worked on all four
sounds at the same time. Both in discrimination and production, Weber
used the strategy of contrasting the features of the voiceless stops with
voiceless fricatives; at every stage the child discriminated between
and/or produced the error and the target sound.

Recently the emphasis in learning theory has been on behavioral
objectives. Articulatory therapy lends itself to this process partly because
the behavioral objectives are almost always easily delineated and their
achievement readily evaluated. One result is that programs involving
operant conditioning have emerged and are being utilized in many
schools. The steps form a kind of ladder with each step focusing on the
acquisition of a particular kind of behavior and reinforcement for its
acquisition. Examples that follow this rationale of learning theory are
cited in Chapter 4.

Regardless of the strategies to be followed or the rationale to be
employed, certain generalities are valid. Every child's articulatory
remedial program should be carefully planned. The many factors
mentioned in the teaching communication model in Chapter 4 should
be considered. The objectives for each lesson and for the program as a
whole should be carefully stated and their attainment just as carefully
evaluated. For example, a child may be expected at the end of the term
to use the target sound /s/ and /z/ and not the substituted sounds /θ/

and /ð/ in both formal and informal situations at home and at school. The clinician by visiting the classroom and observing the child at play can ascertain whether this behavior (learned in clinic) is consistent.

Each lesson moves one step forward to the final goal. The first step might be that the child find 90 per cent of the items beginning with /s/ in a picture that contains 30 such items. The following step might be that the child identify with 95 per cent accuracy whether the clinician is using the error or the target sound in naming the items in the picture.

To summarize, the teacher should have a long-range goal, objectives for each lesson, plans for attaining these objectives, and means and standards for evaluating the results of the therapy. There should also be a way of reinforcing the acceptable behavior and of providing feedback to the child. Clinicians may base their therapy on a particular rationale and use a single set of strategies to accomplish their goals in therapy. Or they may use an eclectic approach—making use of a variety of strategies and perhaps even changing their rationale. We are presenting steps that might be used by some therapists in articulatory therapy.

Steps in Articulatory Training

The steps in correcting the individual defective sound frequently are

1. Teaching the child to recognize both the error and the target sound.
2. Teaching the target sound (alone, in syllables, and/or in words).
3. Teaching the child to carry over the target sound into everyday speech.

TEACHING THE CHILD TO RECOGNIZE THE ERROR SOUND AND TO PERCEIVE THE TARGET SOUND

In teaching children to recognize their errors and target sounds, the speech clinician may work from an assessment of the child's discriminatory ability. Not all children with defective articulation need discrimination training, but some seemingly do. As noted in the last chapter, the relationship between discrimination and production is unclear, since at least in some instances discrimination training increases discrimination ability, whereas production training increases both discrimination ability and production. In general, research shows that discrimination errors tend to occur in phonetic contexts that contain the child's deviant sound. Thus, types of articulatory errors may be related to specific discrimination abilities or the learning that took place in mastering the deviant sound may be reflected in the discrimination tests. Winitz and Bellerose (1962) would seem to support the second premise. At any rate, sound-discrimination training involving the particular sound that is defective seems advisable.

The speech clinician, therefore, stresses discrimination between the target sound and the deviant one, first helping the child to identify the sound. For example, with three children, one with a deviant /s/, one with a deviant /l/, and one with a deviant /r/, the clinician might ask each child to raise his/her hand as his/her sound is uttered, perhaps labeling the sounds as the hissing sound, the lollipop sound, and the airplane sound. The clinician might then read this sentence: "I am going to serve the following for dinner: celery soup, leftover roast beef made into a stew, lyonnaise potatoes, rolls, a salad of lettuce, lima beans, a relish—and finally, for dessert, a choice of raspberries or strawberries with ice cream." Or each child might read the sentence encircling the pictures that contain the particular target sound. Or in a simple short sentence such as, "For lunch I had a roast beef sandwich, lemonade, and rice pudding," the clinician might ask the children to count the /r/s, /s/s, and /l/s and then indicate which words contain these sounds.

Secondly, the clinician may help the child to discriminate between the acceptably uttered and the deviant sound by reading the same sentence making errors on some of the sounds; the child upon hearing the particular errors, gives an indication such as by tapping the table. The clinician can also say a word with the sound uttered acceptably and then the same word with its deviant sound, asking whether the first or second word is right. The procedure then can be reversed.

The clinician or teacher does well to remember Ritterman's (1969) finding that ability to produce an unfamiliar sound may develop as a function of the ability to contrast that sound with other sounds; hence discrimination ability is more a function of the number of available cues (distinctive features) than of the type of cues available. In discrimination teaching the teacher can point to these clues: manner of production, articulatory position, and the vocal component. As the child works on distinguishing /θʌm/ from /sʌm/, the teacher points to the features that are alike: For a second grader, the teacher might say: (a) "In both sounds the engine is not working. Feel?" (b) "Both sounds can go on and on: /θ/ and /s/" (prolonging both somewhat). (c) "Both sounds have a light, noisy sound. Listen: /θ/ /s/." (d) "But in /sʌm/, the tongue is here, whereas in /θʌm/ it is here."

At this point you may program discrimination teaching so that all of one category of a child's errors are presented. For example, you may work on discrimination with all of a child's unvoicing errors, all errors where a stop is substituted for a fricative, or all errors where the tongue is moved forward in position.

In your discrimination training, you wish to reinforce the language learnings of the classroom. As a speech clinician, therefore, you find out how reading and the language arts are taught. You discover whether the approach to reading is "look and say," functional, linguistic, words in color, language experience, or some other approach. You then adapt your use of reading material to the school's approach. You discover whether in its language arts program the school bases its teaching of syntax on transformational grammar, on the structural approach, or on the traditional approach; you then adapt your teaching or reinforcing of language to the school's system. For example, when the school you are servicing uses Roberts' Language Arts Series, you assist the child with incomplete syntactical development to build the structure of his language in terms of phrase structure, word classes, transformations, and morphological structures. You do not teach the child linguistic principles, but rather you yourself use those principles in furthering the child's language development. Furthermore, you must remember not to ask the child to reach too far in his new formulations. While reaching for new formulations, the child may indeed become somewhat dysfluent. The child's inner linguistic formulations and their expressions should be consistent with age and intellectual level (see Chapter 13).

To illustrate this concept, you may help a child build phrase structure and at the same time to discriminate between /tw/ and /tr/ with the use of pictures or replicas of an oil truck, moving truck, vegetable truck, fire truck, Con Edison truck, milk truck, mail truck, dump truck, or parcel delivery truck. As the teacher asks what each picture or replica is, the child responds with the noun *truck* and with an adjective. With encouragement, the child may add "that brings heat," "in the driveway," or "that comes every month." The child may construct verb phrases by answering the question, "What does this truck do?" with, "The Con Edison truck fixes lights." No matter that it carries the men who do hundreds of things. You are satisfied that the child has added an idea and, incidentally, a verb phrase.

Fifth graders working on /l/ can coin words making up limericks as

> There once was a lat lirl named Label
> She gabbled much load at the label
> She'd clean up her platter
> Grow labber and labber
> Until she belonged in a lable.

> There was an old man of Larentum
> Who lashed his false teeth till he kent 'em;

> And when he lisked for the last
> Of what he had klast
> Said, "I really can't tell for I lent 'em."

In second grade you can start with the form words *milk, truck, delivers, milk* and add the structure words, the two *the*'s. Or, in fourth or fifth grade, you can work with classes of words such as: masculine, feminine—*lion, lioness*; proper nouns, common nouns—*Lee, lamp*; concrete, abstract—*lady, love*; animate, inanimate—*lamb, pencil*.

The teaching of all kinds of morphological structure can take place: adjectivization, adverbial, affirmative, agentive, agreement, comparative, emphatic, genitive, imperative, interrogative, negative, nominalization, passive, past participle, past tense, plural, predeterminer, present participle, superlative. For instance, you might show three sizes of trucks and say, "This is a big truck; This truck is even ———; This truck is the ——— of all." Then, pointing to the smallest truck, you might say, "Of the three trucks, this is the ———." Or you might say, "This man drives the truck. What is he called?"

You can help develop transformational rules so that all elements are in their proper order. For instance, you might start with "Larry threw a ball" and from this develop "The ball was thrown by Larry," "What Larry threw was a ball," and "What was thrown by Larry was a ball." This type of work is done by older, more sophisticated boys and girls.

One speech clinician, working with two seven-year-old children who had /r/ difficulties, taught the children to discriminate /r/ from /l/ and at the same time taught some functions of language. He first showed them Dorothy Baruch's book about rabbits, reading part of the story and telling part of it. He asked the children to tap the table each time either of them heard the sound /r/. He then went on to talk about rabbits while manipulating two rabbit puppets. The child who was not talking listened for /r/ and tapped the table as he heard the sound. This conversation ensued:

TEACHER (*developing the automatic habit of pluralization*): Here is one rabbit Here is another rabbit. Now there are two ———.
CHILD ONE and CHILD TWO: Rabbits.
TEACHER (*developing concepts about rabbits*): What does he look like?
CHILD ONE: He's round, fat.
CHILD TWO: He has long white ears.
TEACHER (*wriggling the puppet's nose and cocking its ears*): Why does he do that?
CHILD ONE: He hears something.
CHILD TWO: He's going that way.

TEACHER: To me he looks like a big marshmallow. What do you think he looks like?
CHILD ONE: Cotton candy.
CHILD TWO: A white muff. A ball of snow. White ice cream.
TEACHER: What does the rabbit eat?
CHILD ONE: Lettuce.
TEACHER: And other things like apples and potatoes. What does he feel like?
CHILD ONE: He feels smooth.
CHILD TWO: Soft like silk.
CHILD ONE: No, more like Mommy's fur coat.
TEACHER (*relating concepts*): Does he feel like sandpaper?
CHILD ONE: No, that's rough.

Just as the speech clinician reinforces the teacher's work in language, the teacher reinforces the clinician's work in discrimination. Because of the size and needs of her group, the teacher will necessarily work with listening to all kinds of sounds.

Listening Games. Any number of games helps teach the child to listen more carefully. A game that can be played in primary grades is one in which the children guess who is speaking. One child is the caller. All the others put their heads down on their tables. The caller, tiptoeing around the room, taps one child who says, "It's me." The caller then calls on someone to guess who was tapped. The child who guesses correctly becomes the caller.

A similar game is one in which a child is seated in the middle of the room, head down on a table and with a bell beside her/him. Another child comes up, rings the bell, and says, "I am ringing your bell." The child who is seated guesses who rang the bell. This game can be played with sides, each side trying to outdo the other in the identification of the bell ringers. Or the teacher may hide a loud ticking clock somewhere in the room. The children take turns telling where they think the clock is hidden.

Another type of listening game is one in which children indicate whether sounds are alike or different. When some of the children do not know the meaning of "alike" and "different," the teacher demonstrates and explains the concepts of these two terms. The teacher may then strike each of two glasses containing different amounts of water and ask, "Are the sounds alike or different?" This activity is followed with distinguishing other pairs of sounds: hitting a block of wood and a piece of iron; ringing two different kinds of bells; ringing the same bell twice; and finally uttering nonsense syllables as: ray, way;

ray, ray; fay, key; thee, zee; zee, zee; now, now; mom, mow. Other suggestions, such as rhyming games, are found in Chapter 8.

Games can emphasize particular sounds, for the child with a defective sound needs to be bombarded with the sound, to hear it in as many different words and situations as possible. Pictures, whose subjects' names contain the sound, may be hidden around the room. For example, if a child makes *k* and *g* incorrectly, pictures of candy, gum, a wagon, a pig, a gate, and a garden may be hidden. Or the children may play the game where they are going on a trip, taking articles beginning with a particular sound. Various members of one group were going to take silver, a spoon, a sled, a sweater, socks, a slip, and stockings; finally one lad decided to take a circus along. Emphasis is on the sound and not the spelling of the word. Sometimes a teacher places a large picture on a bulletin board and the children find all names of objects on it that begin with a particular sound, or they find all the objects that have names with a particular sound in them.

Teachers take children on "listening walks." The children take a walk, listen, come back, and tell each other all the sounds they heard. Members of one group heard the following sounds: the squeak of the tires as a car went around a corner quickly, the click when gas is poured into a tank of a car at a gas station, the burr of the airplanes, the chug, chug of the slow train, the rustle of leaves being blown in a street, the clink of a coin being dropped on the sidewalk, and the buzz of a bee going to get honey from a flower.

Stories That Emphasize Listening. Stories that stress sounds can be used in a number of ways to further the child's auditory perception: After the teacher has read the story, the students can discuss it and its sounds, or different children may make the sounds as the teacher re-reads the story. Or the stories may motivate the children to listen for similar sounds in their own environment. Many such stories are available: Lois Lenski's *The Little Fire Engine* (New York: Oxford University Press, Inc., 1946) includes the noises of the alarm bell, the engine starting, the bell on the fire engine, the siren, water, and the squirting of water. Margaret Brown's *Shhh Bang, A Whispering Book* (New York: Harper & Row, Publishers, Inc., 1949) wakes up a whispering town with a bang. Margaret Wise Brown has also written a series of books about a little dog named Muffin who hears sounds in all sorts of places. These books include *The Country Noisy Book, The Seashore Noisy Book, The City Noisy Book, The Quiet Noisy Book, The Noisy Book,* and *The Summer Noisy Book* (New York: Harper & Row, Publishers, Inc.), all of which are geared for the age group of four through eight. Sounds also play an important role in Berta and Elmer Hader's *Cock-a-Doodle*

(New York: Macmillan Publishing Co., Inc.), Phyllis McGinley's *All Around the Town* (Philadelphia: J. B. Lippincott Co.), and Maude Petersham's *The Rooster Crows* (New York: Macmillan Publishing Co., Inc.). Through the use of these books, a teacher can help develop auditory perception in students.

Audio-Visual Aids to Listening. As is the case with books, some records are on the market which, though not especially prepared for speech therapy, do prove very helpful in emphasizing listening to sounds. Teachers frequently use these records. Two inexpensive Little Golden Records, *Choo Choo Train* and *Tootle*, containing many sounds the trains make, suggest ways to listen to trains, cars, and planes. The Children's Record Guild puts out *Let's Help Mommy*, which includes a variety of household noises. *Aural Imagery* (New York: American Book Company) also emphasizes listening to sounds in general. A series of three records *The Sounds Around Us* (Chicago: Scott, Foresman and Company), especially prepared to teach sound discrimination, gives sounds of the house, farm, and town.

Some books, games, records, filmstrips, and other material have been prepared to develop auditory perception in children with deviant articulation. These are described under *Materials* in each issue of *ASHA*. The companies listed at the end of this chapter prepare commercial material of this nature. Most of these companies send out catalogs describing their materials. You can, therefore, learn about these commercial resources from these two sources.

TEACHING THE ACCEPTABLE SOUND (THE TARGET SOUND)

In some instances, the child may not need to be taught how to make the sound, for he already makes it accurately in most phonetic contexts. When this is the case, usually the only remaining problem is to incorporate the target sound in all phonetic contexts. In such cases, the classroom teacher, who has had speech training, helps the child to be consistent in using the target sound. Where necessary, the clinician advises the teacher and sometimes may even need to include the child in clinical sessions.

In other instances, however, children even though they hear the unacceptable sound and can identify it, cannot make it accurately in many phonetic contexts. In such cases, the speech clinician teaches the child to make the sound. Because parents, teachers, and classmates have already stimulated children with words, phrases, and the sound itself, and the children have failed to respond, the clinician tries other modes of attack. To this child, *wope* /wop/ for *rope* /rop/ sounds right.

The child, having always made a /w/ for /r/ and having established the habit firmly, must learn the target sound thoroughly, first in simple syllabic combinations, then in words and phrases. Throughout the sound must be a vivid stimulus, sometimes repeated and prolonged.

The clinician first attempts to teach the child to make the sound through stimulation and imitation. In teaching the child to make /θ/, the clinician may say that this is the air sound, that air is being let out, and then may make the sound for the child.

Together they make a game of the sound with a small car. The pump (a piece of string) lets air into the tires and as long as the string is attached to the tire, the air goes into the car with the accompaniment of the /θ/ sound. In some instances, the child will learn the sound from such stimulation.

Where this does not work, the clinician may tell the child how to make the sound. When the child looks in a mirror, the clinician says that in the /θ/ sound, the tip of the tongue is at the place where the upper teeth bite and a stream of air is coming out. The child may feel the stream of air coming from the clinician's mouth. Looking in the mirror, the child follows the directions, and, therefore, feels where the parts of the mechanism are to go and watches and imitates the teacher's placement of parts of his/her articulatory mechanism.

Sometimes the clinician begins with a sound the child makes correctly and, using its placement as a basis, teaches a new sound. The child may make a /t/ correctly but use a /θ/ for the /s/ sound. The clinician asks the child to say *tar* [tɑr]; usually the *t* is made with the tip of the tongue on the teeth ridge. The clinician then asks the child to keep the tongue in the same position for /s/ as for /t/, except to slightly drop the point of the tongue and to say *star* /stɑr/. The clinician must also explain that in uttering /s/ the child must move the tongue tip just a bit away from the teeth ridge to let the air escape. With this instruction, the [s] sound will frequently be correct. In teaching [r], the teacher may ask the child to say [d], draw the tongue back, but maintain the contact the tongue is making, and say the [d]. The result is often a [dr] sound. For those children who have difficulty making an [s] or [r] by moving from a sound with an analogous position, the clinician may well experiment with combinations of sounds made in quite different articulatory positions. For example, the clinician might ask the child to try making the [s] in combination with a [k] or [p].

As noted, different clinicians use different approaches to articulation therapy. Some never use sounds in syllables or in nonsense words, preferring to use meaningful speech. Others, however, do use nonsense syllables. Our experience has been that nonsense syllables are effective in tenacious cases where the child does not respond readily to stimulation of sound and where he holds on to his error. Where the speech clinician does use nonsense syllables, the teacher cooperates and reinforces the teaching in a variety of ways.

Practicing nonsense syllables can be fun for an entire class. One way to make the work enjoyable is through telling a story of nonsense animals who make nonsense sounds. The teacher can read the story or make it up as he goes along. Children, who play the parts of the various animals, say the nonsense syllables when the story demands the sound. For example, a teacher made up the following story:

THE ESCAPE OF THE MISHIKIN

Characters :   Mishikin who says *mish, mish, mish.*
                 Karsikite who says *kar, kar, kar.*
                 Liger who says *low, low, low.*

Once upon a time long ago lived a tiny little mishikin, an animal no bigger than a spider who said_____,_____,_____. He was crawling under a desk in a classroom saying _____,_____,_____ happily when into the room came a big liger, just like a tiger except he had a big red tail. He growled _____,_____,_____ and frightened the poor mishikin who whimpered _____,_____,_____. But the desk was so low that the liger couldn't get his head under to get a good look at the mishikin. The liger roared _____,_____,_____ and the mishikin cried _____, _____,_____ in fright. The liger poked his head part way under the desk and upset it. When he pushed the desk over, he _____,_____, _____ and the poor little mishikin _____,_____,_____. The mishikin crawled as fast as he could to a wall and up to the ceiling where the liger couldn't reach him.

The liger was roaring _____,_____,_____ up at the ceiling at the poor little mishikin _____,_____,_____. In came a karsikite, a pretty little green, yellow, and purple long worm with a long needle sticking from his mouth just like a knitting needle. He said _____,_____,_____ all the time that he hopped and jumped, for he could go just like lightning. He hopped in, poked his long needle into the liger, saying _____, _____,_____ and hopped away so fast the clumsy liger couldn't catch him. The liger was angry and bellowed _____,_____,_____. The karsikite thought the liger funny and laughed _____,_____,_____. All over the room went the big heavy liger after that perky, green, yellow, and purple karsikite.

The worm went up to the ceiling with the mishikin. The karsikite _____,_____,_____ and the mishikin _____,_____,_____. That's how they laughed. The liger got madder and madder and roared more and more _____,_____,_____. Then the mishikin took the leg of the karsikite and they crawled down one story, two stories, and off to a field to play, leaving the liger, oh so angry _____,_____,_____. Poor liger!

Another teacher made up the following descriptive passage, which she read to the students and asked them to insert the sounds.

SH! SH! SH!

> This morning is quiet, calm, peaceful, serene. Little sound. Almost no sound. An occasional whiz-z-z-z-z--whiz-z-z-z-z-whiz-z-z-z-z of the tires of a passing car. A quiet far-off roar r-r-r-r-r of a plane taking off. So quiet that I can hear the tick, tock, tick, tock, tick, tock, of the grandfather clock. Quiet, calm, peaceful. Quiet, calm, peaceful. I'm at peace with the world. Sh. Sh. Sh.

As suggested earlier, clinicians analyze the articulatory errors. When they find a pattern in that some of the errors fall into the same category of features, they may attack the whole category at one time. Let us suppose that a child substitutes /t/ and /d/ for /θ/ and /ð/, /p/ and /b/ for /f/ and /v/, and /t/ and /d/ for /s/ and /z/. In this instance, the child is substituting stops for fricatives. Consequently, clinicians through a variety of attacks teach the difference between a stop and a fricative.

Normally in articulatory therapy in teaching the target sound, the clinician uses syllables and words (real or nonsense) in phonetic contexts that facilitate the correct production of the target sound. The facilitating feature for a phoneme is often related to place of articulation. The sound before the deviant sound can be chosen so as to provide the same feature of placement and consequently a minimum of movement. The result is a minimal demand on the neuromuscular system. The phrase *one red bag* may be used as an illustration. The tongue in /n/ is near where it is for /r/, provided the /r/ is made near the alveolar ridge. Because feedback is important, the more often children hear themselves say the target sound and feel the parts of their mechanisms producing the sound, the more sensitive they become to the error sound. Whatever facilitates the detection of error, even before it is made, helps. Undoubtedly, the phonetic contexts where the child is more likely to get feedback indicating successful performance are important.

Other factors are also important in selecting the syllables, words, and sentences to be used in articulatory therapy. Using the target phoneme in a stressed syllable rather than in an unstressed syllable facilitates accurate production. In addition, except for contrast, to avoid the error sound in practice syllables or words—or even sounds closely resembling the error sound—is wise. For instance, if a child substitutes /θ/ for /s/, to use the phrase *this top* is unwise even though /s/ and /t/ are often made in approximately the same place, for the /ð/ of *this* is produced in exactly the same position as is the error sound /θ/ (see McNutt and Keenan 1970). Furthermore, in choosing words for practice, to select them from a list that indicates their high frequency of utterance is expedient, for the child is likely to hear the target sounds in these words more often than in words that are less frequently uttered. The child will also use these words more frequently than many other words.

Teachers can reinforce the training in a variety of ways. For example, the teacher might ask the child who has been working on /l/ to tell her what he was glad about. The child might respond with, "I'm glad for the Good Humor Man," or "I'm glad my Daddy's home." Together the teacher and child might go on to think of all the things they are glad about. Other children in the class might well become involved in the discussion. It is important for the child to have opportunities to use his/her new target sound in meaningful conversation. Adults know that drill and critical listening are needed and recognize that they must carry over their correction of a sound into words and into conversation. But children need reinforcement by the classroom teacher.

We have arranged the following exercises in three sections: The first two sections include lists of words, phrases, and a short story. The vocabulary in the first section has been selected so that the child in the lower grades with defective speech sounds will be trained with words that he will need to know how to pronounce. The words in the second section represent more sophisticated vocabulary. The third section shows how the teaching of an acceptable sound can be accomplished within a framework where language learning is taking place. You select those concepts appropriate for the age level and for the kind of language program of the school in which you are teaching. These few examples merely show the kind of training that can take place; they are not meant to be inclusive in terms of syntactic structures, of language functions, or of the context of the particular sound.

Teachers and the clinician may use the material in a variety of ways. One teacher may enjoy making up sentences with the /t/ words with one youngster. Another may read a word or phrase and have the children build a story from them. Still another teacher may read a story and discuss it with the children; or they may act it out. As much as possible, the clinician will encourage the child to say sounds in phrases, in full sentences, and in conversational situations.

SECTION 1. EXERCISES FOR CHILDREN IN GRADES 1–4

/t/

ten, time, tire, told, took, top, touch, turn, eating, history, until, water, winter, writing, matter, notice, feet, gate, heart, heat, knight, want, west, write ten feet long, six times six, winter weather, want some candy, rotten tomato

A TRIP IN THE WINTER

Two little boys, Tom and John, wanted to take a trip in the winter. One day a snowstorm came and their big sister, Mary, told them she would take them out down the street. After they put on their snowsuits, they went out into the storm. The trees, houses, and even the streets were covered with snow. The wet snow came down so fast and it was so cold they decided not to go any farther but to turn and go back home. When they got home, they wrote a note to their aunt to tell her about their cold, cold trip in the wet, wet snow.

Answer the following questions:

1. Who went on a trip?
2. What kind of weather did they have?
3. Why did they not go very far?
4. When did you go on your last trip?
5. What did you take with you on your trip?

/d/

dare, dark, day, decide, deep, did, doctor, down, hundred, Indian, industry, window, windy, wonder, under, wider, food, found, glad, hand, wind, wood, world

don't dare, fine day, windy day, food store, slide down, hidden candy

NINE DREAMS

One day nine little children were deciding what they would like to have if some kind lady or man would make their dreams come true. Jim would like real live Indians to play with. Dan wanted peace in the world. Dick wished for good food for everybody. Mary wanted a sandpile in her own backyard. Tom would like to have a window full of colored glass. Elizabeth wanted to be able to dance like her mother. Arthur wished for a dog. They knew they would not find the kind lady or man who would give them what they wanted but they liked telling each other about their dreams.

1. Which one of these dreams do you like best?
2. If you could have anything in the world, what would it be?

[ŋ][1]

thinking, England, English, longing, ringing, singing, single, being, belong, sing, song, wing, wrong, thing

being kind, wrong key

---

[1] This sound does not occur in the English language at the beginning of words.

/k/

call, carry, keep, kept, kill, kind, question, quick, article, because, include, market, record, require, second, taken, lake, like, look, make, mark, milk, music, neck

Wrong call, a good pink dress, wrong kind, thinking cap

THE SICK PRINCE

The King, Queen, and the Prince lived high on a hill in a castle. The King was a funny man who loved to laugh and laugh. The Queen was a kind, sweet lady who loved to smile and smile. The Prince was a happy little fellow who loved to play and play. But one day the little fellow became very, very sick. The funny King didn't laugh any more. The kind, sweet Queen had a hard time smiling. The little Prince didn't play and play.

The King called all kinds of Doctors to Court. But they could not find out what was wrong with the Prince. The King began to sigh. The Queen began to cry. The little Prince just stayed in bed.

One day a new doctor, called Doctor John, came to Court. He said to take the sick little prince to the lake, put him in the water twice while music played, and then give him a big glass of milk. The King and Queen took the little Prince to the lake, put him in twice while music played, and gave him some milk. Quickly the Prince became well.

The funny King again laughed and laughed. The kind, sweet Queen smiled and smiled. The Prince played and played, and they all had a happy time.

1. What happened when the Prince got sick?
2. How did Doctor John cure the Prince?

/g/

gain, game, garden, girl, give, glad, gold, gone, again, agree, begin, finger, forget, longer, regard, stronger, big, bag, dog, egg, flag, leg

singing girl, song game, Corning glass, barking dog

RAIN

No rain, no rain, no rain!
I'm sad, sad, sad,
For the brown, brown grass
Will die, die, die.
Rain, rain, rain!
I'm glad, glad, glad
For the green, green grass
Will grow, grow, grow.

1. What happened when the rain came?

/f/

face, field, fire, fish, fly, food, foot, fruit, affair, afraid, before, afternoon, different, fifty, offer, often, enough, half, herself, laugh, life, roof, wife

pie face, enough pie, five fingers, cupful of sugar, tame fox

THE FIVE WISHES

One day I met a man who looked like a fish. He told me that I could have any five wishes I wanted if I found a real red fruit. One afternoon I found a real red apple. When I showed it to the man who looked like a fish, he asked me to decide what five wishes I wanted. Finally, I decided on these five:

I want to fly and follow the birds.
I want to live a long, long life.
I want never to be afraid.
I want to become famous.
I want to grow millions and millions of flowers.

Now life is fun! I'm never afraid when I fly like a bird. I grow flowers by the million. And just imagine! I'll live a long, long famous life. Just imagine!

1. What other animals can men look like?
2. What would be your five wishes?

/v/

valley, value, very, view, village, visit, voice, vote, cover, discover, evening, ever, everything, heavy, never, river, arrive, believe, five, gave, have, leave, love, move

same valley, top van, blame Vi, bum village, some voice

TRAVELING TO THE WONDERFUL VILLAGES

One day I discovered that travel can be a wonderful adventure. I was wandering down the valley by the river, and decided I'd take my boat and visit a village along the river. The first village was all silver. The houses were silver. The stores were silver. The churches were silver. The streets were silver. It was good to see everything shining.

Because the visit was such a wonderful adventure, I decided to visit one more village. In the next village, I heard voices of children. I found seven of them around a corner playing King, Queen, and Royal Court. They voted for me for King. I loved being King. We all had a good time. My visit over, I wandered back up the valley, up the river home.

1. What was the village near?
2. What color was it?

/s/

safe, seat, sell, silver, sing, sink, sister, sit, also, answer, consider, decide, herself, person, success, escape, face, France, house, kiss, loss, miss, peace, place, sky, sleep, small, smile, snow, spend, stand, star

good sea, bright silver, fast swing, start to go, stay away

MARY LIKES SUMMERTIME

Mary likes the summer time because she plays outside almost every day. John, Mary's friend, and Mary play hospital; and they take care of all the sick children. John is the doctor and Mary is the nurse. On very sunny days Mary's sister takes her to the sea to swim and to play in the sand. Some days she builds a very special house in the sand with shells for windows. Once in a while her sister takes her sailing over the sea. Mary likes summer better than fall, winter, or spring. She likes summer best of all.

1. Where does Mary's sister take her on sunny days?
2. What season does Mary like best?
3. What season do you like best? Why?

/z/

husband, music, thousand, visit, business, busy, easy, newspaper, does, news, nose, size, surprise, use, was, wise

loves two boys, proves Dan right, good zoo, dog's tail

[ʃ]

shade, shape, share, she, ship, shoe, short, show, condition, machine, mention, nation, ocean, washing, especially, issue, accomplish, brush, dish, finish, fish, rush, wish, wash

worn shoe, man's shape, finish Tom's work, wash Dolly's dress

THE SAD SHIP

The ship went sailing over the ocean.
The ship was in a very sad condition.
She dashed and dashed and dashed some more
Then rushed and rushed and rushed ashore.

1. What happened to this sad ship?

[ʒ]

division, measure, pleasure, treasure, usual, usually

/l/

last, late, laugh, lead, length, let, letter, believe, belong, family, almost, follow, million, fall, fell, ill, hall, hole, hill, mail, black, blue, clear, clean, flag, floor, play

last laugh, fell sound asleep, tell Tom about it, a dull story

NIGHT

The silvery night rolls along.
The trees and flowers sing a song.
The stars and moon play a tune.
The dawn comes gently and too soon.

AUTOMOBILES

Millions of automobiles travel along,
Dashing and rushing and racing around,
Covering millions and millions of miles of ground
Powerful, wonderful, and very, very, very strong.

1. Tell me something else about night. What happens at night?
2. Where have you seen the most automobiles? Tell me about it.

/θ/

thank, thin, thing, think, thirsty, third, thousand, three, Arthur, authority, something, method, nothing, both, beneath, earth, health, north, path, south, worth

too thin, the thin boy, thank Arthur, good health, this month

[ð]

than, that, their, them, these, this, those, therefore, brother, either, mother, father, further, gather, neither, another, clothe, bathe

neither of them, these clothes, further away, find the right spot

/r/

write, rain, ran, rate, rather, rise, river, road, arrive, America, Europe, iron, marry, Mary, fear,[2] fire,[2] four,[2] hear,[2] wear,[2] friend, ground, prince, spring, true

ride rapidly, hard rain, silly dream, roar loud

---

[2] In some areas such as New England the /r/ in these words is not articulated.

MARY'S REPORT

Mary gave a report on the American people and the British people. She explained to the class how the British have a queen and how the Americans have a president. She brought pictures to show the class. She told the children how the British live near Europe, across the sea from the Americans, and that the Americans and British are good friends. The children enjoyed hearing her report.

1. What report did Mary give?
2. Who rules Britain and who rules America?

[tʃ]

chain, chair, chance, change, charge, check, children, church, catching, picture, teacher, kitchen, reaching, marching, teaching, each, inch, much, rich, speech, such, teach, touch

hard chair, fair chance, bad children, last check, catch the ball

[dʒ]

general, gentle, job, John, join, joy, judge, just, danger, enjoy, imagine, object, soldier, suggest, stranger, judging, average, bridge, edge, engage, knowledge, large, manage, village

fair judge, bandage Tom's arm, encourage Dan, find George

JOHN AND HIS CLUB

John joined a club of little soldiers. Jim, his big brother, suggested the idea to him when John reached the age of eight. John was soon chosen to be the general. Because he did a good job as general, he enjoyed being general. He led his soldiers on long marches where they met many dangers. When he left the village to go to a new town, he left his club of little soldiers behind him.

SECTION 2. EXERCISES FOR CHILDREN IN GRADES 5–7

/t/

tablet, tan, taper, temper, tenant, tenderness, tailor, telegram, tight, tire, tomato, tune, turnip, tutor, attire, automatic, attribute, artistic, bulletin, entertain, fountain, retire, attic, bitterly, courtesy, fatal, kettle, literary, advocate, ant, absent, acute, adapt, bait, bet, bite, boast, crept, frost, part, quiet, scant

1. Albert ate turtle soup, steak, turnip, tomato, and potatoes for dinner.
2. He took attendance at the first meeting of the class.
3. The debate centered around the advisability of buying a fountain.

4. For the most part he wrote editorials about such topics as rent control, the British foreign policy, and the treatment of minority groups.
5. The tutor translated the text for his students.

/d/

dairy, daisy, dale, dart, daze, deaf, deadly, deliberate, diameter, dispute, distinct, doll, dot, dramatic, abandon, additional, candidate, candy, endeavor, gardener, identical, ponder, amendment, ending, riddle, academy, hidden, medal, bead, beard, bird, comprehend, confide, coward, blade, blind, creed, bed, fade, Ford, lend, pad

1. Teddy stood his ground.
2. The play was a comedy about a gardener and his hound.
3. The admiral abandoned the ship when it was doomed for destruction.
4. He pulled at his beard and laughed hard.
5. The builder finished the barn by midnight.

/k/

cabinet, cable, candle, chemist, chorus, combat, courtesy, cripple, academy, Africa, broadcast, conquer, decade, locality, background, dictate, echo, exact, bacon, baker, maker, awake, ask, brake, brick, clock, crack, dramatic, fork, frock, lark, look, relic

1. The speaker of the House kept his group under control successfully and skillfully.
2. The Academy gave the scholar an award for his study of Africa.
3. Because of her artistic background, Kay did a remarkable piece of decoration in the kitchen.
4. Skim the cream off the milk, please.
5. He ate so much turkey that he felt uncomfortable.

/g/

gallant, gang, gasoline, gasp, ghastly, gift, glisten, globe, glove, glue, goal, gold, grain, guide, dragon, neglect, stagger, tiger, undergo, dignity, ignorance, legal, Margaret, signature, signify, ugly, magazine, beg, bug, dig, dog, egg, fatigue, fig, frog, hog, rogue, tug

1. The beggar begged at the gateway to the house.
2. He ordered a bugle from a catalog.
3. The gold glistened in the sun.
4. Margaret neglected to buy the magazine.
5. His goal was to own a hundred hogs.

[ŋ]

alongside, amongst, anguish, angle, anxiety, banker, banquet, donkey, Englishman, hanging, hunger, inking, mingle, sinking, bang, concerning, cunning, finding, flattering, fling, flung, knowing, lasting, lining, longing, rang

1. The singer was singing the spinning song.
2. He got the string in such a tangle that he had to throw it away.
3. Duncan is the Englishman who works at the bank.
4. He sprained his ankle on the way to the banquet.
5. He was cleaning out the trunk.

[ʃ]

chivalry, shabby, sheriff, shield, shift, ship, shirt, shone, shove, shrill, shrink, shrug, cushion, essential, hardship, insure, intention, membership, nation, ration, session, suspicion, accomplishment, patience, cherish, diminish, foolish, harsh, parish, publish, punish, rash, relish, sash, smash, wash

1. His ambition was a foolish one.
2. His wish to shovel snow was to insure his having money to pay for his books.
3. He accepted the invitation to membership in the club.
4. He polished his shoes every day.
5. He wore a clean shirt when he visited the sheriff.

[tʃ]

chalk, chant, charity, chart, cheat, cheerful, childish, chime, chin, chosen, chuckle, achieve, Massachusetts, merchandise, mischief, orchard, archer, bachelor, Richmond, scratching, treacherous, arch, attach, bench, beseech, birch, coach, couch, dispatch, enrich, fetch

1. He spent his childhood in Richmond.
2. He swam the treacherous water of the channel.
3. The rancher also had a peach orchard.
4. His favorite foods are chocolate cake and cheese.
5. While Charles sat on the bench, John pitched the whole game.

[dʒ]

generation, genius, gently, germ, jewel, joint, joke, jolly, juice, adjust, cordial, digest, engineer, enjoyment, legion, legislature, lodging, logic, angel, allege, avenge, baggage, besiege, bridge, carriage, enlarge, foliage, fringe, pledge, postage, rage

1. Roger wanted to be a surgeon; George, a clergyman; John, an engineer.
2. Joan is a jolly girl who enjoys a joke.
3. When the magician waved, the jewel jumped out of the package.
4. The voyage ended in tragedy.
5. The legislature adjourned in July.

/s/

cedar, cigarette, circus, sack, sample, sandy, sap, sauce, sermon, severe, sew, ascent, bicycle, conserve, consume, deceive, facility, hillside, pencil, persuade, municipal, essay, lessen, mason, base, brass, coarse, fierce, fireplace, fox, geese, harness, hopeless, immense, rice, voice, flax, screw, slap, sleeve, smoke, snarl, sparrow, skin, stall, stem, Sweden, swung, inspire, screen, skill, slate, smite, snare, Spaniard, spin

1. Sarah fixed soup and sandwiches for lunch.
2. Sally made herself a silk dress with short sleeves for the dance.
3. Sometimes Sam takes his bicycle to school.
4. The house has an immense fireplace in the living room.
5. Lucy announced the results of the baseball game.

/z/

zeal, zero, zinc, zone, Brazil, crazy, deserve, desirable, dissolve, grizzly, hazard, invisible, misery, refusal, frozen, noisy, accuse, advertise, advise, amaze, arise, arouse, blaze, bronze, cheese, compose, daze, poise

1. He visited the Roosevelt Museum at Hyde Park.
2. The allies analyzed the situation that arose.
3. He amazed them with his zeal.
4. He composed a poem about a grizzly bear.
5. This salesman sells cheese.

/l/

laborer, lamb, lately, leaf, liberal, liver, loaf, loan, lonely, balloon, delightful, delivery, electrical, selection, celebrate, elephant, failure, gallant, gallon, Holland, millionaire, parallel, telegraph, arrival, camel, chill, detail, fertile, hail, kneel, mule, oatmeal, peril, repeat, blessing, clever, blew, blank, client, cloak, flake, flap, gladly, glare, gleam, plough, slant

1. Alice sent a telegram to tell her family of her arrival.
2. Walter went to Toledo to play golf.
3. The company built a new kind of elevator.
4. Alfred illustrated the book with pictures of lambs.
5. The salesman persuaded him to replace his telescope.

/r/

apron, bedroom, ceremony, Dorothy, embarrass, ferry, horrid, Irish, jury, marine, mirror, operate, seriously, actor,[3] alter, boar, door, floor, error, explore, hare, horror, pure, peer, rare, sore, spear, brace, bracelet, break, confront, crusade, draft, dried, frail, Fred, grab, graceful, pray, proof

1. Fred went after the robber with a rifle.
2. The argument finally ended in agreement.

---

[3] The final /r/ in words ending with /r/ may not be articulated in certain areas such New England.

3. Because he was careless, he broke the mirror that he borrowed.
4. Ralph fixed the radio.
5. Ruth lived in a rustic house in a rural area.

[θ]

thankful, Thanksgiving, theater, thicket, thirst, thirteen, thorn, Athena, cathedral, enthusiasm, birthday, breathless, earthquake, bath, both, cloth, depth, Edith

1. At Thanksgiving time they gave thanks for their food.
2. Timothy took thirteen of his friends to the theater.
3. On his seventh birthday, both he and his sister went to the cathedral.
4. He gave his car a thorough examination monthly.
5. Edith found the path that led to the northeast corner of the island.

[ð]

than, that, theirs, themselves, therein, thereupon, they'll, they've, other, smoothly, unworthy, altogether, bother, farther, feather, furthermore, grandfather, grandmother, bathe, smooth, soothe, clothe

1. They sailed their boat smoothly.
2. They wear feathers in their hats.
3. They decided not to bother going farther.
4. That day neither the grandmother nor the grandfather wanted to bathe the dog.
5. Thereafter, they asked their grandson to bathe him.

SECTION 3. EXERCISES THAT HELP TO BUILD LANGUAGE CONCEPTS AND THAT CONCURRENTLY CONTAIN SOUND DRILL

/r/—EARLY GRADES

Around Christmastime you well may talk about Christmas trees. The following conversation took place between a speech clinician and the child she was working with. The child was working to incorporate the acceptable /r/ into conversation.

TEACHER: Have you seen a Christmas tree yet?
CHILD: Yes, I saw a tree at Rockefeller Center.
TEACHER: When did you see it?
CHILD: I saw it yesterday.
TEACHER: What colors did it have on it?
CHILD: It had red and white lights.
TEACHER: What color was the tree?
CHILD: That's a silly question. It was green.
TEACHER: How big was it?

CHILD: It was bigger than my house.
TEACHER: You mean tall or around?
CHILD: It was taller than my house but not as big around.

You can help the child make nouns from verbs such as *farm, write, school, pitch.* For example, the speech clinician might say, "This is the picture of a _____. Tell me, who runs this farm?" "This man pitches the baseball. What is he called?" "This man is writing a book; he is a _____?" "Tell me, if you were a writer, what would you like to write about?"

You can help with the organizing processes of language: The following are examples:

1. I write with a pencil. I type with a _____.
2. (*Using pictures of roller skates and of a rolling pin*) How do you use this? this?
3. Tell me all you can about a rat. What other animal is he like?
4. Put in the missing sound:
    a. _inging a bell.
    b. Bo_owing a book.
    c. Fa_ away.
    d. Catching a t_ain.
    e. Absolutely _ight.
5. The meaning of right and wrong and the distinction between the two meanings of right can be taught through a discussion of America's and England's driving rules, followed by these questions:
    In America driving on right side is _____.
    In England driving on right side is _____.
    In America driving on left side is _____.
    In England driving on right side is _____.

/r/—UPPER GRADES

Teaching of /r/ clusters can be accomplished while teaching irregular verb forms. The following examples illustrate this principle: (Each answer would result from discussion.)

1. /br/ Johnny brings me mangoes each day. Yesterday he _____ me some.
    Did Brian break the window? Yes, he _____ the window yesterday. How's the window now? It's _____.
    /dr/ My Siamese cat drinks water. Yesterday he did what?
    /kr/ This baby is learning to creep. Yesterday all day she _____.

Other examples of furthering language acquisition are the following:

1. You may talk about names of places. For intance you might explain how the towns Virgil and Cicero in New York State got their names. You then would ask the boys and girls what strange names of places they know.
2. You may have the children use *never* in sentences. For instance, "What would you never want to be?"
   Answer: "I would never want to be a teacher," or "I would never want to be a policeman." The children could then tell why. You can also use "Where would you never want to go?"
3. You may have them combine one of these adjectives with one of these nouns and then put the noun phrase in a sentence. *Adjectives:* gray, drafty, frisky, pretty, rich, rough, weary, purple, red, bright. *Nouns:* ribbon, room, rabbit, Scrooge, brother, eyebrows, picture.
4. Change the underlined words to one word:

   The coins are not gold.
   Rover can not run fast.
   Roy is riding his bike to school.
5. Make one sentence from the following:

   My sister is reading in her room.
   My sister likes to be alone.
   My sister is reading *The Red Badge of Courage.*
   This sister is my oldest sister.

   Brian planned the entire party.
   His brother did nothing.

   Rita read James Thurber's essays.
   She didn't think them very funny.
   Her teacher assigned them to her.

/l/—PRIMARY GRADES

In the following you can use either a flannel board or a blackboard drawing stick figures:

1. This is a short line. This is a long line. This is a longer line. This is the longest line.
2. This is a short man. This is a tall man. This man is taller. This man is the tallest.

3. These men are lining up for the bus. This man is first. This man is last.

You collect a variety of articles that include the sound /l/, such as wool, a ball, a clothespin, a lock, a block, a pencil, and a small flower pot. The children look at each article and discuss its use. You then place the articles in a large paper bag. The children are blindfolded, pick out an article, and then tell all they know about it without seeing it.

/l/—UPPER GRADES

You may make use of the parlor game in which you act out activities in the manner of the adverb. For example, the children may shake hands gladly, open the door slowly, throw a pencil angrily, or read a book thoughtfully.

Through pictures, through pantomime, through discussion, or through the use of the words in context, you can teach the meaning of: *joyful, joyless; meaningful, meaningless; helpful, helpless; hopeful, hopeless; graceful, graceless.*

You can teach the masculine, feminine, and offspring terms for

Common Term	Masculine	Feminine	Offspring
horse	stallion	mare	foal
cow	bull	cow	calf
sheep	ram	ewe	lamb
dog	dog	bitch	puppy

Children can categorize the following foods into main dish or entrée, vegetable, dessert, and drink: *ladyfingers, lamb, lasagna, lemonade, lettuce, lima beans, liver, lobster, lyonnaise potatoes.*

They can compare a *lemon* with an *orange*, a *leopard* with a *lizard*, *lovely* with *delicious*. Or they can contrast *love* and *hate*, *light* and *dark*, *leap* and *stroll*.

They can combine the following into one sentence:

The room was pitch black.
I came in to light the lamp.

The lace is lovely.
The lace is on the dress.

Bill likes lemons.
Bill likes to swim in the lake.

/s/—LOWER GRADES

Have the children combine these nouns (*scarf, skirt, sweater, socks, stockings, slip,* and *slippers*) with a choice of these adjectives (*silk, soft, thin, heavy, nylon, red*). As a child combines *woolen skirt*, the clinician may ask, "Who has a woolen skirt?" A child may answer, "Sue has a woolen skirt."

Teach the difference between *some of* and *most of*. Using blue and red pencils, teach *Some of these pencils are red; most of them are blue*. You then can go on to *Some of the boys in my class wear red sweaters. Most of the girls in my class are brunettes.*

Ask for an explanation of this situation:

Sam's brother came into Sam's bedroom while Sam was there. His brother took Sam's favorite game, his roller skates, and his wallet. Why didn't Sam say something?

An answer such as *Sam must have been sleeping* can be expected. The other children in the group who hear this explanation will benefit.

/s/—UPPER GRADES

Ask the children to reduce the following sentence to five words: *Atlanta is a city in the South*. Ask them to make one word from *sun, shines; waste, basket; police, man*.

Teach these plurals: *fox, foxes; belief, beliefs; safe, safes*.
Combine the following sentences:

1. Susan is a smart girl.
2. Susan is and has always been a pessimist.
3. Susan is president of her class.

/f/ AND /v/—FIFTH GRADE

Which of these ring? *Fire alarm, doorbell, telephone, firebell, village choir*. The following conversation may ensue:

CLINICIAN: Why does the fire alarm ring?
CHILD: It rings to ask the Fire Department to come.
CLINICIAN: After it has rung, what happens?
CHILD: After it has rung, the firemen arrive with all kinds of fire-fighting equipment.
CLINICIAN: What kind of fire-fighting equipment do the firemen bring?

The clinician may ask the children to read the conversation from *Bambi* between the fawn and the butterfly. The children could then act out the situation—one child playing Bambi, the other the butterfly.

The clinician may ask the child to make a word based on this sentence: *The girl is a friend.* He/she might ask another child to make a noun phrase from this sentence: *The fountain is for drinking.*

/ʃ/—THIRD GRADE

Have pictures of three kinds of food. "This looks delicious; this looks even _____; and this looks _____."

Draw the shape of a bell, a girl, a ship, a shoe, a dish, and a fish. The child then says: *This is shaped like a* _____.

/ð/

Arrange small trucks quite near the child, and big trucks away from the child. "These trucks are _____. Those trucks are _____ _____. This truck is for _____; that truck is for _____ _____. Both of these trucks are dump trucks. They are used for _____."

During these exercises, children can be taught to evaluate each other's utterances. Each member of the group can take turns becoming the judge of a particular aspect. This can be accomplished directly or through a creative drama activity with children becoming the engineer who fixes the train, the judge who makes the decision, or the teacher who is helping the child.

As noted earlier, games must be used judiciously. You make sure that the main goal is correcting the sound, not merely winning the game. Games do supply interest, however. For example, you may play a game similar to Bingo in which the children place beans on cards that contain ten or more pictures. The teacher, who has a duplicate set of pictures, shuffles them, holding up first one, then another picture. The child who has the picture of the object that the teacher holds up on his/her card says its name. Several children with particular sound difficulties can play this game, since the teacher gives them cards with pictures of words that contain their particular sound difficulties. The child who fills his/her card first calls out, "Word!" and wins the game.

A bus route that involves towns with sounds with which the children have difficulty can be arranged. The bus carries a driver who drives the bus and a hostess who explains the points of interest en route. A small toy bus travels over the route, which is drawn on the blackboard or on a large sheet of paper. The driver may either *chug, chug* [tʃʌg tʃʌg], or *bur, bur* [bɝ bɝ], or *si, si* [si si] along while the hostess takes care of the passenger. The driver stops, calls the towns, and assists the passengers on and off the bus. If the *chug, bur, bur,* or *si, si* is incorrect, the inspector sends the bus to the garage to be fixed. When the teacher drives, he/she occasionally says the sound incorrectly so that the children have training in recognizing the incorrect sound.

Another game that children like to play is one for which the teacher has collected pictures of objects the names of which contain the difficult sound. As the child closes his/her eyes tightly, he/she puts his/her finger on one of the pictures, which have been arranged on the table. After the teacher has described the article, the child guesses what it is. For example, the teacher might say to a child in the first grade, "This is something you eat with." After the child guesses a dish, the teacher might respond with, "You often eat ice cream with it." In all probability the child would then guess *a spoon*. The child then becomes the leader.

Children who work with a speech clinician may keep their words, phrases, and sentences in notebooks. They may show their notebooks to the teacher who, on occasion, may remind the child, "Mary, there's a word you can say now. Try it again." The teacher will not interrupt a flow of speech in which the child is interested; the teacher's correction will be easy, natural, and casual. Children cannot watch their speech constantly and will not always incorporate the right sound into words. This process takes time.

TEACHING THE CHILD TO CARRY THE TARGET SOUND OVER INTO EVERYDAY SPEECH

When children incorporate the sounds into words easily, they are ready to begin the transfer of the sounds to their everyday speech. Their clinician, teachers, and parents need to provide as many speaking situations for them as possible. At this stage, teachers are important to the work of the clinician, for they can set up situations wherein the child has many speaking opportunities to incorporate the newly acquired sound. Teachers tell the child to think before making the sound; if the sound comes out inaccurately, the members of the group will wait until it comes out right. After the activity has occurred, the teacher commends the child on the acceptable pronunciations and provides a list of phrases where the substituted sound was retained.

Sometimes the teacher will ask the clinician to work on some words and phrases that occur frequently in the classroom work. For instance, one child, who was working on *s* and at the same time preparing a report comparing a small town in the suburbs to New York City, needed to pronounce these words: *subway, station, supermarket, stores, suburbs, schools, snow, small, success, house, miss, bus, stop,* and *smooth.* Consequently, the clinician helped the child to say these particular words acceptably. Because the child was excited about her research, it also proved a good topic of conversation in the correction session. The classroom work helped to motivate the improvement.

Creative activities, including both puppetry and creative drama, encourage children to talk. To give practice in certain sounds, the clinician may use these activities in a therapy session and the teacher may use them in reinforcing work taught by the clinician. For the puppet play or the creative drama, the teacher or clinician can create a situation or use a story that will involve particular sounds. For example, in guiding a dramatic activity the teacher may suggest articles to build a story that contains many *s*'s: a silver scepter, an evening dress, and a sled.

Other situations for just plain talk arise spontaneously. The teacher takes advantage of these opportunities to promote oral communication. Chapter 8 suggests many speaking experiences for all children.

PARENTAL HELP

When parents are to be used as reinforcers of clinical training, they need to know exactly what to do. Carrier (1970) describes a program that parents could follow successfully. For example, in the first lesson, children have 20 cards with pictures that signify objects where the target sound is in the initial position in ten of the cards and with the target sound in the final position in the other ten. The child is expected to utter all 20 of the words splitting the target sound from the other sounds. When all 20 words are uttered correctly, the child is reinforced with tokens. In the second lesson, the child says the words but with the sounds synthesized. In the third lesson the child responds with words signified by the pictures. In the fourth lesson, the child responds to such questions as, "What do we wear under our shoes?" Such a regime with very specific tasks and very specific behavior requirements and evaluations can be undertaken successfully by parents.

Such training can result from conferences, which may be set up with the teacher, clinician, and parents participating. At these meetings, topics for discussion might well include attitudes of adults toward speech defects, what the parent and teacher can do for the speech-defective child both by way of motivation and correcting the difficulty, and how to handle the handicapped child. Such conferences promote an understanding of the child and the handicap and establish consistency in approach to the child and the child's problems.

We have indicated one set of steps in correcting an articulatory difficulty and noted how the clinician and teacher cooperate to bring about improvement in the child's articulation. Other clinicians and teachers will cooperate differently, because various procedures for correction exist.

Problems

1. Visit a school or clinic where you may observe a specialist working with a child with an articulatory difficulty. Indicate how you can reinforce in the classroom some of the learning that took place in the speech class or clinic.
2. Indicate ways other than those mentioned in the chapter of helping a child to listen to a specific sound.
3. How can you, as a classroom teacher, make use of some of the strategies described in this chapter?
4. Find children's books that emphasize a particular sound. How can each book be used in the classroom? in the clinical setting? (Try to find those books that have particular sounds as well as material that will further some aspects of language development.)
5. Make up a story involving nonsense syllables.
6. Devise a strategy that will contrast an error sound with a target sound.
7. Indicate ways you, as a classroom teacher, could help a particular child with a specific articulatory difficulty.
8. Indicate ways you, as a speech clinician, could seek reinforcement from a classroom teacher of a child with particular articulatory difficulty.
9. Read and report on one of the following: Brown 1975; Fleming 1971; Mowrer 1971; Ringel et al. 1970.

References and Suggested Readings

Arndt, W. B., M. E. Shelton, and R. L. Shelton, "Prediction of Articulation Improvement with Therapy from Early Lesson Sound Production Task Scores," *Journal of Speech and Hearing Research*, **14** (March 1971), 149–153.

Bankson, N. W., and M. C. Byrne, "The Effect of a Timed Correct Sound Production Task on Carryover," *Journal of Speech and Hearing Research*, **15** (March 1972), 160–168. (Investigates the feasibility of a program that would encourage the development of the motor skills necessary to produce sounds with ease and speed and the extent of generalization to spontaneous speech from a particular training task.)

Brown, J. C., "Techniques for Correcting /r/ Misarticulations," *Language, Speech, and Hearing Services in Schools*, **6** (April 1975), 86–90.

Carrier, J. K., "A Program of Articulation Therapy Administered by Mothers," *Journal of Speech and Hearing Disorders*, **35** (November 1970), 344–353.

Carroll, J. B., P. Davies, and B. Richman, *The American Heritage Word Frequency Book*. Boston: Houghton Mifflin Company, 1971. (Based on materials to which children are exposed in grades 3–9. Provides a frequency analysis of five million words sampled from textbooks and other materials currently in use in American schools.)

Edwards, K. J., and J. G. Anderson, "A Factor-Analytic Study of Articulation of Selected English Consonants," *Journal of Speech and Hearing Research*, **15** (December 1972), 720–728. (Gives the results of a factor analysis of speech articulation data for a sample of elementary school children with functional articulatory disorders.)

Elbert, M., and L. V. McReynolds, "Transfer of /r/ Across Contexts," *Journal of Speech and Hearing Disorders*, **40** (August 1975), 380–387. (Points out that training on one specific /r/ allophone may result in transfer to other /r/ allophones without specific training.)

Fleming, K. J., "Guidelines for Choosing Appropriate Phonetic Contexts for Speech-Sound Recognition and Production Practice," *Journal of Speech and Hearing Disorders*, **36** (August 1971), 356–367. (Presents guidelines for formulation of context lists that will enhance or challenge a child's discrimination and production abilities.)

Gray, B. B., "A Field Study on Programmed Articulation Study," *Language, Speech, and Hearing Services in Schools*, **5** (July 1974), 119–129.

Jacobs, R., *On Transformational Grammar: An Introduction for Teachers*, Monograph 11, New York State English Council, Oneonta, New York, 1968.

Kaliski, L., R. Tankersley, and R. Logha, *Structured Dramatics for Children with Learning Disabilities*, San Rafael, Calif.: Academic Therapy Publications, 1971.

Leonard, L. B., and S. I. Ritterman, "Articulation of /s/ as a Function of Cluster and Word Frequency of Occurrence," *Journal of Speech and Hearing Research*, **14** (September 1971), 476–485. (Suggests that inconsistencies of /s/ in consonantal clusters need not be attributed solely to the transitional motor differences in producing one cluster (such as /sk/) as compared to another (such as /st/). These inconsistencies also appear related to the frequency with which these clusters occur, making the more common concatenations more available for the child to discriminate and practice in his language usage.)

Locke, J. L., "Ease of Articulation," *Journal of Speech and Hearing Research*, **15** (March 1972), 194–200. (Asks whether ease of production can account for age of acquisition of sounds.)

Longhust, T. M., and J. E. Reichle, "The Applied Communication Game: A Comment on Muma's Communication Game: Dump and Play," *Journal of Speech and Hearing Disorders*, **40** (August 1975), 315–319. (Shows how theory of interpersonal communication can be used in a clinical setting.)

McCabe, R. B., and D. P. Bradley, "Pre-and Post Articulation Therapy Assessment," *Language, Speech, and Hearing Services in Schools*, **4** (January 1973), 13–24. (Suggests a way to evaluate articulation therapy.)

McGlone, R. E., and W. R. Proffit, "Patterns of Tongue Contact in Normal and Lisping Speakers," *Journal of Speech and Hearing Research*, **16** (September 1973), 456–473. (Notes that lispers possess an inability to use tongue muscles accurately. Suggests that causes could be physiological, neurological, or maturational.)

McNutt, J. D., and R. A. Keenan, "Comment on the Relationship Between Articulatory Defects and Syntax in Speech Defective Children," *Journal of Speech and Hearing Research*, **13** (September 1970), 669–679. (Suggests that therapy take account of the use of facilitating phonemes related to place—or other facilitating features—and avoid the phonemes that are frequently found to be substitutions.)

McReynolds, L. V., and K. Huston, "Token Loss in Speech Imitation Training," *Journal of Speech and Hearing Disorders*, **35** (November 1971), 486–495. (Compares the use of tokens as positive reinforcers for correct responses and no consequences for incorrect responses with the use of tokens contingent upon correct responses and loss of tokens contingent upon incorrect responses.)

Mason, R. M., and W. R. Proffit, "The Tongue-Thrust Controversy: Background and Recommendations," *Journal of Speech and Hearing Disorders*, **39** (May 1974), 115–132. (Reviews oral form and function interactions and provides guidelines for selecting cases and planning treatment.)

Merton, K., "A Self-Directing Approach to Articulation Therapy and Practical Considerations," *Language, Speech, and Hearing Services in Schools*, **3** (July 1972), 24–31. (Discusses therapy based on sounds in successful contexts, practice, feedback, and expansion in systematically successful contexts.)

Mowrer, D. E., "Transfer of Training in Articulation Therapy," *Journal of Speech and Hearing Disorders*, **36** (November 1971), 427–446. (Reviews research having to do with these stages of therapy: (1) discrimination training, (2) sounds in isolation, (3) transfer among words, (4) transfer among sentences, and (5) transfer to spontaneous conversation.)

Mysak, E. D., *Speech Pathology and Feedback Theory*, Springfield, Ill.: Charles C Thomas, Publisher, 1971.

Pollack, E., and N. S. Rees, "Disorders of Articulation: Some Clinical Applications of Distinctive Feature Theory," *Journal of Speech and Hearing Disorders*, **37** (November 1972), 451–461. (Suggests the application of distinctive feature therapy as an approach to articulatory training.)

Powell, J., and L. V. McReynolds, "A Procedure for Testing Position Generalization from Articulatory Training," *Journal of Speech and Hearing Research*, **12** (September 1969), 629–645.

Prins, D. T., "Abilities of Children with Misarticulations," *Journal of Speech and Hearing Research*, **5** (June 1962), 161–168. (a)

———, "Analysis of Correlations Among Various Articulatory Deviations," *Journal of Speech and Hearing Research*, **5** (June 1962), 152–160. (b)

Ringel, R. L., and S. J. Ewanowski, "Oral Perception: 1. Two-Point Discrimination," *Journal of Speech and Hearing Research*, **8** (June 1968), 389–398. (Discusses the concept that knowledge of the perceptual abilities of certain oral structures may yield insights into the role of tactile feedback in the total speech-monitoring system.)

Ringel, R. L., A. S. House, K. W. Burk, J. P. Dolinsky, and C. M. Scott, "Some Relationships Between Orosensory Discrimination and Articulatory Aspects of Speech Production," *Journal of Speech and Hearing Disorders*, **35** (February 1970), 3–11. (Discusses the value of training speech-defective persons in oral-discrimination tasks.)

Ritterman, S. I., *Practice Variables and Speech Sound Discrimination in Learning*, Ph.D. Thesis, Case Western University, 1969.

———, "The Role of Practice and the Observation of Practice in Speech-Sound Discrimination Learning," *Journal of Speech and Hearing Research*, **13** (March 1970), 178–183. (Reports on the effect of learning by participation and learning by observation on the acquisition of a repertoire of phonetic distinctions.)

Ruscello, D. M., "The Importance of Word Position in Articulation Therapy," *Language, Speech, and Hearing Services in Schools*, **6** (October 1975), 190–194. (Evaluates the importance of the position of sounds in words in a typical therapy program.)

Ryan, B. P., "A Study of the Effectiveness of the S-Pack Program in the Elimination of Frontal Lisping Behavior in Third Grade Children," *Journal of Speech and Hearing Disorders*, **36** (August 1971), 390–396. (Presents a particular strategy for eliminating frontal lisps.)

Scott, C. M., and R. L. Ringel, "Articulation Without Oral Sensory Control," *Journal of Speech and Hearing Research*, **14** (December 1971), 804–818. (Shows the effects of articulation without oral sensory control.)

Sommers, R. K., and A. R. Kane, "Nature and Remediation of Functional Articulation Disorders," in S. Dickson, ed., *Communication Disorders: Remedial Principles and Practices*, Chicago: Scott, Foresman and Company, 1975, pp. 106–193.

Van Hattum, R. J., J. Page, R. D. Baskervill, M. Duguay, L. Schreiber Conway, and T. R. Davis, "The Speech Improvement System Taped Program for Remediation of Articulation Problems in Schools," *Language, Speech, and Hearing Services in Schools*, **5** (April 1974), 91–97. (Describes the use of a particular program.)

Van Riper, C., *Speech Correction: Principles and Methods*, 4th ed., Englewood Cliffs, N. J.: Prentice-Hall, Inc., 1972, chap. 6.

Walsh, H., "On Certain Inadequacies of Distinctive Feature Systems," *Journal of Speech and Hearing Disorders*, **39** (February 1974), 32–43. (Describes the inadequacies of distinctive feature systems in diagnosing and treating speech disorders.)

Weber, J. L., "Patterning of Deviant Articulation Behavior," *Journal of Speech and Hearing Disorders*, **24** (May 1970), 135–41. (Indicates how an entire pattern of articulation can be taught at once.)

Webster, E. J., "Procedures for Group Parent Counseling in Speech Pathology and Audiology," *Journal of Speech and Hearing Disorders*, **33** (May 1968), 127–131. (Discusses use of group discussion and role playing in parent counseling.)

Weiss, H. H., and B. Born, "Speech Training or Language Acquisition? A Distinction When Speech Training Is Taught by Operant Conditioning Procedures," *American Journal of Orthopsychiatry*, **37** (January 1967), 49–55.

(Reports on behavior modification in teaching speech to a seven-and-a-half-year-old boy with success in several learning paradigms within limits of circumscribed training sessions, but failure to generalize learned speech patterns outside of experimental settings. Suggests this may be an important distinction between speech and language.)

Wepman, J. M., and W. Hass, *A Spoken Word Count*, Chicago: Language Research Associates, 1971.

Winitz, H., *Articulatory Acquisition and Behavior*, New York: Appleton-Century-Crofts, 1969, chap. 5. (Discusses articulatory programing.)

———, *From Syllable to Conversation*, Baltimore: University Park Press, 1975

———, and B. Bellerose, "Self-Retrieval and Articulatory Retention," *Journal of Speech and Hearing Research*, **18** (September 1975), 466–477. (Gives the results of testing the effect of self-retrieval on articulation recall. Self-retrieval indicates saying the name of the object rather than imitating the examiner's production of the word.)

———, "Sound Discrimination as a Function of Pretraining Conditions," *Journal of Speech and Hearing Research*, **5** (December 1962), 340–348.

Addresses of Companies Supplying Material for Speech and Language Therapy

Academic Therapy Publications, 1539 4th Street, San Rafael, California 94901.

American Book Company, 450 West 33rd Street, New York City 10001.

American Guidance System, Publishers Building, Circle Pines, Minnesota 55104.

Stanley Bowmar Company, Valhalla, New York 10595.

Bureau of Educational Research Services, State University of Iowa, Iowa City, Iowa 52240.

Cebco Standard Publishing Company, Post Office Box 31138, Cincinnati, Ohio 45231.

Childcraft, 964 Third Avenue, New York City 10022.

Chronicle Guidance Publishing Company, Moravia, New York 13118.

Cleo Living Aids, 3957 Mayfield Avenue, Cleveland, Ohio 44121.

Communication Skills Builders, Post Office Box 608, Tucson, Arizona 85716.

Council for Exceptional Children, 1411 S. Jefferson Highway, Arlington, Virginia 22202.

Creative Playthings, Princeton, New Jersey 18540.

The John Day Company, Inc., 62 West 45th Street, New York City 10036.

Developmental Learning Materials, 7440 Natchez Avenue, Niles, Illinois 60648.

Educational Activities, Post Office Box 392, Freeport, New York 11520.

Educational Performance Associates, Inc., 563 Westview Avenue, Ridgefield, New Jersey 07657.

Educational Psychological Research Associates, Post Office Box 614, Verdes Estates, California 90214.

Eye Gate House, 146–01 Archer Avenue, Jamaica, New York 11435.

Fearon Publishers, Inc., 6 Davis Drive, Belmont, California 94002.

Follett Education Corporation, 1018 Washington Boulevard, Chicago, Illinois 60607.

Garrard Publishing Company, Champaign, Illinois 61820.

Ginn and Company, 125 Second Avenue, Waltham, Massachusetts 02154.

Go-Mo Productions, 1906 Main Street, Cedar Falls, Iowa 50613.

Golden Press, 850 Third Avenue, New York City 10022.

Harper & Row, Publishers, 10 East 53rd Street, New York City 10022.

Ideal School Supply, 1100 S. Laverne Avenue, Oak Lawn, Illinois 60453.

Interstate Printers and Publishers, Dansville, Illinois 61832.

Landsford Publishing Company, Post Office Box 8711, San Jose, California 95155.

Language Research Associates, 175 E. Delaware Place, Chicago, Illinois 60611.

The Learning Business, 30961 Agoura Road, Suite 325, Westlake Village, California 91361.

Learning Concepts, Inc., 2501 N. Lamar Street, Austin, Texas 78705.

Love Publishing Company, 6635 E. Villanova Place, Denver, Colorado 80222.

Luxar Corporation, Educational Services Department, 104 Lakeview Avenue, Waukegan, Illinois 60085.

McGraw-Hill, Inc., 1221 Sixth Avenue, New York City 10020.

Mafex Associates, 111 Barron Avenue, Johnstown, Pennsylvania 15906.

Merriman Associates, Post Office Box 899, Waterloo, Iowa 50704.

Miller Brody Productions, 342 Madison Avenue, New York City 10017.

Modern Education Corporation, Post Office Box 721, Tulsa, Oklahoma 74104.

Scott, Foresman and Company, 99 Baver Drive, Oakland, New Jersey 07436.

Simon & Schuster, Inc., 1 West 39th Street, New York City 10018.

Stanwix House, 3020 Chartiers Avenue, Pittsburgh, Pennsylvania 15204.

Steck-Vaughan Company, Post Office Box 2028, Austin, Texas 78767.

Charles C Thomas, Publisher, 301–327 E. Laurence Avenue, Springfield, Illinois 13118.

Western Psychological Services, 12031 Wilshire Blvd, Los Angeles, California 90425.

Word Making Productions, Post Office Box 1858, Salt Lake City, Utah 84110.

Bibliography of Children's Books That Provide Practice
Material for the Indicated Sounds

[k] 5, 9, 10, 13, 20, 27
[g] 5, 9, 10, 12
[s] 1, 3, 5, 9, 10, 12, 13, 18, 22
[z] 3, 10, 15, 17, 18, 32

[ʃ] 6, 18, 21, 23, 28
[tʃ] 4, 6, 18, 23
[dʒ] 4, 7, 12, 19
[f] 3, 18, 22, 30
[v] 7, 23, 31
[θ] 9, 15, 18, 20
[ð] 9, 15, 18, 20
[l] 1, 7, 13, 19, 28, 30
[r] 2, 3, 9, 10, 17, 20, 30, 31
All sounds 3, 4, 8, 14, 17, 21, 24, 25, 26, 29

1. Aliki, *My Five Senses*, New York: Thomas Y. Crowell Company, 1962. (Each sensory organ and its function are presented as "I can see. I see with my eyes.")
2. Bright, R., *My Red Umbrella*, New York: William Morrow & Co., Inc., 1959. (The story of an umbrella that expands in the rain to cover a multitude of animals.)
3. Brown, M., *All Butterflies*, New York: Charles Scribner's Sons, 1974. (Alphabet book with phrases beginning with two sequential alphabet letters as "All butterflies; Cat dance; Elephants fly."
4. ————, *Peter Piper's Alphabet*, New York: Charles Scribner's Sons, 1959. (Tongue twisters that provoke mirth.)
5. Browner, R., *Everyone Has a Name*, New York: Henry C. Walck, 1961. (Clues to the names and characteristics of different animals.)
6. Breinburg, P., *Shawn Goes to School*, New York: Thomas Y. Crowell Company, 1974. (Shawn really wants to go to school but is frightened until the teacher calms him by getting him interested in other children and toys.)
7. Christopher, M., *Jinx Glove*, New York: Coward, McCann & Geoghegan, (Old baseball gloves are best.)
8. Crews, D., *We Read: A to Z*, New York: Harper & Row, Publishers, Inc., 1967. (Concepts that begin with letters; *a* is represented by *almost*.)
9. Dugan, W., *The Truck and Bus Book*, New York: Golden Press, Inc., 1966. (Short descriptions of various trucks and buses.)
10. Fassler, J., *Howie Helps Himself*. Racine, Wis.: Albert Whitman, 1975. (Howie can't run, skip, or ride a bike, for he has cerebral palsy. The story of Howie's going to a special school for the handicapped.)
11. Fife, D., *Adam's ABC*, New York: Coward, McCann & Geoghegan, 1971. (One day in the life of a black child in an urban setting.)
12. Fort, J., *June the Tiger*, Boston: Little, Brown and Company, 1975. (The story of a dog, his old mistress, and the enemy, a bear.)
13. Freeman, D., *The Seal and the Slick*, New York: The Viking Press, Inc., 1974. (Children clean the flippers of a seal who has been caught in an oil slick and who then returns to his family who move to another spot where there is no oil slick.)
14. Gág, W., *The ABC Bunny*, New York: Coward, McCann & Geoghegan, 1933. (The alphabet in rhyme centered around a bunny.)

15. ———, *Nothing at All*, New York: Coward, McCann & Geoghegan, 1941. (The story of three little orphan dogs.)

16. Hoberman, M. A., *Nuts to You and Nuts to Me*, New York: Alfred A. Knopf, Inc., 1974. (An alphabet of poems. Fun.)

17. Holl, A., *The ABC's of Carts, Trucks, and Machines*, New York: American Heritage Press, 1970. (Rhymes about police cars, dump trucks, and the like.)

18. Joseph, S. M., ed., *The Me Nobody Knows*, New York: Avon Books, Inc., 1969. (Poems and essays written by black or Puerto Rican ghetto children. Includes four sections: (1) How I See Myself, (2) How I See My Neighborhood, (3) The World Outside, and (4) Things I Can't See or Touch.)

19. Klein, L., *How Old Is Old?* New York: Harvey House, Inc., Publishers, 1967. (The concept of age is presented using as a base the ages at which different animals are considered old. Ages of people vary, and *how old is old* depends on who is doing the evaluating.)

20. Kuskin, K., *Any Me I Want to Be*, New York: Harper & Row, Publishers, Inc., 1972. (What it would be like to be something other than you— like a bird, a sandwich, or a front door key.)

21. Lear, E., *A Was Once An Apple Pie: A Nonsense Alphabet*, New York: Scholastic Book Services, 1969. (An old favorite in paperback version with delightful illustrations.)

22. Lester, S. A., *Lost*, New York: Harcourt Brace Jovanovich, Inc., 1975. (A little boy gets lost at the zoo but finds another smaller boy who is also lost and whom he helps. Finally the boys are reunited with their families.)

23. Lobel, A., *The Man Who Took the Indoors Out*, New York: Harper & Row, Publishers, Inc., 1974. (Nonsense tale about a man who loved all the things in the house and felt they should have a taste of the outdoors. And so he took outside tables, chairs, dishes, a sink, and so on, which then refused to go back in the house.)

24. Matthiesen, T., *ABC: An Alphabet Book*, New York: Platt & Munk, 1966. (Letters based on everyday experiences.)

25. McGinley, P., *All Around the Town*, Philadelphia: J. B. Lippincott Co., 1948. (A tale of city sights beginning with *A* and ending with *Z*.)

26. Peppé, R., *The Alphabet Book*, New York: Four Winds Press, 1968. (Based on objects familiar to children.)

27. Prelutsky, J., *The Pack Rat's Day and Other Poems*, New York: Macmillan Publishing Co., Inc., 1974. (Fifteen poems about different animals. Fun verse.)

28. Rice, E., *New Blue Shoes*, New York: Macmillan Publishing Co., Inc., 1975. (Rebecca goes shopping for new shoes and really wants blue ones but is persuaded to get the sturdy kind.)

29. Dr. Seuss, *ABC*, New York: Random House, Inc., 1963. (An exciting ABC book.)

30. Simon, M., and H. Simon, *If You Were An Eel, How Would You Feel?* Chicago: Follett Publishing Company, 1963. (The eel, bear, tortoise, bat,

cat, and seal are introduced with "If you were a—". Motivates oral communication.)

31. Sullivan, J., *Round Is a Pancake*, New York: Holt, Rinehart and Winston, Inc., 1963. (Shapes related to children's experiences.)

32. Udry, J., *A Tree Is Nice*, New York: Harper & Row, Publishers, Inc., 1956. (Many concepts about trees are pictured.)

12. *Voice Disturbances*

Before considering voice disturbances, the student should review the material on the vocal mechanism in Chapter 5. As supplemental reading, especially for the student who is concerned about his/her voice, we recommend the chapters on voice in Eisenson (1974, Chaps. 3–9).

The incidence of voice disturbances in school-age children, especially in the primary grades, is much lower than for articulatory defects or for stuttering. For every child with a vocal disturbance we are likely to find from ten to 15 children who have defective articulation or who show signs of stuttering. Thus, the study of voice disturbances is not as important for its total incidence as it is for its possible significance as a reflection of the child's personality, or perhaps of the personality of the individual with whom the child is identifying and imitating. Another reason for us to study voice disturbances is that they may be associated with a physical condition that may require medical attention.

Before considering vocal disturbances, we ought first to appreciate the characteristics and potentialities of a normal voice.

Characteristics of a Normal Voice

A normal voice should be able to communicate reliably the feelings and thoughts the speaker wishes to convey to the listener. When well controlled, the voice should reveal rather than betray the types and shades of feeling that color the speaker's thinking. Through appropriate changes in pitch, force, duration, and quality, a speaker's voice should be able to command attention, maintain interest, and convey changes and emphasis in meaning.

The ability of a speaker to communicate intellectual and affective content will be enhanced if the speaker's voice attracts no attention to itself because of the manner in which it is produced or because of any undesirable characteristics. Vocalization should take place without apparent effort or strain. The acoustic results should be appropriate to the speaking situation. The voice should, in addition, be appropriate to the age and sex of the speaker. Little children may sound like little children, but older ones should not be mistaken for them. Neither should first graders sound like their parents or their teachers.

From the point of view of the listener, a normal and effective voice is one that is *pleasant, clear,* and *readily audible.* It should be heard without listener effort, provided, of course, that the listening conditions are not unfavorable for the purpose.

TYPES OF VOICE DISTURBANCES

The defects of voice most frequently heard are (1) inadequate loudness; (2) faulty volume (loudness) control; (3) loudness inappropriate to the speaking situation or speech content; (4) defects of quality, especially nasality and denasality, breathiness, and huskiness; (5) faulty pitch range or too narrow a range of pitch; and (6) inappropriate rate. Each of these voice defects is considered in some detail in our discussion of therapy for voice disturbances.

CAUSES OF VOCAL DISTURBANCES

It is important that the *diagnosis of a voice disturbance should be made by a specialist.*[1] Where a physical condition may be the underlying cause, treatment should not be undertaken without medical clearance and approval. Fortunately, even where the cause is physical, treatment may help to prevent aggravation of the disturbance and often may improve the condition as well as the voice.

Vocal disturbances may be present for a variety of reasons. Among the most common reasons are (1) poor physical health; (2) anomalies

---

[1] By a specialist we mean a professional person whose training and experience qualify him or her for making diagnoses and for treating persons who present vocal difficulties when speaking. Such persons should have considerably more than the usual exposure to voice problems as part of their general training.

in the structure or condition of the voice mechanism; (3) pathologies in the neurological control of the mechanism; (4) glandular conditions or other physical conditions that may affect the growth or the tonicity and the responses of the muscles involved in voice production; (5) defects of hearing that impair the individual's ability to respond to and monitor his own voice as it is being produced; (6) disturbances of personality that reflect themselves in voice; (7) the presence of poor models that the child is imitating, so that he acquires a vocal defect through normal processes of learning; and (8) poor habits of vocalization.

The speech clinician and classroom teacher are most likely to be directly concerned with the last two of the listed reasons. To a lesser degree, defects of hearing may also directly concern them. Vocal disturbances that have a physical basis, as already suggested, are the therapeutic concern of the specialist in voice problems. The teacher, however, is frequently the first to have an opportunity to recognize that something may be wrong that is causing the child to have a vocal difficulty, and so has a responsibility for bringing the condition to the attention of the parent and speech clinician.

Poor Physical Health

Most of us are able to recognize that "something is wrong" with a friend or relative by the way the friend sounds. Sometimes "what is wrong" may be temporary and a matter of momentary mood; occasionally, it may be physical and a matter of health. The interested and sensitive listener, who may be parent, friend, or teacher, is often the first to suspect that a speaker may not be well. Voice, because it is a product of the physiological as well as the emotional and intellectual state of the speaker, is the mirror that reflects the speaker's state of health. The expert speaker may, with awareness, control his/her voice and so succeed in disguising this condition. School-age children, less practiced in concealment and control, frequently reveal both their affective state and the state of their general physical health through their vocalizations.

Physical Anomalies

Perhaps the most frequent cause of vocal disturbances is the common cold. When we suffer from a cold, any or all of the following modifications of the voice mechanism may be present. The nasal cavities may be filled with mucous and so prevent adequate reinforcement of voice. The mucous membranes of the nose, throat, and larynx may be inflamed, and so modify the normal resonating activity of the voice mechanism. The vocal bands may themselves be inflamed and swollen, and so prevent normal vocal activity. The general "run-down" condition of the individual may impair normal functioning and control of the voice mechanism. If the cold is accompanied by a persistent cough, the general condition may be aggravated by the vocal abuse that is caused by coughing.

Persistent coughing may produce laryngitis. The condition of laryngitis may, however, be caused by vocal abuse not associated with either a cough or a cold. Continued overloud talking, or yelling under conditions of competing noise, may also produce laryngitis.

Sometimes vocal difficulties are associated with abnormalities of the structure of the larynx. The laryngeal cartilages may, for congenital reasons or through injury, be so constructed that the vocal bands may not be able to approximate normally, or the reinforcement of vocal tones may be impaired because of the change in the size and shape of the larynx. More frequently, the vocal bands may have developed nodules on the inner edges as a result of vocal abuse. Sometimes the vocal bands become thickened because of chronic incorrect vocalization. The effect is usually a voice characterized by low pitch, breathiness, and effort in production. Fortunately, these conditions usually improve through a combination of voice rest and a program of training to modify the incorrect vocal behavior of the speaker. Occasionally, the edges of the vocal bands may have slight irregularities, which impair normal activity. Any of the conditions described can be determined only through an examination of the larynx by a competent physician. The treatment of these conditions will call for the active cooperation of the classroom teacher. Voice therapy, if it is indicated, is a problem for the speech clinician working in cooperation with the physician.

HEARING LOSS

Because we learn to vocalize as well as to articulate "by ear," hearing loss, especially in the low-pitch ranges, is likely to be manifest in vocal inadequacies. If the hearing loss is appreciable, and of the type that does not permit the child to check on the voice produced, the child may speak in a voice too loud, or not loud enough, for the specific speaking situation. Sometimes the loss may be temporary, and associated with the effects or aftereffects of a cold. Occasionally, as a result of middle-ear involvement, there may be prolonged hearing loss. With proper medical attention, this situation should clear and the vocal disturbance disappear.

GLANDULAR DISTURBANCES

Thyroid gland deficiency is associated with a falling of the basal metabolic rate. Frequently, though not invariably, decrease in metabolic rate is causally associated with sluggish physical and mental activity, and with a general reduction of body tone. This condition is likely to reflect itself in a colorless, poorly modulated voice.

In contrast with thyroid deficiency, the presence of an excess of thyroid hormone generally results in making the individual hyperactive and "nervous." The condition is likely to be reflected in a rapid rate of speech and in a tense, high-pitched voice.

The teacher and speech clinician who observe what appear to be significant changes in the general activity and mental alertness of a child, in association with vocal changes, should refer the child to the school nurse or physician for a medical examination to determine the possibility of a glandular involvement. Caution, however, should be exercised that no hasty conclusion be made. Comparable changes in the voice of a child may result from conditions not related to glandular disturbances. Vocal changes may sometimes merely indicate a temporary indisposition on the part of the child.

PUBERTAL CHANGES

With the coming of physical adolescence and its associated physiological and growth changes, many children have marked vocal difficulties. These are more likely to be present among boys than among girls. In males, the size and structure of the larynx undergo considerable change, so that boys have to adjust to longer vocal bands as well as a larger larynx. Girls, with a longer and slower pubescent period, and with a smaller amount of laryngeal growth, have less modification and more time for adjustment. The little girl soprano may, during adolescence, become a woman mezzo-soprano or perhaps an alto. The boy soprano may become a tenor or a baritone.

Often the difficulty during puberty is aggravated by problems of social adjustment. The shy youngster may be so embarrassed by his voice "breaks" that he withdraws from his groups or finds excuses for not talking. Some of the difficulties may be related to self-consciousness resulting from a poor skin condition, or an awareness of physical awkwardness. Occasionally, overly passive adolescents may try to vocalize within a pitch range determined for them by their parents or older siblings, or other influential members of their environment. In some instances, dependent and infantile boys and girls may try to maintain their preadolescent voices as an aspect of their general wish to continue to be young children. In other instances, both boys and girls may try to show how mature they are by attempting to establish low, deep-pitched voices incompatible with their own amount of laryngeal growth and general physical change.[2]

The influence of the speech clinician and the classroom teacher in helping adolescents through their period of voice change can hardly be overestimated. The teacher can ward off taunts and help the adolescent build up defenses. If the adolescent has prolonged difficulty in arriving at his/her "new voice," referral to a speech clinician may be of help. If there is reason to believe that psychological problems may be part of the difficulty, referral of the adolescent for proper guidance is in order.

PERSONALITY DISTURBANCES

Few of us question the general observation that the voice is a mirror of the personality. Temporary emotional upsets are likely to be reflected in the speaker's voice. Similarly, chronic emotional disturbances and maladjustments of attitude are likely to be manifest in disorders of voice.

Part of the early and continued experience of classroom teachers is the need to urge a child to "speak up" because of a weak and timid voice. Other children, in sharp contrast, need to be reminded to "tone down" because there is no cause for shouting. Children of both voice types may be revealing attitudes toward their classmates in particular and their environment in general that are suggestive of a significant degree of maladjustment. So does the child whose voice is a constant whine; so also does the child whose breathless voice and breathtaking rate of speaking suggest fear of interruption and apprehension that once interrupted the youngster may not be able to resume talking.

Although the vocal defects described briefly are not important in themselves, they are of importance if they are symptoms of chronic personality maladjustments. Occasionally, the child's voice may be reflecting not only his or her own maladjustments but one of an older member of the environment whom the child is unconsciously imitating. Whatever the case may be for the individual child, appropriate treatment calls for determining and dealing with the underlying cause as well as with the vocal symptoms of the cause. With the young child, the voice symptoms are likely to disappear without direct treatment provided that the basic personality problem is relieved. The older child, who may have established vocal traits that have become habitual, may

---

[2] The junior high school years, usually the 12–15 years age range, is the period for major vocal changes. This period, as many teachers can attest, is also one in which many changes take place in attitude and behavior. Thus, adjustments to vocal change are correlated with other dynamics of adolescence.

need direct treatment for voice even if the personality problem is treated.

IMITATION OF POOR MODELS

The child learns both his language and the manner in which his language is produced by ear. The mother who teaches her child the name of something also teaches the child the manner in which the naming is done. If mother shouts, so will the child; if mother speaks as though she were not worthy of the evocation, the child is likely to develop the same tone. As the child grows up, other models become subjects for imitation. Friends, liked or respected adults, who frequent the home, and teachers, when the child is of school age, become likely models. Usually the imitation is unconscious; occasionally a child's urge or need to identify with another person is so strong that the imitation may be conscious. Imitation that begins early may continue into and beyond adolescence.

Often a parent will be aware that there is something wrong with a child's voice but have no awareness that the fault is parent-centered. We have frequently pointed out to complaining parents that they must have children who love them because the children spoke so much like them. And frequently we have suggested to parents that they accept treatment for their own voices as the best device for improving the voices of their children.

Teachers, obviously, have a great responsibility for the voices of their classroom children. A well-liked teacher is likely to be an imitated teacher. A disliked teacher may be mimicked in manner as well as in voice. So, before a teacher turns to other sources for an explanation of common pupil vocal traits, self-reflection is in order. Beyond this, an objective appraisal by a professionally competent person may go a long way in explaining the positive or negative reasons for common vocal faults among pupils in a given classroom. So, a sudden "epidemic" of hoarseness may be explained by a teacher's hoarseness. Pupil manifestations of breathiness, denasality, or low pitch may indicate the need for teacher correction if the children are to vocalize without these defects.

POOR HABITS OF VOCALIZATION

The professional speech clinician often treats persons whose vocal habits are poor and are not apparently associated with any present disturbance of personality or any specific or general physical condition. It is possible, of course, that the faulty vocal habits have outlived the cause of their origin, that in a given instance the speaker is presenting the residual of an adolescent "crush," or a once-serious personality maladjustment, or a vocal manner that began with an illness and has persisted long after all physical evidence of illness disappeared. Not infrequently vocal habits may be interpreted as lingering memories of what used to be. If, however, "what used to be" is no longer in need of treatment, the vocal symptoms, or the vocal habits with which the symptoms are associated, may be directly treated. Chief among faulty vocal habits are unsuitable pitch level, inappropriate nasal reinforcement, and poor breath control for speech.

Vocal pitch and vocal range are not to be selected by the individual as one might choose articles of dress. Pitch, as pointed out earlier, is determined by the size, shape, and normal functioning of the vocal bands and the resonating cavities. Each of us is potentially intended for a given "optimum pitch" and range of pitch according to individual vocal equipment. Most of us arrive at this without special instruction by doing "what comes naturally." Some of us make the most of our potential by special motivation or by competent instruction. A few of us succumb to pressures to vocalize in a manner not consistent with nature's intentions for us, and difficulties may arise. One of these pressures is the contemporary one of admiring women's voices that are low-pitched and somewhat breathy in quality. The not infrequent result of employing a voice pitched too low for the physical mechanism is hoarseness. Although there is considerable variability in regard to the consequences of the constant use of a voice pitched too low for the mechanism, there is a growing body of evidence indicating that undesirable physical consequences can frequently be expected. Among these consequences are thickening of the vocal bands and chronic irritation of the larynx.

Boys, as well as men, are not at all exempt from the cultural pressure for the low-pitched voice. Unfortunately, just so many women are born to have soprano voices, and only a few to be altos; so it is that many boys and men are by nature intended to be tenors and high baritones, just as some are to be low baritones and basses. The result of confusing physical virility with vocal depth is frequently low pitch and poor quality. On occasion, chronic hoarseness can result from attempts to pitch the voice at a level too low for the optimum functioning of the vocal apparatus. Strain and fatigue may also occur.[3]

Our emphasis thus far has been on the abnormally low-pitched voice. This does not mean that some persons do not speak at a pitch

---

[3] M. Cooper, "Spectographic Analysis of Fundamental Frequency and Hoarseness Before and After Vocal Rehabilitation," *Journal of Speech and Hearing Disorders*, **39** (1974), found that in a population of 155 patients who required vocal rehabilitation, 150 were vocalizing in too low a pitch range. Cooper concluded that "... the use of a pitch which is below the optimal or natural level is a major factor in initiating, contributing to, or continuing most types of dysphonia."

level too high for their vocal mechanism. Among speakers with in-appropriate pitch they are, however, likely to constitute a small minority. Cultural preference in the United States places a premium on the low-pitched voice and is inclined to penalize the high-pitched voices. Unless there is a strong psychological drive to maintain an abnormally high-pitched voice, the individual is likely to yield in the direction of cultural preference. Interestingly enough, persons who persist in vocalizing at high pitch levels, unless they are also shouters, are usually not as susceptible to some of the physical changes that frequently accompany abnormally low-pitched vocalization. We may appreciate some of the reasons for this by intentionally, but briefly, talking considerably below and then considerably above our normal pitch range. In talking at the low end of our range, we will find that it takes appreciably more effort to produce a loud voice than within our normal range, or at a relatively high pitch. Fatigue is likely to set in quickly, and a feeling of vocal strain will follow if vocalization is continued. We are not, incidentally, referring to the use of a high-pitched falsetto or of a pitch range associated with laryngeal hyperten-sion.

Habitual use of pitches much below or above our natural pitch range is often accomplished at the expense of the abuse of the vocal mechanism. We have worked with preschool children who developed nodules on their vocal bands as a result of vocal abuse. Typically, these children were high-pitched screamers (Wilson 1961).[4] There are always, of course, some individuals who are able to vocalize either above or below normal pitch range without suffering physical consequences. Perhaps these persons are kin to those who do not develop calluses despite poorly fitted shoes, or who do not become sunburned despite what would be overexposure to the sun for most of us. Our only sugges-tion is that these hardy persons be considered exceptions rather than models for the more susceptible of us to follow. Most of us do better vocalizing within a pitch range suited to our vocal apparatus. How to determine this range is considered later in the discussion of optimum pitch in the section on vocal therapy.

Caution needs to be exercised when judgments are made about pitch levels and ranges. Schneiderman (1959) found that judgments about pitch, including those by listeners with "trained ears," are not

---

[4] In a survey, E. M. Silverman and C. H. Zimmer, "Incidence of Chronic Hoarseness among School Age Children," *Journal of Speech and Hearing Disorders*, **40** (1975) found that 38 of 162 children in the elementary school grades suffered from chronic hoarseness. A majority of these children were below the fourth grade. Most of them were found to have vocal nodules on otolaryngological examination.

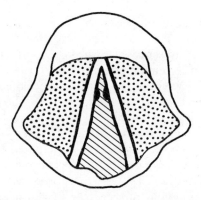

Figure 11. Vocal nodules, often associated with high-pitched shouting. Note typical paired formation in upper (middle third) of vocal folds.

always valid. Other aspects of voice—quality or loudness—may produce an erroneous impression as to the "perceived" pitch. This observation emphasizes the need to determine optimum pitch level and range rather than to make arbitrary judgments as to the appropriateness of the speaker's pitch.

INAPPROPRIATE NASAL REINFORCEMENT

The movements of the soft palate largely determine whether the produced voice is characterized by the presence or absence of nasality. Normally, when vocalization occurs with a relaxed soft palate that permits the stream of breath to enter the nasal cavities, the voice is reinforced there and becomes characteristically nasal. Of course, some nasal reinforcement occurs whether or not the soft palate is relaxed or elevated, so that a degree of nasality is likely to be present even when nasality is not the characteristic quality of the produced voice.

The American-English sounds *n*, *m*, and *ng* are normally produced with a relaxed soft palate and "open nasal cavities." All other sounds of English are normally produced with the soft palate elevated so that the stream of breath is directed and emitted orally. If an individual has a weakened soft palate, he will tend to speak with more than a normal amount of nasal emission, and so has a voice quality characterized by *positive nasality*. The same quality may result from sluggish palatal control and from related activity of the mouth, throat, and nasopharynx in their functions as resonators. Positive nasality may also arise as a result of imitation. The French-speaking child quite properly nasalizes some of the vowels as well as the nasal consonants. The American- or English-speaking child may do the same in imitating the speech of a member of the environment who nasalizes more than most American or English speakers do.

Denasality, or an absence of appropriate nasal resonance, occurs when there is too little reinforcement by the nasal resonators. This may result from a blocking within the nasal cavities themselves, or a partial blocking within the area of the nasopharynx. The result is a pinched, flat quality that suggests the voice of a person with a head cold or an allergic condition involving the nasal cavities. The quality is more than an absence of nasality when it is anticipated in the production of the nasal consonants. It is an overall effect recognizable on sounds that are normally emitted orally. We can produce what approaches a denasal voice by pinching our nostrils in the articulation of such a sentence as "Who is that tall boy with a black coat?" The result even though the sentence does not contain nasal consonants, should be different in quality if the sentence is articulated without pinched nostrils.

Techniques for recognizing and improving nasal reinforcement are considered in the discussion of voice therapy.

BREATHING FAULTS

It is unusual for a physically normal child to breathe incorrectly while speaking unless he or she has somehow been trained to do so. Such training may be the result of a child's efforts to be obedient to the direction, "Take a real deep breath before you begin to speak," or "Raise your chest high and pull your tummy in before you begin to speak." Occasionally, but really rarely, a child may speak with a too shallow breath, or attempt to speak while inhaling rather than, or in addition to, exhaling. In such instances, investigation is likely to reveal that we are dealing with an insecure, apprehensive child who fears that pausing for a normal breath will result in an interruption of thought. Someone will break in, and during the interruption the child will forget and suffer the consequent social penalties. The same factors may operate with the child who attempts to speak on inhalation as well as exhalation, or who tries with effort to speak on residual air after "tidal breath" has been expired. However, we should not overlook the possibility that in some instances we may be dealing with a normal child with normal psychological dynamisms, who is simply imitating a member of the environment whose breathing habits for speech are faulty.

We are inclined to agree with Curtis (1967, pp. 193–194) that it is probably of little importance whether the person's breathing is predominantly abdominal or diphragmatic, predominantly thoracic, or predominantly medial (characterized by activity about the base of the sternum). What seems to be of most importance for almost all speaking occasions is that the speaker have an adequate supply of breath (exaggerated deep breathing is not required) and that he be comfortable while speaking. Most persons who have not been specially trained to emphasize the activity of one part of the thoracic mechanism are likely to do relatively well in coordinated participation of all parts of their respiratory mechanism. For the rare individual who does not have adequate breath for normal speech purposes, attention may be directed to an emphasis on either diaphragmatic action and control, thoracic action, or medial action. Our own preference is for diaphragmatic (abdominal) control, because it is easy, effective, and readily discernible. The individual may be directed to breathe while speaking as he or she is likely to breathe when relaxed, unless tighly girdled or belted. On inspiration of breath the abdominal area will be noted to move upward if the person is lying down, of forward if the person is sitting up or standing. On expiration, the abdominal area should pull in. A gradual, controlled pulling in of the abdominal muscles helps to bring about an upward movement of the diaphragm and so to produce a well-sustained, steady vocal tone if the action takes place during vocalization.

It is probably best to minimize or to eliminate entirely breathing characterized by action of the upper chest (clavicular breathing). Such breathing frequently results in a strained humping of the chest and shoulders, and so interferes with easy breath flow. In this awkward and strained position, which is associated with neck and throat tension, proper reinforcement of tone in the resonating cavities becomes difficult so that voice production becomes unnecessarily effortful. It is apparently also more difficult to obtain an adequate supply of breath with "clavicular breathing" so that the speaker finds it necessary to pause for breath more often than with abdominal, thoracic, or medial breathing.

Generally, we do not consider it either advisable or necessary to stress manner of breathing. As a practical matter, we have found that it is usually possible to modify and improve breath use for vocalization without direct attention to the individual's breathing activity. Correction of posture and attention to the initiation and maintenance of proper vocal tones are usually sufficient and effective.

Therapy for Voice Disturbances

The classroom teacher who suspects that a student has a voice disturbance should first make certain that a personal preference is not being expressed. Second, the teacher should be certain that no physical condition requiring medical attention is present before any treatment is undertaken. It follows also that if a psychological problem underlies the voice defect, the problem and the child rather than the defect should be treated. With these precautions in mind, the classroom teacher with an understanding of voice production may be of real help to those children with defects of quality, pitch, or loudness of voice. The classroom teacher, as well as the speech clinician, will also do well to bear in mind that despite the best of teachings, not all defects are fully remediable. Sometimes the most apparent defect resists specific improvement, but overall improvement may still be attained if other, not so readily apparent, aspects of voice and speech are trained to the fullest extent. For example, a child with a weakened, soft palate may necessarily speak with a characteristic nasal quality. If this child is helped to articulate clearly, but not pedantically, and to have a wide and flexible pitch range reflective of changes in thought and feeling, the overall impression is likely to be favorable despite the persistence of nasality. Similarly, a child with a high-pitched voice, especially if the child is a boy, may not be able to do much about lowering his fundamental pitch if he is one who is intended by nature to have a high pitch. Such a child can still be helped if he learns to make full use of his pitch range, and can produce voice that is readily audible and is meaningfully emphatic according to speech content. With these points in mind, several specific suggestions for dealing with particular aspects of vocal deficiency may be considered.

PITCH LEVEL AND RANGE

As indicated earlier, appropriate pitch for an individual should be determined by factors other than either the listener's or speaker's liking for a given pitch range. The other factors are anatomic, including the length and mass of the individual's vocal bands, the relationship of vocal bands to the laryngeal structure, and the size and shape of the other resonating cavities. We are aware that pitch varies inversely as the length and directly as the tension of the vibrating body. Changes in length and tension enable the speaker to produce a range of normal or natural pitches that comprise a physically appropriate pitch range. The production of vocal tones consistent with the intellectual and affective content of speech comprises an appropriate pitch range for speaking.

The natural or "optimum" pitch is that pitch level at which an individual is able to vocalize most efficiently. This is the level at which good quality, loudness, and ease of production are found. For most persons, natural or optimum pitch level is about one-fourth to one-third above the lowest level within the range of pitch levels at which vocalization can occur.

You can find your own speaking pitch range and optimal pitch by the following procedure:

1. With the musical scale in mind, intone the vowel /ɑ/ at your lowest possible pitch level.
2. Go up the scale, a level at a time, until you reach falsetto.
3. Repeat, using the sound /m/. The two levels should match. If not, take the wider range. Within your pitch range your optimal pitch is about the third or fourth level from your lowest pitch. Thus, if you can intone 12 levels, optimal pitch is about level three or four.[5]

Perkins (1971, p. 354) observes that the idea of optimal pitch is a notion that "seems to have clinical validity but persistently escapes scientific verification."

If a child's habitual pitch is found to be more than two levels below or above the natural or optimal level, then it is advisable to help the youngster to initiate voice at the optimal level. The same advice, of course, holds for adults. It is well to remember, however, that young growing children have changes in their natural pitch as laryngeal growth takes place. After physiological adolescence, growth changes are not so great and natural pitch should become pretty well stabilized.

The determination of natural pitch is a point of departure in the production of an adequate and effective pitch range. For most persons voice will be best produced within that part of the pitch range between the natural pitch and one-third below the highest pitch. Thus, for a child with a 15-level range, pitch levels from five to ten are likely to be produced with good quality and with ease. With training, the child can learn to initiate voice for usual conversational purposes on natural pitch level and to use several levels above it for variety, emphasis, and appropriate expression of feeling. There is no objection to the initiation of voice at a level or two below natural level if the child has a fairly wide range. If the range is narrow, it is probably best to avoid dropping more than one level below natural pitch. The danger of dropping two levels below natural pitch for a person with a narrow pitch range is that

---

[5] W. R. Zemlin, in *Speech and Hearing Science* (Englewood Cliffs, N.J.: Prentice-Hall, Inc., (1968), pp. 182–183 states that "The natural pitch is located one-fourth up the total singing range (including falsetto) when the range is expressed in musical notes."

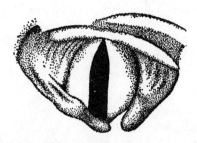

Figure 12. Diagram, adapted from a high-speed photograph, showing vocal bands not sufficiently approximated for good voice production, and too closely approximated for normal breathing.

Courtesy Bell Telephone Company Laboratories, New York.

an effortful, breathy voice may be produced that actually may be harmful to the speaker.[6]

BREATHINESS

Vocal quality characterized by breathiness results from air "leakage" between vocal bands during voice production. The ultimate of breathiness is intentionally whispered speech. Voiceless consonants are, of course, breathy, and appropriately so. Vowels, however, and voiced consonants should be produced without any obvious breathiness.

Breathiness may result from overrelaxed vocalization with associated partial approximation of the vocal bands. If a person's voice is pitched too low in terms of his natural pitch range, the tension of the vocal bands will be less than optimum, and the voice is likely to be breathy. If a person is suffering from laryngitis, attempts at vocalization are frequently associated with pain because of contact between swollen inner edges of the bands. To avoid or reduce the pain, the speaker is likely to keep the vocal bands in a partially approximated position, and so will speak with breathiness. Figure 12 shows the position of the vocal bands when they are not sufficiently approximated for good voice production, and yet too closely approximated for purposes of normal breathing.

Sometimes a breathy voice is associated with shyness or timidity. A child who speaks quietly because of fear of speaking aloud may not bring the vocal bands close enough to vocalize without excessive

---

[6] Alternate methods for determining habitual and optimal pitch and pitch range may be found in J. Eisenson, *Voice and Diction: A Program for Improvement* (New York: Macmillan Publishing Co., Inc., 1974), pp. 88–91.

breathiness. Occasionally a "good" but not necessarily timid child will imitate a teacher's low voice used to keep the class quiet. Such a child, in the attempt to speak "low and quiet" may also speak breathily.

There are several reasons for children to avoid a breathy voice quality. First, the breathy voice is frequently too low in pitch, and vocalization becomes effortful and unpleasant. Second, breathiness is wasteful in terms of length of phrase in speaking. The child, or the adult for that matter, who speaks with excessive breathiness will need to pause for inhalation more often than would otherwise be necessary. In the attempts to establish normal phrasing, the child may speak on residual breath, and the speech efforts will sound strained and be strained.

To overcome breathiness it is frequently necessary to have the child become aware of the difference between a breathy and a normal voice quality. This may be done by having the child place his/her hand in front of his/her mouth while saying a sentence such as "My bunny's name is Lanny." Normally, such a sentence, which has no voiceless sounds and only one voiced stop, should be produced with a very minimum of breath felt on the hand placed a few inches in front of the mouth. The child should then be directed to "feel" the breath accompanying a sentence such as "Polly likes to eat thin crackers," which has both stop and fricative sounds and is, therefore, necessarily produced with accompanying breath. If there is no distinct difference in the child's vocalization of the two sentences, another child whose voice is not breathy should be asked to speak the two sentences while the breathy-voiced child holds his/her hand about six inches in front of the second child's mouth, and notes the difference.

After the concepts and the feeling of breathiness and nonbreathiness are established, other techniques may be employed to produce normal vocalization. A very simple and often effective approach is to direct the child to speak as if breath were precious and to emit as little breath as possible while talking. Then, for contrast, the child may be instructed to be as breathy as possible, so that the difference can be clearly appreciated.

Another helpful technique is to have the child intone a vowel such as /i/ (ee) and to hold the vowel as long as comfortable on a single breath. The vowel /i/, because it is relatively tense and high-pitched, is likely to be produced with a minimum of breathiness even by the child who is inclined to be breathy. If this is done successfully, the child may then be directed to intone /a/ (ah) and to maintain the sound until the child begins to become breathy, or until he/she needs to inhale. Then the effort should be repeated with reduced loudness but without obvious breathiness. In this way the child can learn how "quietly" it is possible to speak without becoming breathy. The same technique may be used with a change in pitch rather than loudness so that the child may learn at which pitch level breathiness occurs, and so avoid that pitch level.

Other recommended exercises include saying as much of the alphabet as possible or counting as long as is comfortable on a single breath. When quantity of production becomes the objective, the child spontaneously is likely to conserve breath. As soon as possible, of course, the child should be given an opportunity to apply what has been learned in the exercises to other situations, such as reading aloud and conversational speech. Although the child should not be interrupted in normal speaking efforts because of breathiness, the clinician should work out a system of signals to tell the youngster whether the effort to control breathiness has been successful. The teacher, working with the speech clinician, may apply this approach in the classroom situation.

ORGANIC CAUSES OF BREATHINESS

Figure 12 shows the vocal bands in a position of incomplete approximation for good voice production. This position would in and of itself produce a breathy or semiwhispered voice. Figure 11 showed vocal nodules that because of their mass would prevent normal approximation of the vocal bands. Pain on contact of the nodules would increase the likelihood of insufficient approximation and consequent breathiness. Any other growth or a thickening of the bands would produce breathiness. Laryngitis, which is accompanied by vocal band thickening and pain on contact between the bands, is thus characterized by breathiness.

Because of the possibilities of organic causes of breathiness, it is important that the child be examined by a physician and cleared medically before any corrective measures are undertaken.

NASALITY

Positive or excessive nasality as a characteristic voice quality, as we pointed out earlier, is associated with a relaxed soft palate during the act of vocalization. In the absence of specific anomaly involving the palate, nasality may occur either because of generally slow or sluggish palatal action or because of specific "retarded" action of the soft palate after the articulation of appropriately nasal sounds. If there is generally sluggish soft palate action, speech as a whole is likely to sound nasal. If there is a limited failure of the soft palate to be elevated quickly immediately following the production of a nasal consonant, the sound or sounds produced after the nasal are likely to be partially nasalized.

In the latter case, words such as *me, many, and, among, nine,* and *mine* are likely to be produced as if all the sounds were nasal.

In some cases, the excessive nasality appears to be associated with a general expression of lassitude and an air of indifference to the environment. Such children, except possibly in their playground activities, seem to lack the energy for any physical effort, including the elevation of the soft palate. We should not, however, overlook the possibility that the expression of lassitude and apparent indifference may have a physical basis. The contrast in the child's playground behavior may be the effect of strong and specific motivation.

Children who have had their adenoids removed frequently change from having markedly denasal voices to having characteristically nasal voices. This change can be appreciated when we realize that when enlarged adenoids are present, a child does not need to elevate the soft palate very much to obstruct the opening to the nasal cavity. After the removal of the adenoidal tissue, the habit of partial elevation of the soft palate may persist, and nasality may then occur during the production of all speech sounds.

Regardless of the cause of nasality, if therapy is in order it should begin with giving the child awareness of how a nasal voice sounds and, if the child is capable of such understanding, how nasality occurs. The child can easily learn to recognize nasality by listening to the teacher intentionally nasalize a sentence such as *The sailor shouted "All aboard!"* or *This is the house that Jack built* and then listening to the same sentences, spoken without intentional nasality. Both of these sentences, incidentally, contain no nasal consonants and so provide no temptation to nasalize because of proximity of a sound to a nasal consonant (assimilation).

The child inclined toward nasality may also learn how nasality feels by pinching the nostrils while speaking one of the sentences that follows. If the child becomes aware of pressure, or a feeling of stuffiness in the nose, or of fullness in his ears, it indicates that breath has entered the nasal cavity that should have been emitted through the mouth.

> Bob took Ted to the zoo.
> Please take care of the kitty.
> The dog chased the bird up the tree.
> Polly likes crackers with cheese.
> Joe played baseball.
> The baby played pit-a-pat with his daddy.

The same sentences may be used to help the child see nasality. This can be accomplished by placing a cold hand mirror under the child's nostrils while he/she repeats one of the sentences having no nasal consonants. Clouding of the mirror by the warm air that escapes from the nostrils is visual evidence of positive and inappropriate nasality.

Once awareness is present in a child, who is not organically involved and is motivated to overcome nasality, the following techniques may be employed:

Raising the Soft Palate

Have the child stand before a mirror and yawn with the mouth wide open. The child should be directed to note that the soft palate tends to lift up. The youngster should learn how this feels as well as how it looks for the soft palate to elevate. The child may also be directed to blow up a previously stretched balloon and note the feeling and movement of the soft palate.

The child may be directed to say [ɑ] (ah) with nostrils pinched. All sound should come through the mouth, and no stuffiness should be felt. Then the child should be directed to produce a nasalized [ã]. The procedure should be repeated with other vowels and for such words as *boy, girl, tree, tall, big, go, bread, hot, skip, stop,* and *dog,* and short phrases such as *go away, pretty girl, big boy,* and *a slice of bread.* Older children, who can understand the difference between nasal and non-nasal sounds, should be encouraged to make up their own list of words and phrases for practice.

Ear Training

Children can be helped to distinguish between appropriate and inappropriate nasality by listening to appropriate articulation of the following pairs of words:

moo	two	an	at	him	hit
me	bee	wing	wig	pen	pet
my	by	I'm	I'll	can	cat
no	go	in	it	bean	beat
may	pay	aim	ape	seem	seat

It may also help if the clinician informs the child that occasionally words in the second column will be intentionally nasalized and the child is to signal his/her awareness of such nasalization. The clinician with good control, who can turn nasality off and on at will, may go beyond single words to pairs of phrases and sentences.

If a recorder and playback equipment are available, ready use may be made of such an instrument in helping the child to recognize his/her own nasality. A sentence or two may be recorded by the nasal child and the same material by another child without the defect. The child "in training" may then hear the difference in voice quality in comparison with a peer. Later, recordings may be used to help the child recognize improvement in exercises and for parts of readings or conversation. Many children enjoy a chance to do intentionally what they are seeking to improve. Permission "to do the wrong thing" should be given so that the child may practice and so gain voluntary control over nasality. The same approach, of course, is also relevant for other aspects of voice therapy as well as for the improvement of articulation.

GENERAL ARTICULATORY ACTIVITY

Often the child who speaks nasally will also be one whose overall articulatory activity lacks precision and clearness. For this child, in the interest of improving articulation in general as well as nasality in particular, more precise and energetic articulatory activity is recommended. With increased activity of the lips and tongue, there will also be a reflexive increase in energetic activity of the soft palate. The child should also be instructed to direct all nonnasal sounds through the mouth and to increase the feeling of front-of-the-mouth activity. Words and phrases such as the following might be used in drill work and incorporated into practice sentences and conversational speech.

two	do	pet
treat	tweet	pit
pooh	boo	step
chew	food	slip
tuck	buck	tent
see	saw	spot
lick	tick	tack
bing	bang	stuck
come along	sing a song	kick the tin can
take some tea	beat the drum	Pat likes to eat
red rose	don't trip	do come soon
all aboard	pickled peppers	see the birds
leave the boat	hit the deck	step lively now
stay away	broken bones	throw the big ball
let's go	pack of sticks	a pack of papers

DENASALITY

Some children speak as though they have either chronically stuffed noses or enlarged adenoids that block the entrance of sound into the nasal cavities. These children need to be helped to become aware of adequate nasal resonance when it is required.

Humming with lips relatively relaxed so that a sensation of tickling is experienced is a recommended technique for establishing nasal resonance. Another useful device is the intentional lengthening of nasal consonants. The child may be instructed to hum and then follow the hum with a vowel. Specifically, the exercise might proceed as follows:

1. Hum gently on a sustained breath, first with the sound *m*, then *n*, and then [ŋ]. Repeat each hum three of four times.

2. Begin a hum and then blend with a vowel.

3. Prolong an initial nasal sound and blend with a vowel as in *mmm-a*, and *nnn-oo*.

4. Begin with a lengthened nasal, blend with a vowel, and end with a lengthened nasal as in *mmmannn, nnnoonnn*.

Other exercises might include articulating such words as *me*, *my*, *moo*, *may*, *meal*, *nail*, *now*, *new*, *never*, *nice*, *sing*, *long*, and *running* with intentional lengthening of the nasal consonants.

Sentences incorporating words with more than a usual number of nasal consonants should be made, and conversation with such words and sentences should be practiced. Whenever possible, the child should be encouraged to make up words and sentences so that he may have the pleasure of creative activity as well as practice.

Following are some additional suggestions for practice:

mine alone	man in the moon
running down	many candies
nine and one	Monday noon
round and round	morning at ten

Amanda ran home.
The moon shines on the barn.
Nine and nine make eighteen.
Only Tom may come.
Molly found a new penny.

INAPPROPRIATE LOUDNESS

Most children whose speech patterns are a result of identification with normal adults speak loudly enough to be heard. Those who speak with inadequate loudness or with a louder voice than the occasion demands reflect either their own personalities or the personalities of the adults with whom they identify. Only in the rarest instances is there an organic basis for either a weak or an overloud voice. The comparatively rare organic causes include hearing loss, weakness of the muscles of the larynx, and weakness of the muscles involved in respiration. Furthermore, it is extremely unlikely that the carrying power of the voice is significantly related to the individual's breath capacity or the manner of breathing while speaking. As Van Riper and Irwin (1958, p. 258) emphasize, "So long as sufficient air pressure is engendered below the vocal folds, it does not matter how it is created, at least so far as adequate loudness is concerned. But we must have a greater air pressure to have louder speech." In the absence of organic pathology, the will to be heard is sufficient to supply the energy to provide for the necessary pressure below the vocal folds so that they are closed firmly, held together firmly for an appropriate length of time, and then blown apart from their occluded (approximated) position to produce a vocal tone that is loud enough to be easily heard.

Occasionally we find children who, because of poor posture, or from anxiety, get in the way of their own efforts of effective breathing for speech. A child with a "caved-in" abdominal area may not be able to breathe comfortably and deeply enough for purposes of speech. Obviously, the slump and the associated cave-in need to be corrected. Similarly, any other postural defect that interferes with adequate air intake and easy control of breath output needs to be corrected. Such correction might well be directed to emphasizing the need for the abdominal area to be relaxed and to "push out" in inhalation and to contract and "pull in" gradually in controlled exhalation.

Another fault found in some children is the attempt to vocalize and speak during inhalation. This fault, in the absence of neuropathology, is usually a result of an anxious effort to continue talking when the child's breath supply has been expended. The creation of awareness of what the child is doing can be established by directing him/her to do intentionally what he/she is doing unconsciously. Such a child is also likely to gain from breathing exercises that emphasize abdominal control of outgoing breath.

THE OVERLOUD VOICE

Aside from the possibility of a hearing loss that prevents proper monitoring of the voice as it is being produced, the overloud voice is likely to be a product of imitation or an aspect of the personality of the speaker. Our experience as clinicians suggests that most children who speak too loudly are either imitating their parents or competing with their siblings for attention from their parents. Some parents, who complained to us about their children's loud voices, presented their complaints in our offices in voices that were loud enough to reach the last row of a 40-row auditorium without electrical amplification.

Children who identify with loud speaking persons, their parents included, speak more loudly than do children who identify with persons who speak with adequate loudness. The overloud voice, expecially if it is accompanied by rapid speech production, suggests excitement, anger, or aggressiveness.

Sensorineural hearing loss is associated with an overloud voice. Such impairment makes it necessary for the speaker to vocalize loudly in order to hear and monitor voice. Occasionally, we find a child with normal hearing who speaks in a way to suggest nerve hearing impairment. Investigation, however, may reveal that the child may have been brought up in a noisy environment, or in competition with siblings who were habitual shouters. The child then may have developed a loud voice in order to be heard and share the attention of the parents. These vocal habits may carry over to relatively quiet noncompetitive situations.

THE WEAK VOICE

In the absence of organic involvement, we may assume that a weak voice is a reflection either of a timid personality or of the reaction of the individual to a given speaking situation. Most children who are unsure of themselves, or of what they have to say, tend to talk with a weak voice. The voice, regardless of the particular speech content, is also saying "Maybe if I don't talk loudly I won't be noticed, or what I have to say won't be heard, and I will be left alone." Occasionally, however, the weak voice may be the result of imitation, and the inadequate loudness has become habitual. The reproduction of such a voice on a playback is a necessary first step in the modification of this manner of voice production.

A possible organic cause of weak voice is the existence of a conductive hearing loss. Persons with conductive loss, in contrast to those with sensory-neural loss, tend to perceive themselves as speaking more loudly than do their listeners. In general, we recommend that any child whose voice is either inappropriately loud or inadequate as to loudness be checked for possible hearing impairment. There may be some value, too, for the parents to have a similar evaluation.

TREATMENT FOR INAPPROPRIATE LOUDNESS

Except for children whose hearing difficulty impairs their ability to monitor their voices, or who have some other organic basis for either their weak or overloud voice, an adequately loud voice should be attainable for all children. Treatment should include the following aspects: (1) an assessment of the voices of the members of the family and other key persons in the child's environment; (2) an evaluation of the personality and adjustment factors that may be associated with the child's manner of vocalization; (3) an evaluation of the specific situations (for example, the child's voice in the classroom compared with the voice in play activity) that may be associated with inadequate voice; (4) an evaluation of the overall characteristics of the child's voice, in addition to the degree of loudness; and (5) an objectification of the voice through recording and playback so that the child may hear himself/herself approximately as others hear him/her.

In many instances, children who have been brought to our clinic for their voice problems have been treated through their parents. We have permitted parents to hear their recorded voices and invited them to accept treatment—*in the interest of their child*. Sometimes we accepted the child for treatment only if the parent or parents accepted concurrent voice therapy. Occasionally, we have encouraged parents to subdue a sibling just enough to give the child concerned a fair chance in the vocal competition. Sometimes, we have had to advise counseling for the parents while the child, *after medical clearance*, was undergoing symptom treatment.

In instances where we felt that an adjustment problem was basic to the voice difficulty, we have recommended treatment by a qualified psychotherapist. Whenever possible, we prefer that the choice of a psychotherapist be made with the help of the family physician. Occasionally, we have found that a child's voice problem was limited to the classroom. For reasons that developed out of the relationship between a child and a teacher—and sometimes it is a previous rather than a present teacher—the child had become anxiously concerned about his/her adequacy as a student. Obviously, in such instances, treatment should be directed at the improvement of the child-to-school relationship rather than to the vocal symptoms.

When, after investigation, we are convinced that there is nothing organically or emotionally wrong with the child who is speaking either not loudly enough or too loudly, direct treatment of the symptoms is in order. As suggested earlier, an overall evaluation of the vocal characteristics of the child is then undertaken. Our experience suggests that the weak voice is often also a breathy voice, and one likely to be too low in pitch. Often, but not always, we find that the loud voice is likely to be too high in pitch. The first order of the procedure for correcting the degree of loudness is to determine the child's normal pitch range and the optimum pitch. When these are determined (see pp. 318–319), the speech clinician should help the child to become aware of them, to initiate voice habitually at optimum pitch, and to vocalize within the optimum pitch range. Breathiness, if it is found to be present, should be treated by procedures indicated in the section on breathiness.

Ordinarily, after following the procedures outlined and after the child has been made aware of the loudness level of his/her voice through playback, adequate loudness is attained. Occasionally, however, old habits are maintained and the child's voice, though appropriate in pitch and not characterized by breathiness, is still not appropriate in loudness. If it continues to be weak, procedures such as the following ones should be productive of improvement.

1. Record successively the voice of the weak-voiced child and a peer with adequate voice. Have the child make the comparisons and make new recording of the voices until both clinician and child are satisfied with the results.

2. If available, employ visual feedback apparatus so that the child may see when his/her voice is at the proper level. Most tape recorders are equipped with "magic eyes," which may be employed for this purpose. An oscilloscope may serve both to impress the child and to provide a basis for visual monitoring. A simpler and more readily available apparatus, though perhaps not quite so impressive, is the raised hand and approving look of the teacher or clinician when the child's voice is at a proper level and the lowered (thumb-down) hand and disappointed (but *not* disapproving) look when the voice level is not loud enough.

3. Emphasis on clarity of articulation with lengthening of the vowels and nasal consonants is often of considerable help. By emphasizing clarity of articulation, the child is likely to use greater energy not only for articulatory activity but also for the accompanying respiratory behavior while speaking. The result is a reflexive increase in air pressure below the vocal folds, and a louder voice.

4. The game of *competitive speaking* or "Who can talk loudest in the group without shouting?" may be employed as motivation and play. It may be of help if some of the competitors are encouraged at the beginning of the game to give the weak-voiced participant a chance to be heard. Later on, the erstwhile weak-voiced member should be permitted free and open competition.

5. The need for the child to adjust his/her voice level to the listener in terms of distance between listener and speaker may need emphasis. A teacher may bring about such an adjustment by asking a child a question when standing close to the child and then intentionally moving away from the youngster. Another technique is to have the child stand in front of the room and speak just loud enough to be heard by the classmates in the first third of the room, then in the second third as well, and finally throughout the room. This procedure impresses the child with the need to change voice level according to the number of

listeners and the distance between himself/herself and the farthest listener.

6. Pretended situations, such as announcing the arrival of a train or plane, giving orders to a military group, or speaking in a crowded and noisy place (a train station or an airport waiting room), can also be useful to help the child to be heard under difficult situations. Artificially competitive noise situations, such as speaking against a masking noise or buzzing noise, may also be used. If these techniques are employed, *care must be exercised that the optimum pitch range is maintained.* We would not want a child to speak loudly at the risk of acquiring vocal nodules.

CONTROL OF BREATH FOR SPEAKING

As indicated earlier in the discussion of breathing faults, difficulty in breathing is not a frequent cause of vocal difficulty for the otherwise normal child. We should be alert to see that the children do not attempt to vocalize while inhaling. Vocalization should occur on an easy, controlled exhalation of breath. Because only a rare and occasional child will attempt vocalization on inhalation, the teacher who has such a child in class should arrange for corrective instruction on an individual basis. It is better for most children to do their breathing while speaking without special awareness or consciousness of the action involved.

If a child shows throat or laryngeal effort in speaking, attention might be directed to abdominal control for expiration. Usually such attention serves to distract the child from excessive tension in the upper part of the respiratory mechanism. Other therapeutic suggestions relative to breathing faults have already been indicated.

Review of Principles for Correcting Voice Defects

1. *Medical clearance is a must* for any child who presents a voice problem and for whom vocal therapy is contemplated. A child who develops a vocal disturbance should be examined by a physician and, if at all possible, by a throat specialist for the detection and treatment of possible physical pathology before consideration is given to voice training.

2. When a child's vocal defects seem to be associated with personality disturbances, referral to a competent counselor or psychotherapist is in order. It should not be overlooked, however, that poor vocal habits may persist after the initial cause is no longer present. This principle holds true for vocal defects of both physical and psychological origin.

3. Often vocal defects are temporary and of short duration and call for patience and understanding rather than active treatment.

4. A voice is a product of the mechanism that produces it. The mechanism belongs to the individual, and the product should be consistent with its features. Neither the professional speech clinician nor the teacher, nor any other person who may influence the child, has a right to decide what kind of voice the child should have. Fundamentally, this decision was made by the way the child was physically endowed. The object of vocal therapy is to help the child to make the best possible use of his vocal endowment.

5. The classroom teacher, especially if he/her is respected and liked, has a personal responsibility that his/her own voice be free of undesirable traits that the children may imitate.

6. Vocal habits, both good and bad, tend to persist. Considerable motivation is necessary to help a child to wish to change a defective voice and to maintain vigilance that the improvements are maintained.

7. The child with a vocal defect should be helped to become aware of what the defect is like acoustically, and how it feels. The child needs to be aware of how his/her voice sounds *and* feels when it it at its best as well as its worst. Objective attitudes and objective listening to one's own voice and comparing one's own voice with others by listening to "on-the-spot" recordings are of help.

8. Often a "negative" approach is helpful. By creating awareness of the nature of the undesirable vocal traits and how they are produced, voluntary control may be established. Thus, a child, by intentionally *doing what is wrong*, learns to know what he/she is doing, and so becomes conscious of what should not be done. By contrast, awareness must be created of the right way to produce voice and to replace the undesirable characteristic with a desirable one. *Negative practice must be replaced by positive practice at the earliest possible time.*

9. Both the classroom and the home situation should be studied for evidence of an atmosphere of undue tension. However, normal enthusiasm and excitement should not be confused with tension. Continued competition for the right to be heard may result in tension and consequent vocal penalties.

Problems

1. Review the section on the vocal mechanism. From the viewpoint of the production and reinforcement of sound, what musical instrument is most directly comparable to the voice mechanism?
2. Good vocalization is the product of *periodic vibration*. What does this term

mean? What kind of human sounds are *complex and aperiodic*? You may consult Curtis (1967, pp. 183–185) for your answer.

3. What are the characteristics of a normal, effective voice?
4. What is the most frequent physical cause of defective voice?
5. Why is puberty often a period of frequent voice disturbance? Why are males more likely to be affected than females?
6. What is the role of identification in the formation of vocal habits?
7. What is nasality? How do you distinguish this characteristic from denasality? How would you check for each?
8. Why is it important that every child who may be considered for voice therapy first be given medical clearance?
9. What is optimum pitch? How would you determine this for a child? Are you vocalizing within your optimal pitch range?
10. What is the evidence that breathing faults are a cause of vocal disturbance?
11. What is negative practice? Describe how the technique of negative practice may be applied to changing an undesirable vocal habit.
12. Read Moore (1971) on environmental factors and voice disturbances. Are there any factors in your home environment conducive to vocal problems?
13. What is the danger of high-pitched screaming in young children?
14. What are two indications of personality disturbances discussed by Murphy (1964)?
15. What are cultural pressures that might be conducive to voice disorders in adolescents?

References and Suggested Readings

Boone, D., *The Voice and Voice Therapy*, Englewood Cliffs, N.J.: Prentice-Hall, Inc., 1971. (A clinical approach to the treatment of common voice problems. Practical and clearly written.)

Brodnitz, F. S., *Keep Your Voice Healthy*, New York: Harper & Row, Publishers, Inc., 1953. (A physician offers suggestions as to how to have a good and "healthy" voice.)

Cooper, M., "Spectographic Analysis of Fundamental Frequency and Hoarseness Before and After Vocal Rehabilitation," *Journal of Speech and Hearing Disorders*, **39** (1974), 286–297.

Curtis, J. F., in W. Johnson et al., *Speech-Handicapped School Children*, New York: Harper & Row, Publishers, Inc., 1967, chap. 4.

Eisenson, J., *Voice and Diction: A Program for Improvement*, New York: Macmillan Publishing Co., Inc., 1974. (Chapters 3–9 are concerned with voice. Contains a considerable amount of practice materials.)

Fisher, H. D., *Improving Voice and Articulation*, Boston: Houghton Mifflin, 1966. (Includes useful practice material that can be adapted for children.)

Greene, M. C. L., *The Voice and Its Disorders*, 2nd ed., Philadelphia: J. B.

Lippincott Co., 1964. (An authoritative presentation for the treatment of voice problems by a practicing clinician.)

Moore, P., *Organic Voice Disorders*, Englewood Cliffs, N.J.: Prentice-Hall, Inc., 1971. (Includes brief but clear and authoritative information on the vocal mechanism.)

Moses, P. J., *The Voice of Neurosis*, New York: Grune and Stratton, Inc., 1954. (A psychiatrist and otolaryngologist describes his approaches to persons with voice problems. Despite the publishing date, still an up-to-date book.)

Murphy, A. T., *Functional Voice Disorders*, Englewood Cliffs, N.J.: Prentice-Hall, Inc., 1964. (A clear introductory consideration of personality disturbances and voice disorders.)

Perkins, W. H., *Speech Pathology*, St. Louis: The C. V. Mosby Co., 1971.

Silverman, E. M., and C. H. Zimmer, "Incidence of Chronic Hoarseness among School-Age Children," *Journal of Speech and Hearing Disorders*, **40** (1975), 211–215.

Van Riper, C., *Speech Correction*, 5th ed., Englewood Cliffs, N.J.: Prentice-Hall, Inc., 1972, chap. 5.

————, and J. V. Irwin, *Voice and Articulation*, Englewood Cliffs, N.J.: Prentice-Hall Inc., 1958.

Wilson, D. K., "Children with Vocal Nodules," *Journal of Speech and Hearing Disorders*, **26** (1961), 19–25.

Zemlin, W. R., *Speech and Hearing Science*, Englewood Cliffs, N.J.: Prentice-Hall, Inc., 1968.

13. *Stuttering*

General Observations

Except for children with articulatory defects, stutterers, if we accept them as a total special population, present the highest incidence among those who are defective in speech. The incidence is close to 1 per cent among children of school age. Thus, it is likely that almost every classroom teacher and certainly every speech clinician with more than a year of experience has had some dealings with a stutterer. These, and other professional workers concerned with stutterers, may have shared their perplexities about the children and their aberrant speech. They may have exchanged observations and opinions about a form of behavior that varies in amount and degree of severity. They may have expressed bewilderment about the comparative ease and fluency some stutterers have for brief or long periods of time, and about their sudden relapses. Those who have made private and comparative observations may have noted that fewer adults stutter than do children, but that almost all adults who stutter began doing so when they were children and almost always before adolescence. They may also have noted that relatively few elderly adults stutter. All of these observations, and some others mentioned later, have been made by professional investigators. They, too, continue to be perplexed about stutterers and stuttering, even though they have strong opinions, if not theories, about the problem.

Much about stuttering is still to be learned. If we cease to regard stutterers as a total and "homogeneous" population, we will begin to learn considerably more in the near future than in the hundreds of years that we have spent in speculations, critical observations, and even carefully designed investigations. For the moment, however, we present several observations that have withstood the test of time about persons whose speech is characterized by rhythm and fluency that are different from most other speakers, who repeat and hesitate, and who prolong sounds, or block on sounds, more than most of us do in our talking.

Tentatively, we define stuttering as abnormally self-interrupted speech flow or utterance characterized by word "fragmentation," excessive sound repetitions and/or prolongations, blockings (maintenance of articulatory positions), and "struggle" reactions. Covertly the speaker usually experiences anxiety or apprehension about speaking. This definition follows closely that of Van Riper (1972, p. 249). However, we are aware that stuttering is otherwise defined by different theorists. For a review of such definitions and theoretical positions, the reader may consult Van Riper (1971, chaps. 2 and 11–15).

Accepted Observations About Stutterers

1. There are more stutterers among boys than among girls. Research on the incidence of stuttering shows a ratio of from two to 10 males for each female stutterer. Probably an average ratio is four male stutterers to each female stutterer. In a survey in England reported by Andrews and Harris (1964, p. 186), a ratio of four boys to one girl was found among children who stuttered. However, a ratio of about eight men to one woman was found among adults.[1]

---

[1] S. G. Andrews and M. Harris in "Stammering," in *The Child Who Does Not Talk*, C. Renfrew and R. Murphy, eds., The Spastics Society Medical Education Association (London: Wm. Heinemann, Ltd. Medical Books, (1964), p. 186) observe, "It is interesting to note that those girls who do stammer appear to have a higher loading of genetic and neurologic predisposing factors." Several references will be made to the Harris and Andrews report. We consider the report of their study of an entire school population of 7,358 children in the nine plus and ten plus age-range in Newcastle, England, to be of especial significance to our understanding of the background history of stutterers (stammerers) and stuttering (stammering). The terms in parentheses are used by the British, where Americans tend to use *stutterers* and *stuttering*. The Newcastle investigators included speech therapists, psychologists, a psychiatrist, and a statistical analyst. Each stutterer (stammerer) was matched for age, grade, and sex with

2. The severity of stuttering tends to be greater among boys than among girls. We are, of course, talking about individuals. We have, in fact, known many severe female stutterers, but not nearly so many—even considering the ratio difference for the incidence of stutterting—as for males.

3. Stuttering tends to be more persistent, to endure for more years, for boys than for girls. This explains the ratio difference noted in our first observation.

4. No stutterer, regardless of the severity of difficulty, stutters at all times. Almost all stutterers have times when their speech is relatively, if not completely, free of significant hesitancies, blocks, repetitions, or prolongations. In group-speaking situations, and in singing, stutterers are likely to do about as well as other children. Similarly, situations that require no on-the-spot formulation or hold little or no communicative responsibility are likely to be relatively easy for most stutterers.

5. Stuttering is more likely to begin in the nursery, kindergarten, and primary grades than in the secondary grades. It is comparatively rare for a child to begin stuttering after age 12. Andrews and Harris (1964, p. 186) report that 50 per cent of the children in their survey were stuttering (stammering) by age five, and 95 per cent were doing so by age seven. "Onset after the age of ten is rare." Van Riper (1971, p. 64), based on a review of the literature of several countries, also concludes that "the overwhelming consensus is that most stuttering begins in the preschool years."

6. Many young children in the kindergarten and first grade seem to have been on the verge of stuttering without becoming stutterers. They were hesitant and repetitous, but apparently had no awareness of their manner of speaking. By the time these children reached the age of eight or nine, their speech seemed to be "normal" again.

These observations are among the relatively few generalizations or "facts" accepted by students of stuttering. Beyond these, there is considerable difference in opinion as to the cause of stuttering, and the choice of treatment. We do not attempt to resolve these differences.

---

a normal-speaking child. Eighty-six stutterers were diagnosed by the speech therapist, of whom 80 participated in the complete study. Thus, the investigation had a population of 160 children and their mothers, who were assessed through interviews and standardized test inventories for clinical background, psychiatric evidence, personality traits, and aspects of intelligence.

The Harris and Andrews observations hold as of this writing.

Instead, we present several of the more prevalent points of view, and suggest what the classroom teacher can safely do about children who are considered stutterers. We also suggest therapeutic approaches that are widely used with some success by speech clinicians in and out of school settings.[2]

The Nature of Stuttering

The hesitancies, blocks, repetitions, and/or prolongations of sounds in excess of normal that characterize stuttering may be referred to as disfluencies. Because many young children of preschool and primary school age have so-called disfluencies, which, according to occasion may occur in as much as 10 per cent of utterance, we should be liberal in our concept of the normal. In addition to disfluencies, the stutterer's voice is likely to be somewhat tense and narrow in pitch range and in modulation. Many children who regard themselves as stutterers also entertain feelings of anxiety and apprehension about some speaking situations or about communicative speaking in general. Some, amazingly, do not! On the other hand, anxiety and apprehension—how stutterers feel—may be the dominant factors in some situations despite overt acceptable fluency as speakers.

The Development of Stuttering

Do stutterers demonstrate any typical histories or stages in development of their speech (language) disorder? We once thought they did. However, the individual histories reveal no reliable developmental stage that permit us to predict that some children with excessive disfluencies and considerable evidence of struggle behavior may spontaneously improve, or change to easygoing repetition and then cease to stutter. Other children may go from "hard" symptoms to "soft" symptoms,

---

[2] One of the confounding observations about stutterers is that a great variety of approaches, some without any apparent rationale, have been used on stutterers with varying degrees of success—at least for a time. Another, as we have noted, is the frequency of spontaneous recovery. So, J. G. Sheehan in "Conflict Theory and Avoidance-Reduction Therapy," in *Stuttering: A Second Symposium* (New York: Harper & Row Publishers, Inc., 1975), p. 187, asserts: "In 80 per cent of the cases in which it begins, stuttering is not perpetuated but disappears without treatment by the time the person reaches college provided he has faced the problem." We assume that facing the problem is a form of therapy that does not always require the help of a professional person who is identified as a therapist.

varying in frequency and degree of severity over a period of weeks and months. Some of these children will become confirmed stutterers. Many will have no memory, unless their parents remind them, that they were ever so disfluent as to be regarded as stutterers. Perhaps the only conclusion we can come to now—and it is still a tentative conclusion—is that the longer stuttering-like behavior persists from early childhood into the preadolescent and adolescent years, the more likely the individual is to become a confirmed stutterer. The confirmation will come from members of the stutterers' environments and from the stutterers themselves. What is confirmed is that the individual identified as a stutterer has difficulty in speaking and usually exhibits some or most of the speech behavior included in our definition of stuttering.

If there are no reliable developmental stages, are there any patterns that occur with sufficient frequency to permit prognosticating about stutterers and their stutterings? At least two respected authorities believe the answer to be "yes" though they are not in complete agreement as to the symptoms and patterns, and whether there is a developmental chronology. We review the positions of Bloodstein and Van Riper as to their respective concepts of *Phases of Stuttering* and *Tracks of Stuttering*.

Bloodstein (1975, pp. 57–84) describes four phases of stuttering, as well as therapeutic approaches for individuals in each of the phases. However, Bloodstein acknowledges that there is considerable overlap in the phases and that some stutterers move back and forth from one phase to another. A few stutterers seem to fit nowhere, moving from one phase to another, and occasionally defying stable description or characterization.

Phase 1. Age range usually between two to six years. The child's difficulty is usually episodic with repetitions being the chief characteristic. Prolongations, forcings, and hard contacts and various associated symptoms ordinarily found among advanced stutterers may also be present. Many of the repetitions occur at the beginning of sentences or other identifiable syntactic units (phrases or clauses). An unusual feature is the tendency to stutter on function words and pronouns.

In general, Bloodstein (p. 57) observes that Phase 1 stutterers appear to do what children might be expected to do if they were fragmentating whole syntactic structures rather than individual words.

Bloodstein notes that children in Phase 1 do not avoid speaking and usually do not show any special awareness or concern about their speech. Some, however, do on occasion show that they are frustrated when blocked in speech and may even ask "Why can't I talk?"

Fortunately, the questions do not deter them in their efforts as speakers. Beyond the questions, "They give little evidence of having formed any distinct self-concepts as stutterers or defective speakers" (p. 57). Bloodstein believes that children in Phase 1 of stuttering are essentially indistinguishable from almost all other children for whom episodes of increased disfluency are transient early childhood phenomena.

The main goal of therapy for the Phase 1 stutterer is the prevention of more advanced forms of stuttering. Basically, this dictates that "We must at all costs prevent the child from developing a self-concept as a defective speaker" (p. 58). Counseling of parents is, therefore, the major therapeutic approach.

Phase 2. Age range: mostly children in elementary school years, but may include adults.

The speaker's difficulty has become fairly chronic though varying in degree of severity. Fragmenting of words rather than of syntactic structures becomes characteristic of the interrupted utterances. Fragmentation and repetition is distributed throughout the sentence or phrase (unit of meaning) rather than occurring on the first word of the unit.

Interestingly, even though the children who are identified as Phase 2 stutterers regard themselves as defective speakers, they do not appear to avoid speaking situations. Bloodstein observes that these children are easy to treat. Moreover, the evidence indicates that "throughout the age range at which Phase 2 stuttering is most prevalent, children recover from stuttering at a very high rate spontaneously." Bloodstein also observes that therapeutically "almost anything works."

From the point of view of therapy, since "almost anything works" the less done the better. Bloodstein suggests that it is important to avoid directing attention to symptoms that might produce anxiety. On the positive side, Phase 2 stutterers should be helped to develop feelings of self-worth. Along this line, parent counseling and teacher cooperation are important.

Phase 3. Age range from about eight years to adulthood; highest incidence during adolescence.

The speaking problems reported by the stutterers begin to be anticipated according to situations identified as difficult. Such situations include talking to strangers and reciting in school, and generally where and when communicative responsibility is involved. Some words and some sounds may be regarded as difficult and approached with anticipation of stuttering. Devices such as word substitutions and circumlocutions may be used to avoid the "bogey" words. Except that stutterers give little or no indication of avoiding involvement in speaking situations, they begin to manifest the speech behavior characteristics of Phase 4 (the confirmed, "chronic" adult stutterer). Bloodstein (p. 67) observes that "In the school environment we soon recognize the Phase 3 stutterer as the familiar boy or girl who seems to have an advanced form of stuttering problem, yet continually volunteers to recite in class and may be communicative and gregarious, even to the point of being 'popular'."

Bloodstein recommends that emphasis in therapy for the Phase 3 stutterers should be on symptom modification and general speech improvement. Because Phase 3 stutterers appear to be free of anxiety about speaking, Bloodstein considers it at best a waste of time to become involved with anxieties and apprehensions that these stutterers, most of whom are adolescents, fortunately do not have. If they were apprehensive and anxious about speaking and about themselves as speakers because of their stuttering manifestations, they would be Phase 4 stutterers.

Phase 4. Age range, approximately ten years to adulthood; mostly adolescence to adulthood.

Phase 4 stutterers are chronic and confirmed about their difficulties. Their speech shows the characteristics of disfluency, blocking, repetition, self-interruption, and the like incorporated in our definition of stuttering. They are anxious and apprehensive about speaking. They have feared sounds, feared words, and feared situations and strategies, usually not effective, to deal with their speech fears.

Therapy for Phase 4 stutterers is directed to reducing anxiety about their stuttering and to a modification of stuttering behavior. Bloodstein (1975, pp. 69–78) pays considerable attention to the treatment of the anxieties of the Phase 4 or confirmed stutterers. Van Riper (1972, pp. 305–327) also appreciates the need to deal with the anxieties of the confirmed stutterer. Both Bloodstein and Van Riper are aware that effective treatment for the confirmed stutterer must include modification of the overt behavior that characterizes the chronic and confirmed stutterer. In his book *The Treatment of Stuttering*, Van Riper (1973) devotes a separate chapter to the treatment of the young, confirmed stutterer—children between the ages of seven and 14 who are of elementary school age. Van Riper points out that children in this age range should not be expected to have the same motivation or trust in therapy or in therapists to improve their speaking or to accept a large measure of self-responsibility for their therapy. On the other hand, because the stuttering has not had as long a history as with adults, the habits and attitudes of these children may not be fixed. Moreover, "The clinician finds that the child's resistances are more open and direct; we do not find the ingenious sabotage which often characterizes the adult stutterer. And perhaps most important, the child has not interiorized the stuttering role to the degree manifested by the adult." All of these are plus factors that permit Van Riper to be optimistic about the treatment of the young, confirmed stutterer.

VAN RIPER'S TRACKS OF DEVELOPMENT

Van Riper (1971, pp. 104–117) describes four tracks in the development of stuttering. Van Riper admits that "Not all of the individuals in any one track followed its sequence exactly in every detail" (p. 104). Nevertheless, he believes that there are four observable fairly consistent major sequential patterns in the development of stuttering. We may note both similarities and differences between Bloodstein's four phases of stuttering and Van Riper's four developmental tracks. However, Van Riper's tracks are routes to fully developed stuttering. Fortunately, no stutterer needs to go all the way from incipient to confirmed stuttering.

Track 1. Age range usually between 30 to 50 months. These children show considerable variation in their speech disfluencies with remission periods that ranged from days to weeks to months. In the early stages, the disfluencies are not differentiated from those of most other children, consisting of effortless syllable repetition of multisyllabic words and whole word repetition of single syllable words. These repetitions are most likely to occur on the first word of a sentence (utterance) following a pause on the most meaningful word of the utterance. The "stutterings" (disfluencies) usually occur on a small but nevertheless very noticeable portion of the child's speech output.

In the later stage of Track 1, Van Riper observes that there is a change in the tempo of the speech output. There is also an increase in the number of repetitions per syllable for the length of utterance. The repeated syllables tend to become irregular and to be spoken more rapidly than the fluent parts of the utterance.

Prolongations of sounds are often a further developmental feature in Track 1. Prolongations are frequently followed by tensions, forcings, and tremors. These, in turn, are followed or accompanied by frustration behavior and other evidence that the child is aware of having difficulty in speaking. Despite such awareness, the stuttering may show remission. If stuttering is resumed, it is usually more severe and of greater duration. The incidence and occurrence of stuttering are likely to be related to degree of communicative stress for the child.

Later developments in Track 1 include struggle behavior that overflows from the speech mechanism to the limbs. Anxiety precedes, accompanies, and follows (and so again precedes) struggle behavior. When this is evident, the child may become a confirmed stutterer. Nevertheless, Van Riper notes: "Remember the oscillatory course of the disorder. We have seen extreme behaviors of this sort disappear a few days later so that the child is stuttering effortlessly again" (1971, p. 106).

Fears of speaking are usually followed by avoidance behavior. Fears may be generalized for sounds, for words, and for types of words. Fears of situations may also be generalized from a person to a kind of person, from a specific circumstance to a kind of circumstance, and so on.

In the final phase of Track 1, patterns of stuttering become stabilized as do the child's attitudes about speaking and the child's self-concepts. Unhappily, the speech disorders become an integral part of the child's existence.

Track 2. Van Riper does not indicate the age range for Track 2 stutterers. We would estimate onset at three or four years of age continuing on into adolescence and adulthood. Van Riper does indicate that usually stuttering begins with the first attempts at connected speech. Furthermore, most of the children are retarded in speech development and do not begin to use phrases or sentences until they are from three to six years of age. According to Van Riper, these children have no usual history of fluent periods. Beyond the single-word stage, the children seem to have difficulty in sequencing, organizing, and constructing syntactic units. Much of the description of the disfluencies of Track 2 stutterers strongly suggests cluttering. So, Van Riper observes that comparatively few of the Track 2 stutterers develop the anxieties and situation fears of other stutterers. Most of them terminate in speech that is mildly stuttered but mainly cluttered. They tend to talk in torrents.

Early training of Track 2 stutterers should emphasize simple syntactic models to shape the children's speech. Patience and generous time and attention are important. Slowing down and learning to self-monitor rate and clarity of articulation helps—as it may with clut-terers.[3]

Track 3. Age of Onset between five to nine. Children in the Track 3 route are described as having a sudden onset of blocking, laryngeal tension, with fixation and prolongation of articulatory position rather than oscillation. Breathing abnormalities appear very soon after the onset, which often become stereotyped and are used as "rituals of attack." Awareness and frustration and struggle behavior are apparent from the start.

In the development of Track 3 stuttering, syllable repetitions follow a period of initial laryngeal tension and sound prolongation. The greatest difficulty for these stutterers is in getting started. Once under-way, they may speak fairly fluently.

Van Riper observes that children who can keep going after getting started have a fairly good outlook for recovery. On the other hand, those who do not all too often become chronic stutterers. They develop avoidance behavior, have nonvocalized blockings, and may cease trying to talk.

Track 4. Age of onset—usually later than for other tracks. As in Track 3 stuttering, the onset of stuttering is likely to be sudden. How-ever, unlike Track 3, the initial stuttering behavior appears to be highly stereotyped and, according to Van Riper, seems "deliberate and contrived." The child seems aware of the problem and aware of the listener's reactions.

Both syllable and whole word repetition occur, including repetition of words and phrases that are produced fluently. Some Track 4 stutterers do not repeat, but instead show stereotyped breathing behavior and oral "postures" such as sobbing, grunting, and protruding the tongue or lip.

Van Riper observes that a major distinguishing characteristic of the Track 4 stutterers is that the stuttering behavior changes very little over the years. They do not appear to develop techniques for avoiding stuttering but stutter openly, with little evidence of concern about their speech or the effects on their listeners.

Van Riper considers Track 4 type stuttering to be relatively infre-quent in onset in childhood and more likely to have onset in the adult years. Our own impression is that such stutterers had episodes

---

[3] See pages 376–379 for a consideration of cluttering.

early in life that may have been forgotten when stuttering was resumed during adolescence or adult years. We tend to agree with Van Riper that the acceptance of the stuttering, the "benign indifference," makes for a poor prognosis for these speakers.

BRUTTEN AND SHOEMAKER: STAGES IN THE DISINTEGRATION OF SPEECH

One way of looking at Bloodstein's phases of stuttering and Van Riper's tracks of stuttering is to see the problem developing as an aspect of difficulty in speech acquisition in children. This position, which happens to be consistent with our own bias and perception, views the stuttering as an inadequacy in the early organization of speech—especially where syntax and appropriate creative communicative messages need to be formulated and expressed to one or more listeners. Brutten and Shoemaker (1967, pp. 31–35) take what may appear to be an opposite position. They postulate stages in the development of stuttering based on their assumption that stuttering is a conditioned (learned) disintegration of speech behavior. Stage 1 is characterized by predominantly fluent speech with occasional fluency failures that may be the result of adverse (noxious) conditions, but not the result of learning (conditioning). Stage 2 is characterized by an increase in fluency failures and qualitative modification "that are indicative of emotional conditioning." Stage 3 is characterized by "the development of conditioned negative emotional reactions to the act of speaking, the words employed, or the speech produced."

It may well be that speech disintegrates in individuals because initially it has not become well organized and well integrated. Thus, the highest incidence of stuttering is in young children. Adults who are identified as stutterers may never have had well-organized speech. Under stress, or under conditions that stutterers respond to adversely, a weakly organized function (oral language) may "disintegrate" and be expressed in the abnormalities of stuttering.

COMMON DEVELOPMENTAL FACTORS

As indicated earlier, stages, phases, or tracks to stuttering represent the judgments of the individual who is concerned with stuttering and its development. We are able to observe considerable overlapping between positions. Perhaps what really matters is the answer to the questions: (1) "Does it really matter?" and (2) "If it does matter, what are the prognostic and therapeutic implications for the individual child?"

Our own view is that it does matter. Further, careful and long-term study of the "developmental" data may tell us whether and when therapeutic intervention is needed, and possibly what the emphasis of the therapy should be.

In reviewing the positions of Bloodstein, Van Riper, and Shoemaker and Brutten, several factors appear to us to be common: (1) Early disfluencies are in excess of normal in most children who are identified as stutterers. (2) There is a difference between children who repeat whole words and those who repeat sounds and syllables. (Children who do the latter are more likely to become stutterers.) (3) The presence of anxieties and fears about speaking differentiate children who are identified as stutterers. The nonanxious children may in fact be clutterers. (4) The individual histories of many stutterers reveal periods of remission ranging from days to years. (5) Many stutterers and most clutterers seem to have difficulty in the early organization of their language. Disfluencies are associated with syntax—with the rules for the production of a sequence of words appropriate to a language system.

Associated Speech and Language Deficiencies

Our review of the overt speech and related behavior of stutterers suggests that though stutterers vary considerably in their individual backgrounds, there are common factors that we enumerated. There are also several associated speech and language differences between most stutterers and most children who are not stutterers and yet not normal speakers. These differences include delayed onset of speech, persistence in so-called infantilisms in articulation (lisping, lalling, sound distortions, and substitutions). Perhaps most important from our point of view is the delay in syntactic proficiency found by both Bloodstein and Van Riper (cited previously) and by Wyatt (1969, pp. 105–106), who regards stuttering "as a disturbance in the learning of speech and language."

Andrews and Harris (1964, p. 191) are impressed with both the late onset of talking, the "poor" talking, and the familial background of stutterers (stammerers) as distinguishing factors. They say:

Late and poor talking and family history together effectively discriminate stammerers from nonstammerers, and as information about these items may be available prior to the onset of stammering, one might well identify the nonfluent preschool children who are 'at risk' of stammering.

Other speech deviances are manifest by stutterers that are probably a reaction to the stuttering. These include defective voice production characterized by tension and narrow pitch range, voice breaks, vocal fry (intermittent weak or absent phonation), speaking with an inadequate breath supply, and "sticky" articulation.

Conditions Associated with Stuttering

We indicated earlier that no stutterer, regardless of the severity of stuttering, stutters with each utterance. Even the most severe stutterers are often free of stuttering, and sometimes even free of anxiety that they may stutter. Parents of stutterers, teachers, and even the stutterers themselves may be aware that they can engage in choral activity without stuttering, that they can talk aloud to themselves with normal fluency, and that they can usually talk to pets or other animals without difficulty. Many stutterers can talk fluently while playing, especially if the talk is on a nonsense level. Some stutterers can talk normally to younger persons, and a few can talk to a selected peer or even an adult without difficulty or with less than usual difficulty. Stuttering, then, may be regarded as a situational problem. We have suggested some situations conducive to relatively free-from-stuttering speech. Are there any general situations that are conductive to stuttering? A review of research suggests an affirmative answer.

Brown (1945), in several studies, found that stutterers tend to have verbal cues or indicators that are related to increased stuttering. These include initial words in sentences; longer words in sentences; more nouns, verbs, and adverbs than other parts of speech; and accented syllables within words.

Eisenson and Horowitz (1945) found that stutterers had increased difficulty with reading material as the intellectual significance of the material was increased.

Lanyon (1969), however, found that the likelihood of a stutterer having difficulty (stuttering) on any given word depends not on how much information the word conveys but on word length and how much speech (articulatory) production is required to say the word.

These and other studies that are available in the literature strongly suggest that two factors or situations are conducive to increased stuttering. These are (1) awareness that what is to be spoken has intellectual content; and (2) awareness of communicative responsibility for the speech content. Conversely, we find that stutterers report that they are relatively free of what characterizes their stuttering when they feel no need to make a favorable impression on their listeners or when they do not feel individually responsible for their utterances. This is in line with the observations of teachers and clinicians who have observed stutterers in their periods or relative fluency and conditions associated with virtually normal fluency.

Beyond these linguistic and environmental situations, which tend to be related to the incidence of stuttering, there are other factors that apparently influence speech control. Most stutterers have increased difficulty when they are fatigued. Stutterers tend to stutter more when they expect to stutter than when such expectancy does not exist. On an individual basis, some stutterers expect to stutter in special situations or with specific persons more than they do in other situations or with other persons. By and large, these expectancies tend to be confirmed by actual experience. Even when other speech and associated stuttering manifestations are not present, stutterers experience feelings of apprehension and anxiety because of their anticipation of stuttering. The result is that they respond to themselves as if they had stuttered even though the listener-observer may have seen no external evidence of stuttered speech.

The last point suggests an aspect of stuttering that is deserving of consideration. Although what the listener-observer hears and sees may be important in the evaluation of stuttering, much goes on within the stutterer that cannot be evaluated by anyone but the stutterer. How stutterers feel about themselves when they anticipate the need to speak is important. How much effort and anxiety do stutterers expect when they are successful in controlling their stuttering? Is it less rather than more than when they stutter? Do stutterers feel better when their speech seems to be normally fluent than when their speech is marked by an abnormal amount of hesitations, blocks, repetitions, prolongations, and any other type of behavior that accompanies or characterizes stuttering? How stutterers feel about their speaking is a subjective aspect of stuttering that may be of extreme importance to the individual stutterer. The overt characteristics affect the listener's responses to the stutterer. The covert feelings, unless directly translated into some form of readily observable behavior, are not likely to affect the responses of the listener. If we appreciate this, we can begin to understand why some adolescents and adults who seem to speak without any of the speech and associated mannerisms of stuttering nevertheless regard themselves as stutterers. They do so, we may conclude, because they feel like stutterers, even though they do not overtly behave like stutterers.

Theoretic Points of View as to the Causes of Stuttering[4]

Theories as to why people stutter are numerous and diverse in their points of view. Many theories that were once influential, if not dominating, have become reduced in importance, not because they have been disproved or discredited but because their proponents have ceased proposing them or have changed their minds. The attempt in this chapter is to present several current points of view This is done with responsible awareness that we are not including many other points of view, which, in a larger or more specialized text, might well be mentioned. The points of view considered in this chapter may be broadly classified along the following lines:

1. Stuttering is a constitutional problem. There are physical reasons that predispose a person to stuttering or that make him/her a stutterer.

2. Stuttering is essentially a learned form of behavior that may happen to anyone.

3. Stuttering is a manifestation of an underlying personality disorder.

STUTTERING AS A CONSTITUTIONAL PROBLEM

The proponents of the theoretical position that there is a constitutional predisposition to stuttering point to research studies to support their stand. Some of the findings suggest that, as a group, stutterers' familial histories include the following incidents as occurring more often than in the population as a whole: (1) more stutterers; (2) more left-handedness; (3) more twins; (4) later onset of speech; and (5) higher incidence of illnesses and traumas that might cause damage to the nervous system. Support for this position comes from some of the older investigations of Berry (1939) and Nelson (1939) and more recently from the findings of the Andrews and Harris Survey (1964, p. 101). The last report includes the presence of significant genetic and neurologic predisposing factors and a higher than usual incidence of birth traumas or evidence of subsequent brain injury. In addition, it reports findings of

---

[4] C. Van Riper in *The Nature of Stuttering* (Englewood Cliffs, N.J.: Prentice-Hall, Inc., 1971) reviews several historical and current theories of stuttering. He also presents his own position on stuttering in his chapter "The Nature of Stuttering: An Attempted Synthesis."

J. Eisenson, *Stuttering: A Second Symposium* (New York; Harper & Row Publishers, Inc., 1975) includes several theoretic positions on stuttering.

delayed onset of speech and a high incidence of speech and language problems other than stuttering, "... but by far the most important predisposing factor is the inheritance from either parent of the genetic predisposition to stammer."

Findings of recent studies by Curry and Gregory (1969) and Perrin (1969) have implications that suggest that stutterers may be different in their neurophysiological organization from nonstutterers. Both investigations employed a special perceptual-listening task (dichotic listening) to compare the responses of stutterers and nonstutterers. The dichotic listening task requires the listener to attend to two different auditory signals presented simultaneously, one to the left ear and one to the right. In essence, the ears of the subject are engaged in competitive listening. Earlier findings indicate an interesting difference in ear-reporting depending upon the nature of the auditory signal. Speech signals, such as digits or words, when presented dichotically are reported by most subjects as being received in the right ear. Nonspeech signals such as clicks, snatches of melody, and other nonspeech environmental noises are usually reported as being received in the left ear (Kimura, 1967, p. 20). The systematic differences between the ears in dichotic listening are interpreted as reflecting the functional differences between the two cerebral hemispheres, consistent with the fact that each ear has its greatest number of connections with the contralateral hemisphere. Findings have been fairly uniform that when the subject reports differences in perception of auditory signals, speech signals tend to be referred to the right ear (processed by the left and normally dominant hemisphere). Whereas nonspeech signals are referred to the left ear (processed by the right or nondominant hemisphere). These findings occur only in binaural competitive (dichotic) listening tasks. This, of course, is a laboratory technique and not the one that pertains to usual listening situations.

Curry and Gregory (1969) and Perrin (1969) found that stutterers did not make the referrals to the right ear for speech signals along the expected lines. Although there was some variation for invididuals, the Curry and Gregory data indicate that taken as a group, "stutterers had smaller difference scores between ears on dichotic verbal scores than did nonstutterers. Seventy-five per cent of the nonstutterers obtained higher right-ear scores on the dichotic verbal task, whereas 55 per cent of the stutterers had higher left-ear scores." Perrin's findings confirmed those of Curry and Gregory.

Specifically, Perrin found that stutterers showed a clear left-ear preference for words and sentences in dichotic reception, whereas nonstutterers showed a right ear preference for such materials. As a group, the stutterers were not different from the nonstutterers in regard to their ear preference for vowels and for noises. As a general observation Perrin (1969) notes, "When a hemisphere exerts some control over speech function in the stutterer, it is the right, which is the reverse of that found in normals." We appreciate, of course, that ear preference is contralateral to cerebral control.

Sommers, Brady, and Moore (1975) compared groups of stuttering children and adults (age range four to 48) with nonstuttering controls on dichotic listening tasks. They found a trend for the stuttering children to show a lack of ear preference for words and digits presented dichotically as compared with nonstuttering children. Further, the study found considerably more left-ear preference by the stuttering children. An additional interesting finding was that the left ear preferences and no-ear preference decreased with the age of the children. In general, the nonstuttering children and adults performed alike on the dichotic tasks. However, right-ear dichotic scores were significantly smaller than those for adult stutterers. The investigators speculate that "the speech perceptual function and/or hemispheric lateralization of speech may continue to develop at a slower rate than in nonstutterers."

A dichotic listening study by Slorach and Noehr (1973) with a group of primary grade children in Brisbane, Australia, showed varying lateralization among stutterers who were compared with children with defective articulation and another group considered to be normal in speech. The dichotic listening task consisted of pairs of three digit series. All three groups showed a right-ear preference but some of the stutterers showed special patterns of lateralization at variance with the other children.

The trend of the findings using dichotic listening studies strongly suggests that stutterers as a total population differ from nonstutterers in their differential cerebral dominance for language. Discussions of cerebral dominance, as related to language functioning, that review techniques other than dichotic listening may be found in Eisenson (1975, pp. 411–416) and Van Riper (1971, pp. 351–359). Our impression is that the findings tend to support the assumption that the cerebral organization of most stutterers for speech (language) control is different from that of nonstutterers.

Van Riper (1971, p. 404), although not certain as to the etiology of stuttering, nevertheless says:

> We should like to suggest that stuttering be considered a disorder of timing . . . when a person stutters on a word, there is a temporal disruption of the simultaneous and successive programming of muscular movements required to produce one of the word's integrated sounds or to emit one of its syllables appropriately . . . or to accomplish the precise linking

of sounds and syllables that constitute its motor pattern . . . . When, for any reason, that timing is awry and askew, a temporarily distorted word is produced and when this happens, the speaker has evinced a core stuttering behavior.

In his chapter "The Nature of Stuttering: An Attempted Synthesis" (1971, 404–441), Van Riper reviews the literature that indicates why stutterers have defective timing behavior for speech, and when they can overcome the effects of this defect. Van Riper does not minimize the psychological factors that may maintain stuttering. However, we believe that the majority of the evidence presented by Van Riper supports a constitutional factor on the etiology of stuttering.

Andrews and Harris (1964, p. 191) suggest a psychobiological theory of stuttering along the following lines:

1. In some instances, a predisposition may be sufficient to initiate stammering (stuttering).
2. "Emotional stress at an age when adequate speech function is precarious may result in a disturbance of this balance of speech maturation and so produce a repetition of sounds and syllables characteristic of stammering. In a child with abnormal speech development, this period of vulnerability will be prolonged. If there is sufficient genetic and neurologic predisposition only minor anxieties will be sufficient, whereas if there is minimal predisposition a more severe emotional stress will be required to initiate stammering."
3. Once the involuntary repetitions of sounds and syllables have begun, the child soon learns to anticipate those words and situations that are difficult for him. "It is this anxiety about specific word and situational cues, and its reduction as they are passed, that results in the development of both the severity and complexity of the stammer syndrome."

This position may explain why all children who may have a predisposing background do not necessarily become stutterers. If a child is fortunate and is free of severe illness, physical, and psychological trauma during the developmental stages of speech, he/she may be reasonably "safe" from becoming a stutterer.

If, however, conditions are less fortunate, and either illness or emotional disturbance upsets the child during the speech-development stage, stuttering is likely to result. In other words, constitutional factors provide a subsoil for stuttering. Stuttering itself is a product associated with the subsoil and the specific environmental, physical, or psychological factors that tend to nurture it.

STUTTERING AS A LEARNED FORM OF BEHAVIOR

The proponents of the point of view that stuttering is a learned form of behavior are, as we might expect, opposed to believing that stutterers as a group are significantly different constitutionally in any way from nonstutterers. Instead, children who stutter are considered to be essentially normal children in regard to heredity, physical development, health history, psychological traits, intelligence, or any other single factor in which the first group of theorists we discussed found important differences. Johnson (1967), who was a leading proponent of "normality of the stutterer" school, held that stuttering is a *speech disturbance which can happen to anyone.* How stuttering has its onset and how it becomes established as a reaction to some but not all speaking situations are explained through principles of learning that apply to behavior in general as well as to stuttering in particular.

The early stages of stuttering are explained as resulting from a misevaluation of the disfluencies normal in young children. Young children of preschool age and in the early primary grades are inclined to be repetitious and hesitant when they talk as well as in other forms of behavior. Parents, teachers, or other adults who mistake these disfluencies for stuttering symptoms, and who show concern or anxiety about them, are likely to transmit this attitude to the child. When a child becomes aware of adult anxiety and permits it to affect him, he may approach a speaking situation with an attitude of apprehension. It is not the hesitation or repetition but the speaker's reactions to them and to the reactions of other persons to which he, in turn, reacts that make the child into a stutterer.

In another publication Johnson (1961, p. 138) explained that:

> The problem called stuttering begins, then, when the child's speech is felt, usually by the mother, to be not as smooth or as fluent as it ought to be. There seems as a rule to be a quality of puzzlement mixed with slight apprehension and dread about the mother's feelings. She uses the only name she knows for what she thinks must be the matter with her youngster's speech, and that word is "stuttering"—or, if she has grown up in England or certain other parts of the world, "stammering."
>
> . . . She may not be sure of herself at first in deciding that her child is stuttering, but her use of the word crystallizes her feelings and serves to focus her attention on the hesitations in the speech of her child.

Johnson emphasized that the mother's feelings and apprehensions tend to become apparent to the child and in time the child "takes from the mother the feelings she has about his speech."

Eisenson (1966) "tested" Johnson's assumption that stuttering is a result of maternal reaction to the child's speech by investigating the incidence of the disorder among preschool and primary-grade children brought up in kibbutzim (communal organizations) in Israel. Children in these settings were cared for by nurse-teachers throughout the day. They saw their parents in the late afternoon and on some holidays. They slept, ate, were trained and taught in cottage facilities by the nurse-teachers. There was no conscious differences in the treatment of the children along sex lines. The incidence and sex distribution for the presence of stuttering in children brought up in kibbutzim were essentially the same as those found in the United States and those reported by Andrews and Harris in England. The total incidence was about 1 per cent, with a sex ratio of about four boys to one girl.

To return to Johnson's position, stuttering may be considered a learned and specific anxiety reaction associated with speaking situations. But stuttering and its consequences seem to be unpleasant and apparently more penalizing than rewarding. Normally, behavior that persists is behavior somehow rewarded. Are there any rewards or pleasant aftereffects (reinforcers) in stuttering? There are, if we look for them. One of the possible reinforcers is the attention a child may receive that may not otherwise be available. Stutterers may learn to enjoy the intensity of reaction, and the disturbance they cause by their speech. If they need such reactions more than they do normal speech, stuttering is likely to persist. In the classroom, stutterers may be excused from recitations or win sympathy that they may learn to enjoy. A stutterer may become a "special child" and be reluctant to give up that status. Until ready to do so, the child who began to stutter through no fault of his/her own is likely to continue to stutter. Unfortunately, when the penalties of stuttering begin to exceed the rewards, the habits and attitudes of the stutterer may persist, and many stutterers need help in overcoming them. A few, however, seem able to stop without outside help. These children may have taken an accounting of the assets and liabilities associated with stuttering and reached a conclusion that became translated into self-modified behavior. Certainly, many experienced teachers know youngsters who stuttered in the early grades and who became normal speakers in later grades without any outside help.

For those stutterers who do not or cannot stop, a theoretical explanation for the continuance of stuttering can be made along these lines: Stutterers continue to fear that they will stutter in a given situation or on a given word. They become tense and apprehensive in anticipation of the situation or word. If, with great effort, they finally manage to speak despite the initial tension and anxiety, this brings about a momentary reduction in the anxiety-tension state. This brief period of relief may be sufficiently pleasurable to reinforce and to perpetuate not only the stuttering but also the entire attitude and pattern of behavior associated with it.

In *Stuttering: A Second Symposium* (Eisenson 1975, ed.) essays by Brutten, Ingham, Shames, and Sheehan represent related but somewhat different views of how stuttering becomes a learned (conditioned) form of behavior. Therapeutic approaches that are compatible with conditioning theories are also explained. Gray and England (1969) also present several conditioning theories and therapies for stutterers. Gregory (1968) edited a monograph on *Learning Theory and Stuttering Therapy*.

STUTTERING AS A PERSONALITY DISORDER

The position that stuttering is primarily a manifestation of an underlying neurotic personality is not as widely held as it was up until the 1960s. Nevertheless, many psychologists and psychiatrists, mostly those who are identified as psychoanalysts, still emphasize the maladjustment and do not appear to be concerned with the possibility that stutterers are constitutionally different from normal speakers. They regard stuttering as a manifestation of personality disorder and are inclined to agree that the stutterer speaks as he does because of some psychological need that is better satisfied through stuttering than through normal speech. Stutterers are likely to be characterized as infantile, compulsive, dependent, ambivalent, regressive, anxious, insecure, withdrawn, or by some other adjective or combination of adjectives consistent with the specific theoretic formulation or bias of the theorizer. For example, the psychoanalyst Coriat (1943) viewed stutterers as "... infants who have compulsively retained the original equivalents of nursing and biting." The equivalents, we might note, are the specific oral characteristics of the stutterer, the way in which he repeats, hesitates, blocks, or prolongs on the sounds he utters or stops himself from uttering.

Travis (1971, pp. 1009–1033), in an essay entitled "The Unspeakable Feelings of People with Special Reference to Stuttering," traces the development of neurotic behavior and the responsibility as well as the fear of speaking in stutterers. "Stuttering is the consequence of the young child speaking with his mother and father. In his utterances he asked to be known and be understood. In their reply they told him of his unacceptability in his current verbalized forms" (p. 1009). Travis uses learning theory to explain how stuttering behavior becomes reinforced. Basically, however, "stuttering is a manifestation of a fear to speak the truth to oneself or about oneself to another. It occurs most frequently in those families that place a high premium upon the truth and then punish its verbalization. To the extent that a child can be self-conscious comfortably, he will not stutter."

Therapy for Travis emphasizes the need to help stutterers accept their feelings, however hostile and "unspeakable" they may be. Most of the stutterers were adults by the time they were seen by Travis for psychotherapeutic help, and so were able to express their feelings. There is a note of preventive therapy in the Travis position. It is for parents to learn to listen so that their children's feelings may be expressed and not become repressed and "unspeakable."

Van Riper (1971, pp. 265–284) reviews the literature on "Stuttering as a Neurosis." We agree with Van Riper's conclusion (p. 277) that "The case for stuttering as a neurosis and only a neurosis has not been made."

Theorists who believe that stuttering is a manifestation of a personality disorder are able to point to a large number of studies to support their position. The results of many, but by no means all of these studies, suggest that adolescents and adults who stutter are, on the whole, not as well adjusted as nonstutterers. We might add, however, that seldom do the studies provide evidence to indicate whether the stuttering is the cause of, or is caused by, the maladjustment. The possibility that the stuttering preceded the maladjustment must be considered by those who look objectively on the overall problem of the stutterer and his stuttering.

MULTIPLE ORIGIN VIEWPOINTS

The points of view just presented each sought to explain stuttering as having a single cause. Obviously, theories that are inconsistent with one another cannot all be correct at all times. There is a possibility, however, that each of the theories, and the theorists, is correct at some times—often enough, we would gather, to satisfy himself, but not often enough to persuade those holding opposing or even supplementary viewpoints. Before leaving the discussion of theories as to the cause of stuttering we consider two points of view of practicing speech clinicians who currently believe that stuttering may have multiple causes. Why any given individual stutters can best be estimated by his individual clinical history and the cause that seems most likely to fit his case.

STUTTERING AS A MANIFESTATION OF PERSEVERATION

Eisenson (1975) believes that persons tend to persist in a given mode of behavior even when such behavior is not appropriate, when they are confronted with conditions that call for more rapid change than they are capable of making. The tendency for an individual to resist change, and for a mental or motor process to dominate behavior after the situation that originally evoked it is no longer present, is termed *perseveration*. The perseverating phenomenon is normal for all of us. Most often we experience it when we are tired or sleepy, or under conditions of pressure or tension. We do the same thing or feel the same way even when we are able to recognize that the cause for the doing or feeling has ceased to exist. So, minutes after we have gotten off a bicycle, we may still feel that we are riding on it. When we are tired, and required to talk, we tend to repeat utterances more often than the intellectual aspect of the situation requires. If we do not become anxious or apprehensive about our normal inclination to perseverate, we are not likely to fear recurring or similar situations because we have perseverated. There are, however, physiological and psychological conditions that are conducive to more than a normal amount of perseverative behavior. Among these conditions are brain damage, brain difference, lowered vitality, the after-effects of physical or mental shock, and emotional tension and anxiety.

According to Eisenson (1975), if an individual is required, or feels required, to speak under a condition conductive to perseverative behavior, the perseveration will be manifest in his/her speech. Unfortunately, the awareness of blocked or repetitive tendencies in speech may increase the individual's apprehension about speaking and so aggravate the condition that was initially responsible for the speech perseveration. The result is a generalized reaction toward speaking that transforms what might otherwise be hesitation, block, repetition, or prolongation (perseverating manifestations) into stuttering.

As indicated earlier, speaking conditions that are associated with a feeling of responsibility are more likely to be associated with perseverative speech than speech that is devoid of responsibility. Communicative language content is also associated with perseveration in speaking. Persons who find themselves pressed by their environment, or by their own inner compulsions, to speak (communicate) on an intellectual level when they have nothing to say, or are not completely prepared to say what they would like, are likely to perseverate in speech. In general, these speech situations are all productive of some degree of anxiety.

It is also possible that some persons with atypical neurological mechanisms are unable to respond with spoken language as rapidly as some speech situations require. In such situations, and for such persons, perseveration in speech tends to occur. These may be the persons with a constitutional predisposition to stutter.

As noted, most stutterers have periods of relative fluency, and others in which they are normally quite fluent. Such conditions include speaking to animal pets, responding as a member of a group (where communicative responsibility is shared, reduced, or lacking), speaking nonsense intentionally, singing (singing is not really speaking because it is devoid of responsibility either for the formulation of the word sequences or its "communication"), and often reciting memorized material. All of these conditions share a common feature—the lack of formulating and the responsibility of uttering a thought, or a propositional statement (it may be a question) to which an answer might be expected. Stuttering, unless it is patently of neurotic origin, almost always occurs when a speaker is engaged in propositional talking. It has its parallel with the normal hesitations of nonstutterers who are talking about something of importance, even if only of momentary importance, while they are thinking of how to say it. These are normal hesitation phenomena.

In summary, most stuttering behavior is expressed when the speaker is engaged in propositional or communicative interchange. At such times, either because of an anxiety specific to the situation, or a more generalized anxiety about speaking when there is any degree of communicative responsibility, perseveration in speech tends to occur. Only a neurotic individual who feels that he has a commitment to stutter whenever and to whomever he talks or nontalks is likely to stutter in many other situations. Normal speakers, and stutterers when not under stress, may engage in normal hesitations. However, despite superficial resemblances, normal hesitations, regardless of who produces them, should not be confused with stuttering.

In essence, according to Eisenson, stuttering as a manifestation of perseveration may take place whenever the speaker finds himself inadequate or unequal to the demands of the speaking situation. The perseverating tendency may have a physiological cause, a psychological cause, or a combination of both. Initially, the onset cause for most stutterers is a neurologial difference along lines considered in our discussion of cerebral dominance for language. Early stuttering is a manifestation of difficulty some children have in the organization of language for purposes of the communication of their thinking.

VAN RIPER'S ECLECTIC POSITION

In our consideration of Van Riper's tracks of stuttering, it is evident that he does not believe we know enough about stuttering to assign a single cause to the disorder. Van Riper emphasizes that there are multiple routes or tracks to stuttering and so possibly multiple causes. Elsewhere he says:

> What is a student to believe when so many different explanations exist? Our own resolution of the problem is an eclectic one. We feel that stuttering has many origins, many sources, and that the original causes are not nearly so important as the maintaining causes, once stuttering has started. We can find stutterers who partly fit any one of the various statements of theory and some stutterers who fit several. All stutterers are not cut from the same original cloth. It is important that we know these various explanations because the problems of some of the stutterers we meet can thereby be best understood. The river of stuttering does not flow out of only one lake. (Van Riper, 1972, p. 263).

Van Riper acknowledges that all stutterers do not go through all the stages within any track. There are differential characteristics in the behavior of the stuttering—the onset of speech symptoms and the associated behavior—that require differential treatment. In some instances, the psychodynamics that may be maintaining stuttering also require treatment. Some of the approaches recommended by Van Riper and others that we endorse are now considered.

Therapy for Stutterers

Although the burden of therapy for stutterers is one that should be carried by the professional speech clinician, the classroom teacher is necessarily an important member of the therapeutic team. In the following discussion, we consider the objectives of therapy for the beginning stutterer and the confirmed stutterer as well as the specific role of the classroom teacher in regard to each.

OBJECTIVES FOR THE EARLY (INCIPIENT) STUTTERER

In characterizing the early (incipient) stutterers, we stressed that their disfluencies, even though they may be excessive, occur without evidence either of awareness or special effort in speaking. Emphasis in the treatment of the early stutterers is to prevent them from becoming aware that their speech is in any way different from that of others around them and a cause for concern. Awareness of difference, whether it be of speech or any other form of behavior, arises from observed reactions. Young children will have no way of knowing that their speech is atypical unless some person important to them says or does something to direct their attention to the difference. A child who is disfluent is not likely to compare himself/herself with other children until after some older person has made or suggested a comparison. Disfluencies become something for a child to be concerned about only if he/she has responded to another person's concern. To prevent the child's awareness and concern, we must somehow control the reactions of persons who may show and so create such awareness. Essentially, therefore, the early stutterer if not of school age is to be treated through the parents. If the stutterer is of school age, the child's teachers as well as parents become the recipients of direct treatment. The early stutterer should be given no direct speech therapy or any other form of therapy that can be related to the production of speech. Nothing should be done or said to the child that suggests that his/her speech is in any way in need of change. If the early stutterer is to be involved in therapy, it is only to permit the trained speech clinician to observe what possible pressures exist in the child's environment that disturb his speech production. For this purpose, a permissive play group is recommended, in which a clinician is able to observe conditions that are conducive to increased disfluency. The clinician's observations are, of course, later discussed with the parents with a view toward modification of comparable home conditions so that pressure and excessive disfluencies can be reduced, or, if possible, eliminated. Some of these specific aspects of treatment, and some of the information to be given to the parents of the early stutterer, or to the child believed by the parents to be a stutterer, are now considered. Many of these aspects, incidentally, are also relevant for the classroom teacher.

DISTINGUISHING BETWEEN DISFLUENCY AND EARLY STUTTERING

Often parents are unduly sensitized about stuttering because of their own family history. One or both of the parents may have stuttered or may still be stuttering. Older children or relatives may be stutterers. Perhaps the parents are being pressured by their own parents to "do something" about the child's speech. The parents, understandably concerned, are "doing something" about what they believe to be stuttering.

A first step in the direction of treatment of the parents is to determine whether the child's disfluencies are within the limits of normal or, in terms of incidence and situation, in excess of normal. Are we, in other words, dealing with normal disfluency, which includes some amount of so-called disfluency, or early (incipient) stuttering? Information is obtained from the parents' description and, if possible, imitation of an actual tape recording of the child's speech. The parents are asked to recall when disfluencies most often occur and when they are least likely to occur. The child's speech should be observed when talking to the parents, with a special note made as to whether there is any difference in ease of speaking when the response is made to the mother or to the father. The child should also be observed in a play situation when away from the parents as well as in their presence. If the total observed speech behavior adds up to normal speech flow—normal ease of speech disfluencies included—this should be stated and explained to the parents. We have found that parents are frequently able to understand and accept hesitancies and repetitions in speech when these are compared with hesitant and repetitious nonspeech behavior. We are usually able to get from parents their observations that not only their child but most children repeat activities when at play, that young children enjoy hearing the same song or the same story repeated many times. We try to make parents realize the normality of repetitions in all aspects of a young child's behavior so that repetition does not seem abnormal when it occurs in speech.

We have found effective the technique of recording and playing back part of the interview held with the parents about the child. In listening to the playback, parents are able to hear their own hesitations and repetitions as well as those of the interviewer. If they do not consider themselves stutterers, the parents are then able to compare their own speech with that of their child in regard to the incidence of "disfluencies." If the parents are disturbed about their own hesitant speech, they should be assured that few if any persons are always fluent, except possibly when they are reproducing memorized material. Even actors, it can be pointed out, have occasional "disfluencies," so that nonprofessional speakers should certainly be permitted some of their own.

Nothing in the interview with the parents should suggest, by words or manner, that the parents were either foolish or overanxious or in any way exercised poor judgment in coming for help about their child's speech. We believe that parents have a right, if not an obligation, to be concerned. We also believe that each child has his/her right not to be concerned about all things that may concern the parents. The child's hesitations, if they are normal in frequency and not excessive for the situation, are among those things about which the child should not be concerned. We think that parents are usually able to appreciate that most disfluencies are normal. Furthermore, the difference between normal hesitation and stuttering may lie in the matter of awareness and anxiety that young children who are not indifferent to their parents may get from them. Stuttering is frequently the sum of disfluency, plus awareness plus anxiety, whereas disfluency alone is developmentally normal speech behavior.

It is possible that in some instances the child may really be disfluent, more than normally hesitant and repetitive in speech. The advice, nevertheless, still holds. There is much greater likelihood that a child will reduce this manner of speaking without direct attention being paid to it, than with intervention. The only positive suggestion we would make for "correction" is to observe whether a child is trying to arrive at a new, more mature, and syntactically more complex way of saying something than he/she did before the occurrence of the hesitations and repetitions. For example, a child at age three might say "Johnny is my brother. Johnny and I go to school together." The same child when a year or so older might try to indicate the same meanings with a single sentence formulation such as "My brother Johnny and I go to school together," or "I go to school with my brother Johnny." While trying to figure out the new "grown up" way to say things, hesitations and repetitions may well take place. If this seems to be the situation, then the mother or the nursery school teacher should give the child a "model" sentence to imitate. The model sentence should not be too obvious or too directly offered. We would suggest that the parent or teacher might take an opportunity to make a parallel statement for the child. If our little Johnny's brother is bright, he will get the idea. If not, no harm will be done.

What we are suggesting has more general implication. We believe that most adults have hesitations in speaking when they try new formulations. Certainly observers of the speech of children may readily note this phenomenon. Most children develop control of new formulations such as embedded phrases and clauses, for example, "Mary, my very dearest doll, broke her arm today." While "reaching" for this new formulation, this new way of saying two sentences (thoughts) in one, the child may indeed become somewhat disfluent. So may the child in trying out a "big" word, or the expression of any new "big" thought. Hesitations, repetitions, and even backing up and starting again, are all quite normal for adults. Certainly they should be considered normal for children. To repeat an earlier observation, normal fluency should include an amount of so-called disfluencies, which are really normal hesitation phenomena. However, it is possible that in some instances, which we believe include most young children with a constitutional predisposition toward at least incipient or early stage stuttering, children may be delayed in their ability for syntactic development. Their inner linguistic formulations, and so, of course, their expressions may be inconsistent with age and intellectual level expectations. So, they have difficulty in "mature" expressions of their thoughts.

The child who is found to be delayed in language development, and particularly in syntactic competence, deserves and should be given help in how to say a few words well. The child at the outset needs many models of simple but "complete" language formulations. When these formulations of from three to five words are mastered, then more elaborate constructions should be provided. These constructions may be incorporated and practiced in play situations. At first it may be a role-playing situation in which a child talks to a doll, a stuffed animal, or some other toy object. Ultimately, of course, we want communicative interchanges with a peer or an older person. Give the child ample time to formulate and produce the utterances. Interchange roles with the child so that "grown-up talk" and "grown-up behavior," even though it is play behavior, will go together in a mutually enjoyable situation.

INFORMATION ABOUT LANGUAGE DEVELOPMENT AND SPEECH FUNCTIONS

Many parents become anxious about their children's speech because they are either uninformed or misinformed about how speech and language develop in children. They are likely to have some vague notions that children begin to talk somewhere about the time that they begin to walk. Most parents have heard about children who talked reasonably plainly at one year of age and may show disappointment if their own children seem slower. We believe that properly informed parents are likely to be less anxious parents, and so, either in an interview situation or in a larger parent group situation, we inform the parents about the normal expectancies in regard to language development, speech proficiency, and the function served by speech. Among the points we emphasize for parents are the following:[5]

1. Every child has his/her own rate and pattern of language and speech development just as he/she has an individual rate and pattern of physical growth and motor development. A slower than "normal" developmental pattern does not necessarily mean that the child is retarded.

2. Language and speech development are related to some factors over which the child has no control. These include the position and number of children in the family, the linguistic ability and intelligence of the parents, the child's sex, and the appropriateness of motivation and stimulation for the child to talk. A first child tends to begin to talk

---

[5] The teacher or clinician might at this point review Chapter 7 on the development of language in children.

earlier than a second, and a second earlier than a third. Girls, by and large, talk somewhat earlier and more proficiently than boys. The child who is urged to talk too soon may be more delayed in beginning than the child who begins to talk when ready and needs to talk.

3. Attentive and available parents are much more helpful for the development of speech than are either anxious or nonavailable parents.

4. Language is not likely to be used unless its use is associated with pleasure.

5. Children should enjoy making sounds before sounds are used as words. Even after children begin to use words, they continue to enjoy making sounds even when they have nothing to communicate.

6. Many children do not establish articulatory (speech sound) proficiency until they are almost eight years of age. A young child is entitled to lisp, hesitate, and repeat without being corrected except by good example.

7. Children must hear good speech if they are to become good speakers.

8. Fluency does not become established all at once, if indeed it is ever established. Most preschool children speak with some amount of hesitations and repetitions much of the time. Hesitations and repetitions, even up to 10 per cent of utterance are not abnormal provided they do not abruptly interrupt or fragment the flow of speech. In very young children who are just beginning to speak and in many three- and four-year-olds who are striving for grown-up sentence formulations, so-called disfluencies may exceed 10 per cent of utterance.

9. Absence of speech fluency becomes important and a matter for concern when it is associated with specific recurring situations or events. Parents should note whether the child becomes increasingly hesitant when frustrated, when fatigued, or when talking to particular persons. If the child's disfluencies increase sharply in these situations, control of the situations, if possible, is recommended. Control may take place either by avoiding the situation or by doing nothing that requires the child to communicate in these situations. By communicating, we mean having to answer questions that call for precise answers. Nothing, however, should be done to give the child a feeling that he/she is not to speak if the wish to speak is present.

Parents should also note whether the child becomes increasingly disfluent when bidding or competing for attention. If this is so, parents should be alert to give the child quick attention when the child is normally fluent. This is important so that increased disfluency by the child does not result in greater satisfaction than normal fluency.

Parents should know that children do not always want to say something specific or communicative when they talk. They may wish to use words as they once used sounds, merely for the sake of the pleasure derived from utterance. Adults also do this when they sing nonsense songs or talk nonsense words to their children.

Parents should be on guard to watch how often they unconsciously or consciously interrupt their children. Interruption may produce frustration, and frustration, in turn, produces disfluency. The child who is brought up to become silent when an adult wishes to talk may interrupt speech attempts and become hesitant in fear of talking out of turn.

MODIFICATION OF REACTIONS TO THE CHILD'S DISFLUENCIES

If the child is in an early phase or stage of stuttering, or is showing any of the speech characteristics associated with stuttering, it is essential that parents avoid revealing their anxiety. First, of course, we try to assure the parents that despite our acceptance that the child may be in the first stage of stuttering, later phases or stages are by no means inevitable. By relieving parental anxiety, we hope to reduce the occurrence of displays of anxiety. Parents are encouraged to listen patiently and without tension when the child speaks. They are instructed not to do or say anything that may be interpreted by the child as a sign that his/her speech is not acceptable. Among the important *do nots* are the following:

1. Do not permit the child to hear the word *stuttering* used about his/her speech. This holds for any synonym or euphemism for stuttering.
2. Do not tell the child to speed up, slow down, think before speaking, start over again, or do anything that makes it necessary for the child to inhibit speaking or to conclude that he/she is not speaking well.
3. Do not sigh with relief when the child speaks fluently, or look with wide-eyed fear that the youngster may speak hesitatingly.
4. Do not show impatience if the child blocks, hesitates, or repeats.
5. Do not ask the child to speak in situations where disfluencies are likely to occur.

Among the important *positive suggestions* for the parents of the early-stage stutterer are the following:

1. Establish as calm a home environment as can be achieved. Try to avoid exposing the child to situations that are overexciting, embarrassing, or frustrating.

2. Encourage the child to talk, but do not demand talking even in situations where the child is usually fluent and at ease.

3. Listen to your child with as much attention as you would like shown to you when you are talking.

4. Speak to your child in a calm, unhurried manner, but not in a way that is so exaggerated as to be difficult to imitate.

5. Keep your child in the best possible physical condition and check for possible ailments if he/she suddenly shows excessive hesitations and repetitions.

6. Expect that your child will sometimes begin to say things he/she cannot finish. If the child seems to be groping for a word to complete the thought, offer the word. Do not, however, anticipate what the child may want to say by completing the thought in your own words.

7. Do all you can to make speech behavior pleasurable. Tell amusing anecdotes and read stories that you know the child enjoys. If you note that a certain time of day your child has an increase of disfluencies, try to make that the time in which you do the reading. This reading has two results. It removes the opportunity for the practice of disfluent speech, and with it the possibility that the child may become aware of disfluencies. It also affords the child an opportunity to be passively engaged in an enjoyable speech activity.

8. Assure your child, if he/she asks you whether there is anything wrong with his/her speech, that you think the speech is just fine. If he/she tells you that sometimes he/she has trouble getting words out, make him/her understand that everybody has such trouble at some time so that there is nothing to worry about. Avoid overexplaining and overtalking your assurance, or your child, as a wise child, may suspect that you do not really mean what you say.

THE ROLE OF THE CLASSROOM TEACHER

Virtually all that has been outlined or suggested as appropriate attitude and behavior for the parents of the early stage stutterer may be applied to the classroom teacher. The problem of an early stutterer is one that the teacher is likely to meet in the nursery and kindergarten grades and in the first two grades of school. In these grades, the teacher has an opportunity to observe the pressure situations that are conducive to increased disfluencies and to control them in the child's behalf. The teacher, by being a patient and attentive listener, can help the child considerably. The child who shows signs of early stuttering should not be corrected in his/her articulation or have any other aspect of defective speech called to his/her attention. The teacher should avoid calling upon the child when it is likely that the child will be disfluent and go out of the way to call upon him/her when relatively fluent speech may be expected.

The attitude of calm recommended for the early stutterer's home should also prevail in the classroom. This applies to all children and, of course, to the teacher. A teacher, who shows ready anger, ridicules a child for an error, or permits children to ridicule one another, creates an attitude of apprehension. On the other hand, the teacher who accepts error as a normal way of life and indicates that it is better to try even though a mistake may be made sets a tone that most children will accept with pleasure. If any child responds to a mistake with ridicule, the child should be corrected in a private session.

The teacher should be generous with praise for any special abilities shown by the early stutterer. If no special abilities are apparent, praise those abilities that are the child's chief assets.

If the child has been teased because of his/her speech, or dubbed a stutterer by the classmates, the teacher should assure him/her that the classmates are mistaken. The early stutterer should be told that everyone has the same kind of speech trouble at some time just as all children stumble occasionally when they walk or run. It might help considerably if the teacher, in a not too evident way, does some intentional hesitating or repeating. Beyond this, the teacher should explain to the class that teasing and name calling are not permitted and that some privilege will be denied to any offending member of the class.

Perhaps the teacher's role can best be summed up in a single directive. Be accepting, permissive, and kind; do only those things to and for the early stutterer, or any other child in your class, that you would want another teacher to do to and for your own child—or for any child you may love. Beyond this, special language instruction is in order if it is evident that the child has difficulty with learning how to combine words into acceptable constructions (syntax).

OBJECTIVES FOR THE CONFIRMED STUTTERER

Confirmed stutterers, as noted previously, are aware that their speech is atypical and react to themselves and to their environment in terms of their awareness and evaluation of their speech. Therapeutic objectives, therefore, include a modification of the speech pattern as well as a modification of the attitudes that the stutterers have developed toward themselves, their speech, and their environment. How much can be done depends upon the professional resources that are available to the stutterers and their readiness for making use of the resources. In some instances, little more than superficial treatment of speech symptoms can be attempted. Unfortunately, this is not enough for many confirmed stutterers, especially for those who have evident personality maladjustments associated with their stuttering. In some settings, psychotherapy as well as speech therapy is available, and more than speech modification can be attempted in a treatment program. When the family of a confirmed stutterer has no financial problem, private help can be sought outside of the school.

Where the confirmed stutterer shows no evidence of significant maladaptive behavior of attitudes requiring modifications, treatment may be limited to the speech symptoms. The assessment of what is needed should be made by a psychologist, speech pathologist, or other professional worker trained in personality evaluation. The clinician should undertake the assessment of the patient with an objective attitude without assuming either (1) that every stutterer, by virtue of his/her stuttering, necessarily has a personality disorder; or (2) that stutterers need treatment only for their speech symptoms to become wholly normal persons.

One basic understanding must be established with the confirmed stutterer if treatment, either for stuttering symptoms or for behavioral maladjustments, is to be successful. The stutterer, at the outset, must accept himself/herself as a person who stutters and is in need of treatment. The stutterer must not try to conceal stuttering or fight against the notion that he/she is a stutterer. When control over stuttering symptoms is established, and attitudes and behavior are modified, the once confirmed stutterer can then discard this label along with the speech characteristics, attitude, and associated traits.

Another area of understanding that stutterer and clinician must establish is one of possible gains or values that may have grown out of stuttering. The stutterer must be helped to ask, and to answer honestly and objectively, the question, "Am I getting anything out of my stuttering that I don't want to give up?" If the stutterer realizes that his/her speech may serve as an excuse from social situations that may not be enjoyable, from running errands when there are other things to do more to his/her liking, or from preparing for daily recitations because he or she is not called on in school, then he/she will be in a position to weigh the advantages as well as the disadvantages of the speech defect and be prepared for further therapy. When the stutterer ceases to entertain and never uses stuttering as a ready-made alibi for what he or she might do, or might have been, except for the speech difficulty, then he/she has traveled a long way toward achieving the objectives of therapy.

Treatment for the Family

Often the parents of the stutterer are in need of counseling if the stutterer is to obtain maximum help from therapy. In some instances, the attitudes of the stutterer's parents are characterized by high aspiration, rigidity, and unconscious rejection of the child. If the study of the familial picture shows this to be the case for the individual stutterer, appropriate treatment should be undertaken. Our experience indicates that parental resistance to treatment must be anticipated. Often parents want and expect their children to improve without their active participation in a therapy program. Parents must be made to realize that their participation is essential. The aims of therapy for parents are to give them an understanding about the problem of stuttering in general, their child's stuttering in particular, and the relationship of their evaluations and attitudes toward their child's speech, and to reduce their own anxieties and possible guilt feelings about their child's speech difficulty. Parents must be helped to appreciate that stuttering does not disappear all at once. Frequently, in fact, speech becomes apparently worse rather than better in the early stages of treatment.

Speech Goals

Stutterers as well as their parents must accept the virtual certainty that stuttering will not stop with the beginning of therapy. The immediate objective for stutterers is to encourage them to speak more rather than less despite their stuttering. While speaking more, stutterers need to be helped to take an objective view of their difficulty so that the following intermediate objectives may be attained:

1. A weakening of the forces and pressures with which the individual stuttering is associated.
2. Elimination of the secondary, accessory symptoms of stuttering.
3. Modification of the form of stuttering so that relatively easy, effortless disfluencies replace the specific blocks, marked hestitations, strained prolongations, or repetitions.
4. Modification of the faulty habits directly associated with speaking such as improper breathing, rapid speaking, or excessive tensions of the speech mechanism.
5. Modification of the attitudes of fear, anxiety, or avoidance associated with the need for speaking or that occur after speech is initiated.

THERAPEUTIC APPROACHES FOR SYMPTOM MODIFICATION AND CONTROL: THE ROLE OF THE SPEECH CLINICIAN

Some of the objectives of an overall therapeutic program for stutterers, regardless of the possible etiology for the individual stutterer's difficulty, should include modification with an ultimate hope of elimination of the major speech symptoms manifested by the stutterer. Although the rationale for the use of the specific approach may vary considerably with the theorist or the clinician, a number of approaches are widely used with a considerable degree of success. We review those we have used and that have wide application.

Negative Practice. We have previously referred to the principle of negative practice, an approach in which an individual learns to control a habit he or she would like to discard by practicing intentionally and purposefully that very habit. For a stutterer this would mean that the clinician will direct him/her to become aware of the particular manner of stuttering and to practice one or more of the features of the manner. Thus, a stutterer will practice blocks by imitating his or her own particular way of blocking. When he or she learns this technique of self-imitation, modification of the blocks may be achieved through one or the other approaches we discuss. Through the technique of negative practice the stutterer is helped to undo by consciously doing what he or she presumably prefers not to do. This approach may be employed to overcome facial or bodily tics, faulty breathing, or any other mannerism that characterizes the speech behavior of the individual stutterer.

Voluntary Stuttering. This approach in effect helps stutterers to learn a new, easier way of stuttering so that they can get on with the business of saying what they have to say with a minimum of blocking or spasm. One technique is to direct the stutterer *voluntarily to repeat* the first sound or the first syllable of each word. At first the stutterer may repeat the sound or syllable two or three times, or as many times as necessary to complete the rest of the word. The repetitions should be easy and "nonsticky." Stutterers usually find it easier to engage in voluntary repetition in material read aloud while observing themselves in a mirror. With practice, the number of repetitions are reduced to the minimum needed to enable him/her to feel prepared to move along and to finish the utterance. Finally, the stutterer reduces the repetitions to the sounds of the words on which a block is anticipated. We usually proceed with the stutterer from reading to paraphrasing and then to a conversation that incorporates the words that carried the key ideas in material previously read. Ultimately, the technique of voluntary repetition is applied in free conversation. This technique is particularly useful in group sessions in which stutterers observe how successful the members of their group are in their efforts at voluntary, easy repetition. A good repetition (easy and "nonsticky") is given a positive value; and involuntary repetition earns a minus score.

Prolongation. Prolongation or the intentional *lengthening* of initial sounds that are capable of being lengthened (vowels, diphthongs and continuant consonants) is another approach to voluntary stuttering. The lengthened sound must be produced in an easy, relaxed manner. The stutterer must use the lengthened sound production as a preparatory set to move into the next sound and so to complete the utterance. The modifications from reading to free speaking may follow the sequence suggested for voluntary repetition.

Easy Articulation. Though clarity of diction may suffer somewhat, many stutterers find it helpful to learn a relatively lax, "nonsticky" manner of articulation. This is especially helpful in the production of stop sounds. With reduced articulatory tension, it may become possible for some stutterers to move from sound to sound and word to word without abrupt pauses that suggest mild spasms.

Articulatory Pantomiming. Some stutterers need to be convinced that there are no real difficult sounds but only "bogey sounds" that the individual has somehow come to believe are difficult for him. For such stutterers, initial pantomiming of words or phrases—going through the articulatory activity without uttering the words aloud—may be of considerable help. After pantomiming, the stutterer is directed to add voice and to speak (read or engage in free conversation) what had previously been pantomimed. In the second phase, ease of articulation and moving through the utterance are stressed.

Fake Stuttering. A useful group technique is to have a stutterer imitate a speech feature of another stutterer. Many can do this with considerable success. For those who can, a feeling of control is achieved. Such control may then be used to imitate speech free or relatively free of stuttering mannerisms.

Imposed Rhythm and Timing. Speaking to an imposed rhythm has long been known to facilitate speech flow in stutterers. However, there is no encouraging evidence that normal fluency is maintained with the benefit of rhythmic pattern that is not consonant or relevant to the contents of the utterance.[6] A modification of imposed rhythm is syllable timed speech.

In syllable timed (ST) speech, the subject (stutterer) is taught first to speak each syllable of an utterance to the accompaniment of a metronome. When the subject is able to speak (syllabicate) without stuttering, he/she is encouraged to speak *as if* to a metronome in comunicative situations. At this stage speech is slow, monotonous, and far from normal. In later stage of ST therapy, the stutterer is encouraged to speed up the rate, add syllable stress, and phrase pauses more in the manner of normal speech flow.

Ingham (1975, pp. 354–379) describes a program of syllable timed speech employing operant procedures in a population of 16 adults. Ingham reports improvement with nine of the 16 nine months after the end of the treatment program. However, Ingham has considerable reservation about the long-term implications of ST therapy, and just what aspect of the program brought about the demonstrated improvement.

Delayed Auditory Feedback (DAF)

Nonstutterers can be made to stutter by having them listen to themselves after an imposed delay in auditory feedback. Interestingly, a delay in auditory feedback improves the fluency of stuttering when the delay is about one quarter of a second and speech rate is slowed to about 30 words per minute.

At the present time, we consider DAF an experimental laboratory approach and not one we recommend for use with school-age children. Reviews of DAF experiments may be found in Van Riper (1971, pp. 382–403) and Sheehan (1970, pp. 216–217).

Operant Conditioning and Behavior Modification

An approach that has come into increasing use by clinicians working with confirmed stutterers is operant conditioning. Stuttering is viewed as behavior that is subject to modification (conditioning or recondi-

---

[6] Evidence and arguments for and against imposed rhythm are reviewed by R. J. Ingham in *Stuttering: A Second Symposium*, J. Eisenson, ed. (New York: Harper & Row Publishers, Inc., 1975), pp. 346–347.

toining). The underlying principle of operant conditioning is stated succinctly by Shames and Egolf (1976, p. 3).

"Specifically, it refers to a process of reinforcement whereby the frequency of a particular class of behaviors can be increased or decreased or maintained at a designated level by presenting or withdrawing certain stimuli immediately after a designated response has been emitted."

The use of operant procedures may be applied directly to the speech behavior of stutterers or to an aspect of behavior associated with stuttering. Wolpe (1969 (a) and 1969 (b)) assumes that when dealing with stuttering of long duration, regardless of the causes for the onset of stuttering, the stutterer eventually develops a neurotic anxiety about his speech. This anxiety maintains stuttering, and thus must be treated. Specific techniques for the modification of anxiety include encouraging the patients to talk about their feelings, and so reduce their strength. Relaxation based on Jacobson's *Progressive Relaxation* is taught to stutterers and they are "trained" to assume the posture and recognize the feelings of relaxation. When one shows evidence of tension associated with anxiety, the stutterer is trained to relax voluntarily, so that relaxation replaces the tension state. In effect, the awareness of tension cues a state of relaxation. The stutterer is asked to list anxiety-producing (stuttering-producing) situations in order of severity (hierarchies). Each state is then a subject of therapy.

> When relaxation has become adequate and when the hierarchies are ready, one begins the central procedure, which is to present the weakest scene from a hierarchy to the *imagination* of the deeply relaxed patient for a few seconds, repeating presentations until the imagined item no longer evokes any anxiety at all. At each presentation the weak anxiety evoked by the scene is to some extent inhibited by the relaxation so that at the next presentation its evocation is weaker still, until it is eventually zero. The therapist then proceeds to the next scene, and so on, until the whole anxiety has been dealt with (Wolpe, 1969(a), p. 19).

Wolpe observes that almost always there is complete transfer of the anxiety from the imagined situation to the corresponding real-life situation as reported by the patient.

A variety of behavior therapy techniques are based on these general approaches. Several of these techniques are presented in the monograph by Gray and England (1969). Another behavior therapy approach, more elaborate than the one that we have described, is presented in detail by Brutten and Shoemaker (1967) and by Shames and Egolf (1976). Most behavior therapists report good success in the modification of stuttering symptoms after relatively few sessions as compared with other approaches. Perhaps the success is related to the readiness of the stutterers to do whatever they need to do to put an end to or at least to reduce the overt symptoms of stuttering. Behavior modification approaches require considerable training for the clinician. We recommend that they not be undertaken without such training.

ULTIMATE OBJECTIVES FOR THE STUTTERER

We should like to be able to recommend that a legitimate, ultimate objective for every confirmed stutterer is the establishment of normal speech and a well-adjusted personality. Such a recommended objective, however, cannot be made in the light of our experience with many stutterers. Perhaps a more reasonable and more moderate objective may be speech that is relatively free of the more severe characteristics of stuttering, and a relatively normal adjustment. We should not expect stutterers, not even ones who are having psychotherapy, to become better adjusted than most of their peers because most of their peers have some traits that can stand improvement.

Many stutterers are able to free themselves of their significant aberrant speech symptoms. Some, however, continue to have excessive disfluencies under conditions of fatigue, ill health, or stress. For some, also, it is possible that disfluencies are likely to persist on a constitutional basis. For these, the acceptance of disfluency without accompanying apprehension and struggle behavior may be all that can be achieved. If this attitude can be established, the characteristics of stuttering that generate from anxiety and apprehension are removed and the overall occurrence of abnormal disfluencies is, therefore, reduced.

THE ROLE OF THE CLASSROOM TEACHER

The task of helping the confirmed stutterers toward better speech and the improvement of their associated adjustment problems are, as we have indicated, primarily for the speech clinician and not for the classroom teacher. There are, however, a number of ways the classroom teacher can be of appreciable help to the stutterer in his improvement program.

The teacher should make note of the class situations that appear to be conducive to stuttering. Unless the child volunteers, he/she should not be called upon to speak in these situations. If he/she does speak, the stutterer should not be stopped regardless of the severity of difficulty. If at all possible, however, the stutterer should be called upon for short replies rather than for ones that require lengthy communications.

If many children are to be called on during a recitation period, the teacher should call upon the stutterer early. Waiting induces anxiety and anxiety induces an increase in stuttering. The stutterer should know that participation is expected, but that he/she will not have an indefinite period of anxious waiting for the moment of active participation.

The teacher should also note the conditions or situations when the stutterer is likely to have least difficulty with speaking and invite active participation when these situations are present. For example, if a stutterer can recite memorized poetry without difficulty, he/she should be given an opportunity to recite. If the child can read aloud much better than recite impromptu, he/she should be called upon to read aloud.

The teacher can get considerable information from the stutterer as to both easy and difficult speech situations. In most instances, an understanding can be reached with the stutterer as to participation in class recitations. We recommend a basic principle to be followed in regard to oral recitations: If the stutterer is exempt from any oral activity, he or she must compensate by some other form of activity. This may call for additional written work done at home, or for board work done in class. Exemption without compensation gives stuttering a positive value that may be difficult to surrender. The teacher should not become a partner to the creation of gains to be derived from stuttering; neither, of course, should the teacher become part of any classroom attitude that inflicts punishment on the stutterer because of the stuttering.

The teacher should try to reward the stutterer for fluent speech, but to do so without readily apparent fuss. "Very good, Johnny" is much better than a lengthy response of praise because Johnny has been fluent. If the teacher looks pleased, Johnny is likely to get the idea even without a verbalization of the pleasure. There is a very real danger that a remark intended as a verbal reward may actually backfire and become an implied penalty. For example, "You spoke very well, Johnny" may be interpreted to mean that in most instances Johnny does not speak well, hence the need to point out the occasions when speech is good. As a general procedure, the teacher should try to avoid directing attention to good speech as well as to poor speech. The nature and form of the reward should depend upon the intellectual and emotional maturity of the child. Rewards should be given for good speech as for any other worthwhile performance. They should come quickly and inconspicuously.

The teacher should help to create a classroom atmosphere that will encourage the stutterer to talk. Such an atmosphere exists when any child, whether he/she stutters, has no defect in speech, or has some form of defective speech other than stuttering, feels free to volunteer to speak without fear of penalty or criticism. It may help to explain to the stutterer's classmates, *at a time when the stutterer is out of the classroom,* how they can be of help. Nothing said to the classmates should suggest that the stutterer is in need of pity or excessive sympathy. Instead, the teacher should emphasize that what the stutterer needs is a group of patient listeners when he or she talks and be given opportunities to talk. If the stutterer is excused from any recitations, the classmates should be informed that the child is doing other work to make up for it. In this way the classmates will not feel resentful that the stutterer is a privileged member of the group. Rather they will feel that the stutterer is a member of their group who has a problem that all are helping to solve by their understanding.

Luper and Mulder (1964, chap. 8) sum up approaches for the treatment of the stuttering child in a school setting, with special emphasis on the interrelated roles of the speech clinician and the classroom teacher. Johnson (1967, pp. 297–307) describes the special concerns of the classroom teacher related to the stutterer's adjustments in school.

Cluttering

Cluttering is usually included among disorders of rhythm and fluency. By some authorities (Weiss 1964), it is considered a forerunner of stuttering. Yet were cluttering to be designated as an articulatory disorder, or as a language disorder, it would be so based upon verifiable observation. A description of cluttering should indicate why all of these designations might well be correct and why, therefore, it deserves its own classification. We are discussing cluttering at this point in our considerations because of its superficial resemblance to stuttering, from which, nevertheless, it needs to be differentially identified.

Superficially, cluttered speech suggests a torrent of words, poorly or partially articulated, with repetitions of monosyllabic words and first syllables of longer words. It is a "hot potato in the mouth" speech, with morphemes falling where they may. Cluttered speech spurts rather than flows, then stops and spurts again. Behind the speech is the clutterer who, unlike the stutterer at any stage, seems unaware of his perpetrations. Objectively, we may characterize cluttering as repetitious, poorly articulated utterance produced at a rate incompatible with the speaker's ability to speak intelligibly. Part of the lack of intelligibility is the clutterer's loose and poorly organized phrase and sentence

Summary of Similarities and Differences Between Clutterers and Stutterers[7]

	Clutterers	*Stutterers*
Family history	May be present, especially on the male side	May be present, much more often in the males than females
Onset of speech	Often delayed	May occasionally be delayed, but not as often or as long as for clutterers
Likelihood of awareness	Usually unaware	Often aware to level of anxiety
Feeling about own speech	Indifferent	Fearful, anxious
Likely result of (a) speaking after instruction to be careful	Improves	Increase of stuttering symptoms
(b) Interruption and reminder to slow down	Improves	Worsens; anxious, tense, blocked speech
Speaking with awareness of importance of situation	Usually improves	Usually worsens
Speaking when relaxed, at ease	Worse	Improves
Reading new material aloud	Better at outset	Worse
Reading familiar material aloud	Worse	Improves

[7] This summary table is adapted from D. A. Weiss (1964, p. 69).

structure. These last features make it difficult for a listener to anticipate and so comprehend or guess what the speaker is trying to say. Weiss (1964, p. 24) believes that clutterers may well be at a loss for the words to express their thoughts. "Because the clutterer is inept at finding the necessary words to express his ideas, his speech is studded with clichés and repetitions of words and phrases." We accept this position, with emphasis on the notion that the clutterer does not really have more than a vague idea of what he/she wants to say, along with an apparent compulsion to say it.

When the clutterer slows down, both articulation and intelligibility improve. Perhaps when a clutterer speaks slowly, at a rate compatible with his/her neuromuscular system when it operates efficiently, the clutterer also gives himself time to think and to formulate the utterance.

The table on p. 377 presents similarities between clutterers and stutterers and how different situations affect their speech and language productions.

BACKGROUND HISTORY OF CLUTTERERS

Clutterers often present a history suggestive of minimal brain disfunction and minimal brain damage (see Chapter 16). Weiss (1964, p. 51) reports a familial history of speech disorders other than but also including cluttering, especially on the paternal side. He views it, as do we, as a *central language imbalance* (*disorder*) that includes such features as delayed language onset, retarded language development, delayed articulatory proficiency, and vocal monotony. We would add to these characteristics slow development of vocabulary and syntax. As they grow older, clutterers are likely to have reading and writing difficulties, the latter both for legibility and sentence structure. Behaviorally and motorically, the clutterer is likely to show impulsiveness, late laterality development, and ambinondexterity. The clutterer gives the impression of being a loosely assembled person, who is awkward and imprecise.

DIFFERENTIAL DIAGNOSIS: STUTTERING AND CLUTTERING

Most stutterers tend to speak better when they are relaxed and when they give minimal attention to their articulation. In contrast, clutterers tend to improve when they direct conscious attention to their utterance. Stutterers, especially in later stages, show apprehension and anxiety about their speech, and tend to have difficulties that are directly related to their apprehensions. Clutterers, as indicated, show a benign unawareness about their speech. With awareness, they tend to improve. Finally, the marked difficulties of clutterers in all language functions, written as well as spoken, distinguish them from most stutterers. Thus, though there is some evidence that stuttering has a familial, constitutional basis, the evidence of such etiology for the clutterer is clear.

CLUTTERING AS A TRANSITIONAL STAGE TO STUTTERING

Whether cluttering is a transitional stage, an early stage in the progression toward stuttering, is a moot point. It is possible that when some clutterers are directed to attend to their speech, they may develop anxieties and frustrations growing out of the awarenessses, and begin to speak like stutterers. Van Riper (1972, p. 263) observes "There are clutterers who do not stutter, stutterers who do not clutter, some stutterers who have cluttered, and some who still do." Thus, though some stutterers may begin as clutterers, most do not show the early characteristics that we have described. However, we have known families that included both stuttering and cluttering siblings and a cluttering father. We have also known individuals who shifted periodically between cluttering and stuttering.

THERAPY

The treatment for clutterers is implied in the differential diagnosis. Clutterers do tend to improve when they slow down and "mind their speech." They also tend to improve by being urged to formulate, to think through in words, before they begin to speak. Unfortunately, in conversational give-and-take we cannot ordinarily preformulate our utterances. Most of us have to learn to talk as we think. The best we can do for clutterers is to remind them to slow down, and cue them when their speech begins to accelerate, and so becomes unintelligible. These external controls must, with practice, become habitual. Clutterers must, therefore, be taught to observe their listeners for indications that they may be talking too rapidly and are failing to make themselves understood. Rewards in the form of verbal and facial approval by the teacher, the clinician, and the family members when the clutterers do mind their speech should reinforce such behavior. Practice in making short announcements before the class and in therapy sessions with the speech (language) clinician are of help. Finally, we wish to re-emphasize that the clutterer's primary problem is with language. Each clutterer needs help in verbal expression, both oral and written. Clutterers need, to begin with, to learn to make simple statements simply. They need to learn to become slow and considered speakers. Most clutterers, we believe, will enjoy such a reputation if it can be achieved.

Problems and Projects

1. Define stuttering. Distinguish between early and confirmed stuttering.
2. What is meant by normal hesitation phenomena?

3. Observe two or three speakers in a conversation. Note evidence of normal hesitation phenomena. How does this differ from stuttering?

4. What is the difference between a nonstutterer's "Well, well . . ." and a stutterer's postponement devices?

5. Briefly describe Bloodstein's phases of stuttering and Van Riper's tracks of stuttering. How are they the same? How are they different?

6. Talk to two or three stutterers about their feared word or speaking situations. Are there any common factors? Do they resemble yours?

7. Outline your own theory about the onset of stuttering.

8. Read J. Sheehan's essay on stuttering in J. Eisenson, ed., *Stuttering: A Second Symposium*. Why does Sheehan regard stuttering as a learned form of behavior? What does Sheehan mean by his observation that stuttering is essentially an expression of an approach-avoidance conflict?

9. What is the evidence to support the position that stuttering is a manifestation of constitutional predisposition?

10. What is the evidence that the predisposition to stuttering may be inherited? What is a predisposition?

11. Read W. Johnson's position on stuttering in *Speech-Handicapped School Children*. How does Johnson explain the evidence of the heredity of stuttering on a nongenetic basis? Do you agree?

12. Which of the positions on stuttering presented in this text best reconciles the therapeutic approaches with the onset causes?

13. Suppose a four or five-year-old child is sent to you by a parent with the complaint that the youngster is a stutterer. How would you go about determining whether the child has "normal disfluencies" or is *normally expressing* normal hesitations and repetitions? What would you tell the parent?

14. Why do most stutterers have less difficulty in reciting memorized material than in explaining or paraphrasing it?

15. What is meant by "secondary gains?" What are some possible secondary gains, other than those mentioned in this chapter, that stutterers may entertain? How would you deal with them?

16. What is conditioning? What is deconditioning? How do they relate to therapy for stutterers?

17. What is meant by "desensitization" for stutterers? Can you give any examples of how you or a friend were desensitized against an anxiety or fear-producing situation?

18. Why should the treatment of an early stage stutterer be directed toward the parent? Outline such treatment.

19. What is meant by "negative practice?" How does this relate to stuttering therapy?

20. Distinguish between cluttering and stuttering.

21. How is the treatment of a young clutterer different from that of a primary stutterer? Of an adult clutterer and a confirmed stutterer?

22. Check the literature on delayed auditory feedback (DAF). How are the effects of DAF in most stutterers different from what they are for most nonstutterers? How is DAF used in therapy?

References and Suggested Readings

Andrews, S. G., and M. Harris, "Stammering," in *The Child Who Does Not Talk*, C. Renfrew, and K. Murphy, eds., The Spastics Society Medical Education Association, London: W. Heinemann Medical Books, 1964.

Berry, M. F., "Twinning in Stuttering Families," *Human Biology*, **9**, 3 (1939), 329–346.

Bloodstein, O., in J. Eisenson, ed., "Stuttering as Tension and Fragmentation," in *Stuttering: A Second Symposium*, New York: Harper & Row, Publishers, Inc., 1975, pp. 1–95.

Bluemel, C. S., *The Riddle of Stuttering*, Danville, Ill.: Interstate Publishing Company, 1957. (A psychiatrist's exposition about the nature of stuttering as an underlying language disorder.)

Brown, S. F., "The Loci of Stuttering in the Speech Sequence," *Journal of Speech Disorders*, **10** (May 1945), 181–192.

Brutten G. J., and D. J. Shoemaker, *The Modification of Stuttering*, Englewood Cliffs, N.J.: Prentice-Hall, Inc., 1967.

Brutten, E. J., in J. Eisenson, ed., "Stuttering: Topography Assessment and Behavior Changing Strategies," in *Stuttering: A Second Symposium*, New York: Harper & Row, Publishers, Inc., 1975, pp. 199–262.

Coriat, I. H., "The Psychoanalytic Concept of Stammering," *The Nervous Child*, **2** (1943), 167–171.

Curry, F. K. W., and H. H. Gregory, "The Performance of Stutterers on Dichotic Listening Tasks Thought to Reflect Cerebral Dominance," *Journal of Speech and Hearing Research*, **12** (March 1969), 73–82.

Eisenson, J. ed., *Stuttering: A Second Symposium*, New York: Harper & Row Publishers, Inc., 1975. (Six points of view are presented on the nature of stuttering with suggested therapies for stuttering consistent with the theoretic position. Van Riper provides a separate essay on "The Stutterer's clinician." The contributors are O. Bloodstein, G. J. Brutten, J. Eisenson, R. J. Ingham, G. H. Shames, E. J. Brutten, and C. Van Riper.

——, in J. Eisenson, ed., "Stuttering as Perseverative Behavior," in *Stuttering: A Second Symposium*, New York: Harper & Row, Publishers, Inc., 1975.

——, "Observations of the Incidence of Stuttering in a Special Culture," *ASHA*, **8** 10 (1966), 391–394.

——, and E. Horowitz, "The Influence of Propositionality on Stuttering," *Journal of Speech Disorders*, **10** (March 1945), 193–198.

Goldman-Eisler, F., "Hesitation, Information, and Levels of Speech Production," in A. V. DeReuck, and M. O'Connor, eds., *Disorders of Language*, Ciba Foundation, 1964.

Gray, B. B., and G. England, eds., *Stuttering and the Conditioning Therapies*, Monterey, Calif.: The Monterey Institute for Speech and Hearing, 1969.

Gregory, H. H., *Learning Theory and Stuttering Therapy*, Evanston, Ill.: Northwestern University Press, 1968.

Ingham, R. J., "A Comparison of Covert and Overt Assessment Procedures in Stuttering Therapy Outcome Evaluation," *Journal of Speech and Hearing Research*, **18** (June 1975), 346-354.

Johnson, W., in W. Johnson et al., *Speech Handicapped School Children*, 3rd ed., New York: Harper & Row, Publishers, Inc., 1967.

Kimura, D., "Functional Asymmetry of the Brain in Dichotic Listening," *Cortex*, **3** (1967), 163-178.

Lanyon, R. I., "Speech: Relation of Nonfluency to Information Value," *Science*, **164** (April 3, 1969), 451-452.

Luper, H. L., and R. L. Mulder, *Stuttering Therapy for Children*, Englewood Cliffs, N.J.: Prentice-Hall, Inc., 1964. (Addressed to public school speech clinicians and emphasizes therapeutic approaches for stuttering children that the authors have found to be practical, operational, and effective.)

McDearmon, J. R., "Primary Stuttering at the Onset of Stuttering: A Re-examination of Data," *Journal of Speech and Hearing Research*, **11** (September 1968), 631-637.

Murphy, A. T., and R. M. FitzSimons, *Stuttering and Personality Dynamics*, New York: The Ronald Press Company, 1960.

Nelson, W. E., "The Role of Heredity in Stuttering," *Journal of Pediatrics*, **14** (1939), 642-654.

Orton, S., *Reading, Writing and Speech Problems*, New York: W. W. Norton & Company, Inc., 1937. (A pioneer but still highly relevant consideration of organic factors underlying language disorders.)

Perrin, K., *An Examination of Ear Preference for Speech and Non-Speech in a Stuttering Population*, Ph.D. dissertation, Stanford University, 1969.

Shames, G. H., and D. B. Egolf, *Operant Conditioning and the Management of Stuttering*, Englewood Cliffs, N.J.: Prentice-Hall, Inc., 1976. (Intended for clinicians; describes how operant procedures can be used in the treatment of stutterers, including young ones.)

————, and C. E. Sherrick, "A Discussion of Non-Fluency and Stuttering as Operant Behavior," *Journal of Speech and Hearing Disorders*, **28** (February 1963), 3-18.

Sheehan, J. G., *Stuttering: Research and Therapy*, New York: Harper & Row, Publishers, Inc., 1970.

————, "Conflict Theory and Avoidance-Reduction Therapy," in J. Eisenson, ed., *Stuttering: A Second Symposium*, New York: Harper & Row, Publishers, Inc., 1975.

Slorach, N., and B. Noehr, "Dichotic Listening in Stuttering and Dyslalic Children," *Cortex*, **9** (1973), 295-300.

Sommers, R. K., W. A. Brady, and W. H. Moore, "Dichotic Ear Preferences of Stuttering Children and Adults," *Perceptual and Motor Skills*, **41** (1975), 931-938.

Travis, L. E., "The Unspeakable Feelings of People with Special Reference to Stuttering," in L. E. Travis, ed., *Handbook of Speech Pathology and Audiology*, New York: Appleton-Century-Crofts, 1971, pp. 1009-1033.

Van Riper, C., *The Nature of Stuttering*, Englewood Cliffs, N.J.: Prentice-Hall, Inc., 1971. (A major contribution in the area of stuttering. Van Riper reviews the litterature on stuttering to provide a comprehensive view of the disorder. A monumental work!)

————, *Speech Correction*, 5th ed., Englewood Cliffs, N.J.: Prentice-Hall, Inc., 1972. (Chapter 7 presents Van Riper's revised and practical considerations of the nature and treatment of stuttering. The treatment is both objective and sympathetic, strongly recommended for teachers and clinicians.)

————, and J. V. Irwin, *Voice and Articulation*, Englewood Cliffs, N.J.: Prentice-Hall, Inc., 1958, chaps. 7–13.

Weiss, D. A., "Therapy for Cluttering," *Folia Phoniatrica*, **12** (1960), 216–228.

————, *Cluttering*, Englewood Cliffs, N.J.: Prentice-Hall, Inc., 1964.

Wingate, M. E., "Evaluation and Stuttering, Part I: Speech Characteristics for Young Children," *Journal of Speech and Hearing Disorders*, **26** (May 1962) 106–115.

Wolpe, J., "Behavior Therapy of Stuttering: Deconditioning the Emotional Factor," in B. G. Gray, and G. England, *Stuttering and the Conditioning Therapies*, Monterey, Calif.: The Monterey Institute for Speech and Hearing, 1969 (a).

————, *The Practice of Behavior Therapy*, New York: Pergamon Press 1969(b).

Wyatt, G., *Language Learning and Communication Disorders in Children*, New York: The Free Press, 1969.

14. Speech and Impaired Hearing

It is a rare teacher who has not had some experience with a hearing-impaired child. Most observant teachers have probably dealt with a Tommy or a Mary who earnestly look as if they are listening, and may in fact be listening "hard," yet fail to understand even a simple direction unless it is accompanied by a gesture or some visual cueing. A child may return to school after a brief absence with the residuals of a cold, ears still "stopped up," and have difficulty understanding the teacher unless in direct view. Occasionally, the difficulty continues after the cold has completely cleared. If there is evidence of chronic difficulty in comprehension unless the teacher is talking from the front of the room, there is a fair likelihood that Tommy or Mary may have a slight hearing loss that becomes worse with a cold and the aftereffects of even a slight cold.

The alert and observant teacher should recommend that the child be seen by a school nurse or school physician, if either is available, and confer with the child's family about an examination of the child's hearing by their own physician or by an otolaryngologist or an otologist, medical specialists who are concerned with problems of hearing.

Any teacher who has taught 100 or more different children is likely to have at least one with some degree of impaired hearing. In some instances the child's articulation was also defective, and perhaps so was the extent of the child's vocabulary and competence for producing conventional syntactical sentences. Generally, the degree of the hearing impairment will be related to the presence and severity of the speech problems. A child may produce a voice that is either lacking in adequate loudness or, less frequently, overloud. Conductive losses, which are discussed later, are associated with inadequate loudness. In contrast, a nerve (sensorineural) loss is associated with an overloud voice.[1] We expand later on the types of speech problems associated with impaired hearing. First, however, we consider briefly some aspects of sound and the reception and perception of speech sound by the hearing mechanism.

Sound and the Speech Range

Sound for our purposes may be considered the result of energy applied to a body capable of vibration in a manner that produces waves (disturbances of air) at a rate and in a manner that makes them perceptible to the human ear. Normal, young persons can hear sounds between 20 to 20,000 Hz (cycles per second or cps).[2] Older persons, above age 30 or 40, tend to lose hearing in the upper ranges, above 8,000 or 10,000 Hz. However, since most of the sounds of speech lie within the range 250–4,000 Hz, adults of "middle age" suffer no impairment of hearing for speech.

The decibel or dB is the unit of intensity of sound. Very simply stated, intensity varies directly as the amount of energy applied to the body capable of vibration. However, sounds of different pitch are discernible to us at a different intensity levels. This, we believe, is related to the differences in the sensitivity of the endings of the auditory nerve in the cochlea of the inner ear. Thus, we may hear sounds within one part of our pitch range at a relatively low intensity, as compared with sounds within a different part of the pitch range that may be perceived (heard) only at higher intensity levels.

The Hearing Mechanism

THE EXTERNAL AND MIDDLE EAR

The external ear, or pinna, is part of the auditory mechanism that most of us refer to as the ear. Its function which is, to a limited degree, to

---

[1] The relationship of voice disturbances to hearing was briefly considered in Chapter 12 on voice disturbances.

[2] The letters cps for cycles per second are now represented by Hz or "Hertz."

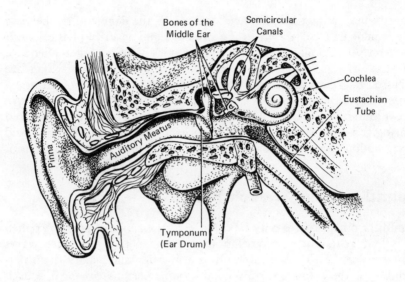

Figure 13. A sectional view of the ear.

help us to gather in sound, may be enhanced by using a hand to cup over the ear. The pinna includes a skin-lined canal leading to the eardrum or tympanic membrane (see Figure 13).

The middle ear is a small cavity on the inner side of the eardrum.

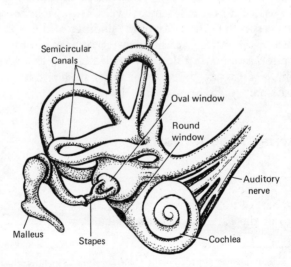

Figure 14. Enlarged representation of the middle and inner ear: the ossicles, cochlea, and semicircular canals.

The middle ear includes three tiny bones, or ossicles: the malleus (hammer), the incus (anvil), and the stapes (stirrup). The named designations correspond to their resemblance to the objects (see Figure 14). The malleus is directly attached to the eardrum. The incus constitutes a connection or bridge between the malleus and the stapes. These ossicles are connected but normally *not rigidly fixed* to positions within the middle ear by attachments of ligament and tiny muscles. Thus, the ossicles are able to move whenever the eardrum moves, as it does whenever it is stimulated by sound waves (air vibrations). The movements of the ossicles transmit the vibrations of the eardrum from the middle ear to the inner ear.

THE INNER EAR

The inner ear includes (a) the semicircular canals, (b) the cochlea, a snail-shaped structure that contains tiny hairlike structures of varying length, which are in fact the sensitive endings of the auditory nerve, and (c) the vestibule, a connecting area between the semicircular canals and the cochlea.

When air vibrations cause movements of the eardrum, the impulses are transmitted to the stapes, which in turn produces movements of the fluid that fills the vestibule. These vestibular-fluid movements stimulate the nerve endings in the cochlea. The stimulations received from the auditory nerve endings are carried by way of the auditory (eighth cranial nerve) to the temporal area of the brain cortex, producing the experience we refer to as sound perception or hearing.[3]

Hearing Impairment

CLASSIFICATION AND INCIDENCE

Although "functional" definitions of hearing loss are presented in this section, it is essential to appreciate that the effect of hearing loss is variable. In some instances, what may be regarded as a relatively small amount of hearing loss may be associated with greater impairment of hearing in particular and adjustment in general than a measurably greater amount of hearing loss for other persons. Even among persons born with severe hearing loss, some are able to make considerably better

---

[3] See the discussion of the speech mechanism in Chapter 5 for the function of the left temporal cortex in the analysis of speech sounds.

use of a small amount of residual hearing than others. With these reservations in mind, "practical" definitions are offered.

The *deaf* are those for whom the sense of hearing is so impaired as to have precluded normal acquisition of language learning. Somewhat more broadly, the deaf are those for whom the capacity to hear is so limited as to be considered nonfunctioning for the ordinary purposes of life. Children who are deaf either (1) are not able to learn speech through the avenue of hearing or (2), if their hearing impairment was acquired shortly after "natural" speech was learned, have lost their speaking ability or have become severely impaired in it.

The deaf may be divided into two subgroups according to onset of impairment. The *congenitally deaf* are those who are born without hearing. The *adventitiously deaf* are those who were born with hearing sufficient for the acquisition of speech but later, as a result of illness or accident, suffered severe hearing impairment.

The *hard of hearing* are those for whom the sense of hearing, although defective, is functional with or without a hearing aid. Hard-of-hearing children, although frequently with considerable defects, learn to speak essentially through the avenue of hearing.

Northern and Downs (1974, p. 32) classify hearing loss into four groups that are associated with common descriptive terms as follows:

> 15 to 30 dB—mild loss
> 31 to 50 dB—moderate loss
> 51 to 80 dB—severe loss
> 81 to 100 dB—profound loss

Northern and Downs (1974, p. 32) observe that the effects of hearing loss vary considerably according to whether it is unilateral or bilateral. "The child with a totally dead ear on one side but with a normal ear on the other side may function quite well in most situations. . . . This youngster's auditory abilities will be lacking in circumstances where sound localization is needed or in instances when noise exists to compete with the signal of interest."

The practical and fundamental criterion for the distinction between the deaf and the hard-of-hearing is *in the manner in which* the child acquires speech. The deaf then include those who require specialized instruction to learn to talk, or to acquire a substitute (visual) system for the normal oral/aural system. The hard-of-hearing are those who learned to speak essentially in the normal developmental manner of hearing children.

Many deaf children are educated in special schools or in special classes, and some in residential schools. Most hard-of-hearing children are educated in "regular" schools and usually attend classes with hearing children.

Incidence

It is difficult to arrive at "hard" figures for the incidence of hearing loss even in the school-age population on whom figures are relatively easy to gather. Silverman (1971, pp. 402–403) notes that on the basis of mass-testing surveys among schoolchildren, reported percentages of findings of hearing loss range from 2 to 21 per cent. "This great variability in reports of hearing impairment is undoubtedly due to differences in definitions of hearing impairments, in techniques, apparatus and conditions of testing, and in the socioeconomic status and climate of the communities in which the surveys were carried out." Silverman accepts that about 5 per cent of school-age children have hearing levels at least in one ear that is outside of the normal range.

The 1969 report of the Subcommittee on Human Communication and Its Disorders to the National Institute of Neurological Diseases and Stroke (1969, p. 15) includes an estimate of hearing loss in the United States. According to the report, about 250,000 children of school age have hearing losses of sufficient severity to impair their communication ability and their social efficiency. Approximately 40,000 children are deaf.

TYPES OF HEARING LOSS AND RELATED SPEECH IMPAIRMENTS

CONDUCTIVE LOSS

Conductive loss is associated with external or middle ear abnormalities that impede the transmission of energy (vibratory energy producing sound) to the middle ear. Abnormalities may include an accumulation of hardened wax (cerumen), the presence of a foreign body, and structural malformations, such as an incomplete canal or an exceedingly narrow ear canal. The external ear may be inflamed by disease processes that may affect other skin surfaces. Except for the structural abnormalities, the resultant hearing loss is likely to be temporary, that is, lasting only as long as the abnormal condition persists.

Middle-ear involvements include conditions that impair the vibratory-transmissive functions of the ossicles, infections of the middle ear, which are often associated with upper respiratory disease (the common cold), or excessive fluid, often associated with inflammation in the middle ear, and enlarged adenoidal tissue growth in the area of the nasopharynx.

Because conductive losses are usually the result of temporary pathologies, most children with such impairments are likely to have normal speech. Chronic involvements may be associated with an inadequately loud voice. This, as suggested earlier, may be the result of the child's hearing his own voice louder than he is able to hear the voices of other speakers. He assumes, therefore, that he is speaking loudly enough to be heard, even though he may be barely audible to others. This interesting phenomenon takes place because the child with conductive loss hears himself through the vibrations produced by his vocalization by way of the bones of his head. If his inner ear is normal, the nerve endings will respond to these vibrations. However, the child's hearing of himself is not modified by the vibrations that normally would also come to him through air vibration by way of his external and middle ears. The child with conductive loss also hears the voices of others as less loud than they sound to normal ears.

Denasality is also likely to characterize the voice and the nasal consonant sound production of the child with respiratory infections or with enlarged adenoids. Speech, as far as articulation in general is concerned, is likely to be unaffected in children with mild conductive loss of hearing. Chronic conductive hearing impairment, if more than of mild degree, is likely to be associated with distortion and omissions of speech sounds.

Sensorineural Hearing Loss

Sensorineural hearing loss results from involvements of the inner ear or those of the eighth (auditory) nerve. Reception and perception (discrimination) of sound are impaired. Such losses, especially if they are congenital or had their onset before speech was acquired, are associated with vocal, articulatory, and linguistic defects. Children with severe degrees of nerve involvement may make little or no sense out of the speech to which they are exposed because they will have difficulty in the analysis of the complex sounds that constitute speech. Usually, high-pitched sounds, including those that comprise most of the consonants of speech, are within the range of impaired hearing. Voiced and vowel sounds, if produced with sufficient loudness, are usually heard and perceived. Some children may speak excessively loudly in order to hear themselves. They may produce vowels acceptably but have difficulty with consonants, especially the high-frequency sibilants and the velar stops, which are not readily visible. They may confuse voiced and voiceless cognate sounds. With severe impairment, children cannot readily hear functional words (prepositions, conjunctions, articles)—which normally are not given much emphasis in running speech—or grammatical markers (plurals, tense endings). Their verbal productions may also be characterized as ungrammatical or agrammatical. They will, therefore, be linguistically deficient.

Some bright children who are skilled in visual speech (lip) reading, which they may learn without direct teaching, may have good comprehension of speech and may themselves have fairly good articulation. Children who are not skilled in visual reading may have severe difficulty in comprehending speech. With the usual reservation for the exceptional child, the severity of speech and language impairment is generally related directly to the severity of the sensorineural loss. Usually the age at which the hearing loss, if progressive, became severe is another factor affecting the quality of speech. As a rule, the later the age after speech onset, the better is the overall speech quality.

Mixed Hearing Loss

Mixed hearing loss combines the impairments of conductive and nerve loss. The cause is the existence of both conductive (transmissive) and sensorineural pathology. In effect, the child with such combined pathology will have difficulty in receiving a sound signal as well as difficulty in analyzing (perceiving) those signals that—however weakly—are received. Unless the conductive condition is chronic, the speech characteristics of the child will be related to the factors associated with sensorineural loss.

Central Auditory Impairment

Some children, fortunately few in number but complex in the severity of their impairments, may be able to respond to nonspeech auditory signals as most children do, but are still unable to make sense out of speech sounds. These children hear spoken language but have severe difficulty in interpreting what they hear. We consider these children—tentatively diagnosed as aphasic—in a later chapter.

MEASUREMENT OF HEARING LOSS

Hearing loss is objectively measured in terms of decibels. From our point of view, we may consider a decibel the minimum unit of intensity necessary for us to appreciate a difference between the loudness of sounds.

The pure-tone audiometer, which is widely used as an objective instrument for measuring possible hearing loss, is an electrical instrument designed to produce a number of tones of discrete or individual frequencies at intensity levels that can be controlled. Most modern pure-tone audiometers cover the frequency range between approximately 125 and 12,000 Hz (cycles) per second. Many audiologists in their examinations, however, do not consider it necessary to go beyond 8,000 Hz. On a pure-tone audiometer the weakest sound that can normally be heard is considered as zero decibels.

Losses are measured in terms of the normal threshold of hearing for tones at specified pitch levels and are stated in decibels. The following tables suggest how we would evaluate the results of a pure-tone audiometric examination. We should always bear in mind, however, that many factors other than the "objective" amount of hearing loss enter into the effect of the loss for the given individual.

We strongly recommend Newby's (1972, p. 114) observation as to the need for assessing functional hearing as well as the results of pure-tone audiometry. Says Newby:

> Although the audiogram yields important information concerning the rehabilitative needs of patients, it is most valuable when the information it conveys is combined with the results of clinical speech audiometric tests, which measure directly a patient's ability to hear and understand speech. After all, the measure of the handicap of a hearing loss is how one's communicative ability is affected. Whereas predictions of how communication is affected can be made from the pure-tone audiogram with some certainty, actual measures of the communicative ability can be derived through speech audiometry.

IDENTIFICATION AUDIOMETRY

Identification audiometry signifies the application of appropriate hearing test procedures leading to an initial discovery of a hearing loss.[4] In the ordinary school situations, a screening test rather than a complete audiometric examination is likely to be given as the first step in the evaluation of a child's hearing. An early and still widely used screening device is the fading-numbers test. A recorded voice is played back and listened to through earphones, either by a single child or by a group of children. The usual recording is of a sequence of numbers, which fade out at the end of the sequence. The results provide information *under the conditions of testing* about the intensity levels at or above which a selected speech sample—a sequence of numbers—can be heard.

---

[4] See ASHA Committee on Audiometric Evaluation, "Guidelines for Identification Audiometry," *ASHA* (February 1975), pp. 94–99.

Table 1
Classes of Hearing Handicap

dB	Class	Degree of Handicap	Average Hearing Threshold Level for 500, 1,000 and 2,000 in the Better Ear*		Ability to Understand Speech
			More than	Not More than	
25	A	Not significant		25 dB (ISO)	No significant difficulty with faint speech
40	B	Slight handicap	25 dB (ISO)	40 dB	Difficulty only with faint speech
55	C	Mild handicap	40 dB	55 dB	Frequent difficulty with normal speech
70	D	Marked handicap	55 dB	70 dB	Frequent difficulty with loud speech
90	E	Severe handicap	70 dB	90 dB	Can understand only shouted or amplified speech
	F	Extreme handicap	90 dB		Usually cannot understand even amplified speech

* Whenever the average for the poorer ear is 25 dB or more greater than that of the better ear in this frequency range 5 dB are added to the average for the better ear. This adjusted average determines the degree and class of handicap. For example, if a person's average hearing threshold level for 500, 1000, and 2000 Hz/s is 37 dB in one ear and 62 dB or more in the other his adjusted average hearing threshold level is 42 dB and his handicap is Class C instead of Class B. (After Davis, 1965.)

Source: Lee Edward Travis, *Handbook of Speech Pathology and Audiology*, (c) 1971, p. 402. Reprinted by permission of Prentice-Hall, Inc., Englewood Cliffs, New Jersey.

Unfortunately, as Newby (1972, p. 225) points out, a fading-numbers test is not an accurate indicator of a child's ability to hear normal running speech. The test does have a merit as a rough screening device that permits relatively quick assessment of the hearing of many children. Unhappily, as the *ASHA* Guidelines point out, the fading-numbers test often passed children with hearing losses in the range above 500 Hz.

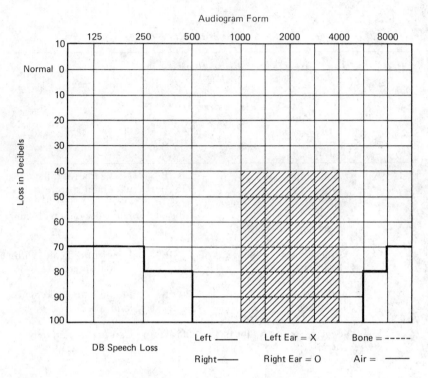

Figure 15. Audiogram Form. The shaded area indicates the hearing range most critical for the reception of speech.

Another technique that permits screening of children on a group basis is the Massachusetts Hearing Test.[5] This is a pure-tone rather than a speech-hearing test which was devised to permit screening testing of as many as 40 children at one time at three critical frequencies within the range of normal speech. The usual frequencies tested are 500, 4,000, and 6,000 Hz. Each of these frequencies is presented at sensation (loudness) levels of 20, 25, and 30 decibels, respectively. Responses are ordinarily entered on a prepared test blank and consist of a "Yes" or "No" to indicate whether the child who is being examined does or does not hear the spurt of pure-tone sound produced by the test instrument. An audiometrist signals the individual child or children when the

[5] This and other testing techniques specially suitable in the school situation are described in some detail in Chapter 8 of H. Newby's *Audiology* (New York: Appleton-Century-Crofts, 1972). See also J. Northern and M. P. Downs, *Hearing in Children* (Baltimore: The Williams & Wilkins Co., 1974), chap. 4 for an in-depth discussion of the purposes and types of identification audiometry for children beginning in early infancy.

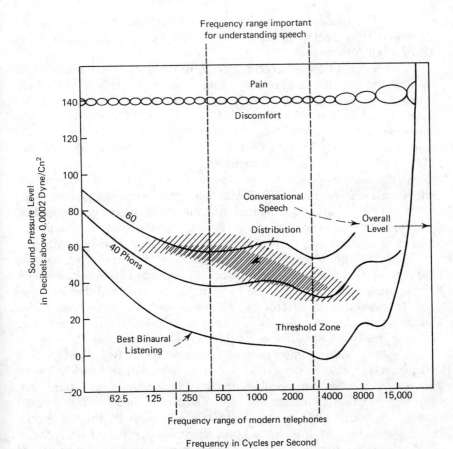

Figure 16. The Speech Area. Speech is a mixture of complex tones, wide band noise, and transients. Both the intensities and the frequencies of speech sounds change continually and rapidly. It is difficult to measure them and logically impossible to plot them precisely in terms of sound pressure levels.

response to the sound is expected. According to a prearranged plan, the audiometrist may not always present a tone and signal for a response. Through this procedure, some "No" responses are expected and such entries should appear on each test blank.

Another approach for screening employing pure-tone audiometry is the *sweep test*. This testing is done with a pure-tone audiometer, and results are obtained in a very few minutes. In sweep testing the dial is set at a critical point, with allowances made for the room and the "free-floating" noise in the surroundings. The most usual setting is 15 decibels. The examiner then "sweeps" through the frequency range. The child is instructed to signal whether or not the tone produced is heard at each frequency.

A recent addition to screening tests utilizing standard audiometric equipment (pure-tone audiometry) and headsets is described by Hollien, Wepman, and Thompson (1969). Up to 40 children at a time can be screen-tested in about 15 minutes. This test can be administered by a classroom teacher, a school nurse, or any trained adult. The frequencies employed are 500, 1,000, and 4,000 Hz; the hearing levels used are 35, 25, and 20 decibels. ASA standards are used.

As the name suggests, the purpose of screening tests is to single out individuals who may have significant losses of hearing at the time of the testing. Final evaluations should include more thorough individual pure-tone testing as well as speech testing through speech audiometry. In addition, of course, an otological examination should be routine.

In many public schools, the responsibility for discovering hearing loss among the children has become an integral part of the overall health conservation program. The development of this aspect of the detection and treatment of children's health needs has received considerable impetus from the availability of instruments and techniques for assessing hearing loss that can easily be used in school settings.

School hearing conservation programs have two fundamental purposes. The first is the earliest possible detection of hearing loss so that children, whenever possible, may be referred for medical treatment in the hope that in many instances permanent hearing impairment may be prevented. The second purpose is to provide for the special needs—educational, speech, and audiological—of children whose hearing may not be directly subject to improvement but who can be helped to conserve and make maximum use of their hearing capacities.

Responsibility for the actual asssessment of hearing loss varies considerably among school systems. Many large school districts conduct their own hearing testing and conservation programs. Some smaller school districts may contract for hearing services with professional agencies or audiology clinics assocated with colleges or universities. In some school districts, audiologists or audiometrists are engaged whose responsibilities include the assessment of the children's hearing throughout the grades.

The concentration, as Newby (1972, p. 221) points out, should be in the primary grades. Children in these grades are likely to have a higher percentage of upper respiratory ailments and other conditions associated with temporary hearing loss that may become chronic if untreated. Fortunately, most of these conditions respond favorably to medical treatment. As a result, the discovery of treatable conditions that produce hearing loss will appreciably reduce the incidence of hearing impairment and associated educational and social problems in the upper school grades.

In many schools, including those that provide organized audiological services, the detection of possible hearing loss continues to be the responsibility of the classroom teacher or the school nurse. The nurse may note a child's difficulty in hearing in her routine examination of the children. The classroom teacher, however, has a daily opportunity to detect whether a child, habitually or occasionally, seems to have difficulty in hearing. The child who frequently misunderstands directions, or who asks that questions directed to him be repeated, or who looks blankly at the teacher talking to him or to the class should be checked for possible hearing loss. The teacher should also watch for the child who seems to hear only when spoken to from one side of the rooms but fails to hear what is said when spoken to from the opposite side. Some children unconsciously turn their heads to favor the better ear. If these habits and manifestations are associated with poor articulation and with voice production that is inappropriate in quality and loudness, hearing loss should be suspected. Additional significant signs of hearing loss include poor coordination, poor balance, occasional dizziness, and complaints of earaches and of running ears. A child suspected of hearing loss should be referred to the school physician for further examination. If the school has no physician, the possibility of the child's hearing loss should be discussed with the principal and, of course, with the parents, and then referred to a physician.

Therapy for the Child with a Hearing Impairment

HEARING AIDS

Many children whose hearing losses range from moderate to severe are able to get considerable help from a properly fitted hearing aid. The decision whether a hearing aid is needed should be made by the otologist, a medical specialist. The actual fitting of the hearing aid may be done either by the otologist or a properly trained audiologist.[6] Although many individual factors enter into the usefulness of hearing aids, experience indicates that hearing aids are usually indicated for children when

---

[6] Many college and university clinics, as well as medical centers, provide services for the selection of hearing aids.

the hearing loss is between 35 and 70 decibels in the pitch range most important for speech. This range is roughly between 200 and 4,000 Hz (ASA standard). For children with more severe hearing losses, exceeding 70 decibels in the pitch range, the help to be derived from a hearing aid is limited. In some instances, only the awareness that there is noise and activity about is made available to the user. This may be important, however, in preventing the child from feeling isolated by inner silence if a hearing aid is not used. To be able to anticipate that someone is about to enter a house because a doorbell ring is heard is often considerably better than to be caught by surprise, or to fail to answer a doorbell because it is not heard.

If a hearing aid is indicated, training in its care and proper use is in order.[7] Such training may be provided by the otologist or by the audiologist associated with a medical center, college, or university speech and hearing clinic, or in private practice.

It is important to appreciate that a hearing aid does not serve to give the user normal hearing in the same sense that properly fitted eyeglasses give most users essentially the equivalent of normal vision. The hearing instrument, as its name suggests, is only an aid. It helps the wearers make more complete use of the hearing they have. If the hearing loss is moderate rather than severe, and an individual learns how to employ the aid effectively, hearing that is functionally close to normal may be achieved. If, in addition, the individual learns speech reading (lip reading), comprehension close to normal may be achieved. For the severely impaired, speech reading is of greater importance than for those with moderate hearing loss. The hearing aid has more limited application and value for the deaf, but together with speech reading, it can be of significant help.

Speech reading implies the use of all visual cues in interpreting (decoding) what a speaker says. Speech reading entails more than the reading of lips. It requires that the listener be attentive to all of the visible movements of the speaker that are involved in the communication of a message.

SPEECH AND HEARING THERAPY

Proper medical attention may help many children as well as adults to conserve whatever hearing they have. Proper speech and listening

---

[7] Criteria for determining the need for a hearing aid are considered by H. A. Newby, *Audiology*, 3rd. ed. (New York: Appleton-Century-Crofts, 1972), pp. 110–111 and by J. Northern and M. P. Downs, *Hearing in Children* (Baltimore: The Williams & Wilkins Co., 1974), pp. 225–227. Both of these sources emphasize the need for flexibility and the responses of the individual child rather than fixed audiometrically determined level of hearing loss.

training should help them make the maximum use of their hearing and conserve the quality and intelligibility of their speech.

The hearing therapist helps the child to make maximal use of residual hearing as well as effective use of the hearing aid, if one is used. In addition, the child is made aware of all the aspects of sound production so that tactile as well as auditory and visible cues are recognized and utilized. In this way, the child not only becomes more completely responsive to how other persons speak but also responds to his/her own speech with greater awareness. The result is better articulation, better voice, and improved intelligibility. In working with the schoolchild, specific instruction is correlated with academic subject matter. The vocabulary of a new subject is introduced and becomes the core of the speech and hearing instruction.

Newby (1972, p. 342) summarizes the goals of an auditory training program along the following lines:

1. Persuade the child to accept the hearing aid.
2. Teach the child to operate the hearing aid so effectively that he/she will not want to do without it.
3. It may be desirable in early stages of training to prevent the child from observing visual cues so that concentration and attention may be given to auditory signals. However, the long-range objective is to help in the development of the child's overall communicative abilities to their fullest extent. "Therefore, auditory training should usually be combined with speech reading, and while the comprehension of speech is being taught emphasis must also be placed on helping the child to improve his own speech."

The Role of the Classroom Teacher with the Hard of Hearing

The classroom teacher has social and educational responsibilities for the hard-of-hearing child that are like those for other children in the classroom, but just more so. The teacher can help the child to obtain a sense of social competence and to function normally in a school setting. Hard-of-hearing children are inclined to withdraw and isolate themselves from others, especially when the going is rough. The teacher must be on the alert for such signs and behaviors, and attract the child to group activities. Through the assignment of regular as well as inspiration-of-the-moment responsibilities, the teacher can help the hard-of-hearing child to feel and be accepted as a fully participating member of the group.

Perhaps more than anything else, the teacher should encourage oral language through recitation activities in class as well as in less formal discussion and conversation. Reading is of especial importance for the hard-of-hearing child. Through reading, grammatical markers, functional words, and syntactic structures may become more readily apparent than in heard speech.

The physical placement of the hard-of-hearing child in the classroom is particularly important. The following suggestions will enhance the likelihood that the child will have full awareness of what is going on in the classroom:

1. Make certain that the child is seated where speakers are best seen and heard.
2. Seat the child where there is the least amount of interfering noise. A seat up front in the aisle farthest from the window should accomplish this objective. However, the child should be permitted to move as freely as space permits if the teacher needs to move to another part of the classroom.
3. Make certain that there is no light glare in the child's eyes.
4. When addressing the hard-of-hearing child, speak naturally but somewhat more loudly and slowly than otherwise might be necessary.
5. Use appropriate gestures freely, especially if the word or idea is new.
6. Emphasize the use of prepared visual materials. Use the blackboard for writing words, phrases, and sentences associated with the essential material of the oral presentation.
7. Remember to observe the child for signs of lack of comprehension or confusion. If material is repeated, it should as closely as possible be an exact repetition. If rephrasing is in order, provide cues that you are indeed rephrasing and not repeating. Something such as, "I will say it another way." should do. The "other way" should be in clear syntactic structures.
8. If the child is using a hearing aid, make certain that it is operational, batteries are on and working, and ear piece is properly fixed.

Many of these suggestions, though intended primarily for the hard-of-hearing child, are not without value for other children who may have learning difficulties. What the classroom teacher does for the hearing-impaired child will often make it possible for other "special" children to be better school achievers. The payoffs in sensitivity to the teacher will not be purely incidental.

Education for the Hearing Impaired: The Deaf

LANGUAGE AND LEARNING PROBLEMS

Many school-age children with moderate or greater hearing loss who have skill in speech reading are able to be educated in classes with normal hearing children. Some children with severe hearing loss who are designated as deaf are nevertheless able to be absorbed and educated in classes for the hearing. Silverman (1971, p. 407) reports that some deaf individuals attend secondary schools and colleges for the hearing. We assume that the age of hearing loss, the acquisition and competence of the individual before becoming deaf, the skill in speech reading, and highly individual factors of personality and intellect account for the ability of some deaf persons to be educated in school settings for the hearing. However, most deaf children are educated in either day or residential schools for the deaf (see Silverman, 1971, pp. 407–408 and Northern and Downs, 1974, pp. 274–248 for statistics on the distribution of deaf children in schools in the United States).

A recent and important movement in the education of deaf children is the development of nursery school programs. Earlier (see chapter on Development of Language) we emphasized that language acquisition is critical in the preschool years as a foundation for cognitive and social development. Even though the language training may not be auditory, it is vital that language behavior including appropriate syntax be established as early as possible. Silverman observes "Formal and informal intercommunication (by whatever means) tend to lessen the child's feeling of apartness and hence make him feel wanted and significant" (Silverman 1971, p. 408).

If, as indicated previously, some children whose hearing loss is so severe they are considered deaf can be educated with hearing children, why can't many if not all deaf children be educated? This question suggests the nature of a controversy among educators of the deaf that at long last may become resolved. The controversy is among advocates of the oral method and those who believe that the primary and more "natural" approach for deaf children is through manual (sign) teaching. There are probably fewer strict oralists and strict manualists in practice than there are in theory. Before outlining the arguments on either side of this controversy, and describing briefly the "total" method, we review a few observations on the educational achievements, and particularly the language achievements of the deaf.

With some important exceptions, and possibly without regard to the method taught, deaf children do not learn at the same rate as hearing children. Silverman explains (1972, p. 411), "With the need to master new vocabulary and language, it takes about two or more years to achieve second grade level and an additional one and a half to two years to complete third grade." Silverman points out that though this slow rate is discouraging, neither the deaf child or the teacher is at fault. "It can be attributed to the time necessary to build a foundation for future progress."

Beyond the primary grades, we still find a slow rate of educational achievement for deaf children. By age 16, an age at which most hearing children who attend school are in the third year of high school, the majority of deaf children are at about the level of the eighth grade. Based on measurements of standardized tests, Silverman (1971, p. 411) reports that "Deaf children do not score equally well on all tests. The poorest scores are found in reading tests (paragraph meaning and word meaning) and in arithmetic reasoning or problem solving. The best scores are obtained in arithmetic computations and spelling."

Wiley (1971, pp. 422–428) reviews some of the pertinent literature on the language deficits of the deaf. The essential finding is that deaf children as a special population are generally deficient in language development. In regard to English, the deaf are particularly deficient in learning and applying syntactical rules and word-order sequences.

THE ORALISTS, THE MANUALISTS, AND TOTAL COMMUNICATION

ORALISM

The proponents of *pure oralism* (*auditory stimulation*) recommend that from the beginning—when a child is identified as deaf—the child should be exposed to environmental sounds and spoken language at all possible opportunities. If possible and as early as possible, the deaf child should be fitted with a hearing aid. Northern and Downs (1974, p. 250) explain the rationale of the oralist/auralist approach:

In theory, the deaf youngster is to "hear" everything he might be exposed to, only the auditory stimulation must be conducted with more deliberate action and intensity than usual circumstances might dictate.

The oral method, as developed and practiced in the Clarke School for the Deaf in the United States, discourages the use of all signing. Lip reading (speech reading) is emphasized, progressing from the recognition and imitative production of isolated phonemic elements, sound combinations, words, and finally speech utterances.[8]

As of 1970, Silverman and Lane report that 85 per cent of deaf children who were enrolled in schools for the deaf were, at least in their early schooling, instructed by the oral method. The basic argument of the proponents of the oral method is that every deaf child deserves and should be afforded an opportunity to learn to communicate by speech. Proponents of the oral method also argue that an early use of signing will create a dependence on this (manual) approach and the deaf child will not readily or willingly accept the more strenuous demands of the oral/aural approach. Consequently deaf children will be limited in their social world and in vocational situations to the nonoral deaf. In effect, they will be socially and vocationally isolated from the hearing world.

The opponents of pure oralism point to the low language and educational achievement of most deaf children as an argument against the method. Further, they argue that it is simply not natural for a deaf child to learn an oral/aural system of language. They point out that most deaf children, when left to themselves and presumably unobserved by their teachers, resort to signing because it is a natural mode for them. Other arguments to which we are sympathetic are that the oral method is a slow one and tends to retard language comprehension and production in the early critical years of life when such acquisition is readily and easily established. Specifically in regard to English, lip reading as a mode of speech reception has too many "invisible" sounds and others that are so closely alike in manner of production as to cause confusion. At best, few persons become sufficiently skilled in lip reading to be at ease in conversation. Even those who do become skilled in lip reading need ideal environmental situations of light and distance, and a speaker who articulates carefully.

The Manual Method

A fundamental question in regard to the manual method (signing) is whether sign language is, in fact, a natural language or a limited and artificial one, comparable to pidgin.[9] The answer, at least since the late

---

[8] For a brief review of the "pure oralists'" approach and other related methods and a critique of these methods, see J. Northern and M. P. Downs (*Hearing in Children*, Baltimore: The Williams & Wilkins Co., 1974), pp. 250–253.

[9] Pidgin, by definition, is a simplified language used for special purposes and situations by speakers who are primarily speakers of different languages.

1960s, as signing has been developing in the United States, is that whatever sign systems may once have been, some sign systems now incorporate all the essential features and functions of a natural language. Perhaps the most widely used of the sign languages in the United States is the *American Sign Language* or *Ameslan*. A variant of *American Sign Language* is *SEE* (*Seeing Essential English*). The *SEE* system employs morphemes, English word order, and syntax. Still another system based on *Ameslan* is *SEE* 2 (*Signing Exact English*).[10]

It should be apparent that critics of the oral method recognized the limitations of older manual methods. The newer sign systems are attempts to provide a natural language system for the deaf that will permit communication comparable to the oral/aural systems of hearing persons.

Total Communication

The total approach to language education for the deaf combines manual, auditory, and oral methods. Children who are identified as deaf are exposed to this total approach as early as possible in their own homes. Hearing parents of deaf children are themselves encouraged to learn signing and finger spelling and to use these visible methods along with oral speech.

Northern and Downs (1974, pp. 262–265) review some early demonstration studies in which parents employed the total approach with their deaf children. The results are encouraging. The reports indicate that preschool deaf children are acquiring words and syntactical features of language at a rate comparable to hearing children. Beyond this, parents are able to communicate with their children without the barrier of a lack of language.

The Total Communication approach is now being used experimentally in classes for the deaf in public schools. We earnestly hope that investigation can be carried on that will provide objective evidence of the values of each approach and what kind of deaf child can best be taught by one of the approaches. It is also possible that an issue we may need to assess is *when* one approach may be more effective than another.

Problems and Topics for Papers

1. Why is it not advisable to assess the effects of hearing loss solely in terms of the percentage of loss below normal hearing?

---

[10] See J. Northern and M. P. Downs, *Hearing in Children* (Baltimore: The Williams & Wilkins Co., 1974), pp. 253–262 for descriptions and critiques of the "new" manual sign systems.

2. Distinguish between the deaf and the hard-of-hearing.
3. What are the most frequently used nonobjective techniques for detecting the presence of hearing loss?
4. Define or explain each of the following: (a) cps or Hz, (b) decibel, (c) pure tone, (d) audiometer, (e) audiogram, (f) sweep test, (g) hearing aid, (h) residual hearing.
5. Does a hearing aid give the same assistance to its user as properly fitted glasses do for most persons with visual impairment? Justify your answer.
6. What does *identification audiometry* mean? Describe three techniques commonly used in identification audiometry.
7. Why does Newby (1972) recommend testing for functional hearing, as well as pure-tone audiometry, in the assessment of hearing loss?
8. What specifically can the classroom teacher do for the child known to have a hearing loss?
9. What is the implication of age and acquisition of speech in relation to an acquired hearing loss?
10. What are the characteristic speech defects of a child with sensorineural hearing impairment?
11. How are children with hearing loss educated in your school district?
12. What are the objectives of an auditory training program?
13. What are the basic philosophical and methodological differences between oralists and manualists? In effect, can there be any *pure oralists?*
14. Describe some recent advances in sign languages. Which sign language meets the criteria of a natural language?
15. Why was a sign language (The American Sign Language) chosen to train chimpanzees in the use of a linguistic system? Why wasn't an oral/aural system selected?

References and Suggested Readings

ASHA Committee on Audiometric Evaluation, "Guidelines for Identification Audiometry," *ASHA*, **17**, 2 (1975), 94–99.

Davis, H., and S. R. Silverman, *Hearing and Deafness*, New York: Holt, Rinehart and Winston, Inc., 1970. (A lucidly written survey of research, including some of their own investigations, on problems of hearing.)

Eagles, E. L., W. G. Hardy, and F. Catlin, *Human Communications*, Washington, D.C.: U.S. Dept. of Health, Education, and Welfare, 1968.

Hollien, H., J. M. Wepman, and C. L. Thompson, "A Group Screening Test of Auditory Acuity," *Journal of School Health*, **39**, 8 (1969), 583–588.

Newby, H. A., *Audiology*, 3rd ed., New York: Appleton-Century-Crofts, 1972.

Northcott, W. H., *The Hearing Impaired Child in a Regular Classroom: Preschool, Elementary and Secondary Years*, Washington, D.C.: The Alexander Graham Bell Association for the Deaf, 1973. (Emphasizes the kind of planning needed by teachers, audiologists, speech pathologists, social workers, psychologists, and administrators in planning for the teaching of hearing-impaired children in integrated school programs.)

Northern, J. and M. P. Downs, *Hearing in Children,* Baltimore: The Williams & Wilkins, Co., 1974.

Silverman, S. R. "The Education of Deaf Children," in L. E. Travis, ed., *Handbook of Speech Pathology and Audiology,* New York: Appleton-Century-Crofts, 1971, 399–430.

———, and H. S. Lane, "Deaf Children" in H. Davis. and S. R. Silverman, eds., *Hearing and Deafness,* 3rd ed. New York: Holt, Rinehart and Winston, Inc., 1970.

Subcommittee on Human Communication and Its Disorders, *Human Communication and Its Disorders: An Overview,* Washington, D.C.: National Institute of Neurological Diseases and Stroke, U.S. Dept. of Health, Education and Welfare, 1969.

Van Riper, C., *Speech Correction,* 5th ed. Englewood Cliffs, N.J.: Prentice-Hall, Inc., 1972, chap 9.

Wiley, J. "A Psychology of Auditory Impairment," in W. M. Cruickshank, ed. *Psychology of Exceptional Children and Youth,* Englewood Cliffs, N.J.: Prentice-Hall, Inc., 1971, chap. 8.

15. Facial Clefts: Cleft Lip and Cleft Palate

A facial cleft is any opening in the oral cavity, lips, or nasal cavity that may be caused either by developmental failure (prebirth), or accident or disease at or following birth.[1] The vast majority of facial clefts are developmental failures. That is, during the embryonic state of fetus, parts of the facial area failed to fuse and develop normally. Facial clefts may involve the palate as a whole, or be limited to parts of the hard or soft palate. Clefts may also involve the upper gum ridge (alveolar process), the upper lip, and one or both of the nares (the passageway from the nostril to the nasal cavity). Extensive clefts may involve any two or more of the parts of the oral cavity or upper lip. An insufficient palate, though not technically an oral cleft, is believed to be associated with the anomaly. An insufficient palate is one that does not have a normal amount of soft palate. The uvula may be missing or be shortened, and part of the soft palate anterior to the uvula may be smaller than is normal.

Although the specific cause of congenital facial cleft is not known, there is little doubt that heredity plays an important role in its etiology. Other factors that may be associated with congenital facial clefts are believed to be the diet and health of the mother and intrauterine pressure on the developing fetus.

---

[1] We are using the term *facial cleft* to comprise what is frequently included in the terms *cleft lip* and *cleft palate*.

Incidence

The incidence of facial cleft varies somewhat according to geographic distribution. Surveys record ranges from one in about 600 to one in 1,000 in the population. Probably a moderate estimate is that one child in 800 is born with some form of facial cleft that will require special care and training.[2] Among cleft-palate children the likelihood is that there will be more boys than girls.

Voice and Articulation Characteristics

From the description of the inadequacy of the mechanism, the speech difficulties are readily discernible. In the speech of the child with a palatal cleft, all sounds pass directly into the nasal cavity where normal oral reinforcement is not possible. Therefore, all the vowel sounds are nasalized and most of the consonants have nasal characteristics. For example, $[b]$, $[d]$, and $[g]$ take on the characteristics of $[m]$, $[n]$, and $[ŋ]$. Other articulatory difficulties are obvious. The stop sounds $[p]$, $[b]$, $[t]$, $[d]$, $[k]$, and $[g]$ are defective because they are emitted nasally rather than orally. The fricatives $[f]$, $[v]$, $[s]$, $[z]$, $[ʃ]$, $[ʒ]$, $[θ]$, and $[ð]$ are also defective, because the air stream coming through the mouth cannot be controlled adequately. Because s and z require the direction of an air stream down a narrow channel, they are likely to be the most seriously affected of the fricative sounds. Other distinctive traits include frequent inhalation and considerable use of the glottal stop, particularly before vowels. The resulting speech of a child with a severe cleft-palate condition may be a series of snorting sounds.

Westlake and Rutherford (1966, p. 30) make an interesting observation in regard to the sound substitutions made by young cleft-palate children. They point out that normal children tend to substitute [w], [f], [t], [d], [b], [θ], (th), and [tʃ] for the sounds they are unable to make. In each instance, the sound substituted is one that requires articulatory adjustments similar to the appropriate sound. Thus, we may say that normal sound substitution is close to the required sound and the articulation, and the child with "infantile" speech is moving toward his target. In contrast, cleft-palate children produce substitutes that are quite different from the correct ones. "More than half of their

---

[2] *Orofacial Anomalies*, *ASHA* Report No. 8 (Washington, D.C.: American Speech and Hearing Association, 1973), p. 3.

substitutions are glottal stops and pharyngeal fricatives. These sounds, in addition to the [m], [n], and [ŋ], and nasal emissions, account for three fourths of cleft-palate substitutions." Thus, the cleft-palate children are far from the target sounds in their defective articulation.[3]

RELATED PROBLEMS

Certain facial mannerisms are frequently associated with cleft palate. Some children seem to engage in nasal twitching; others look as if they are habitually sniffing. The alae, the winglike structures of the nose, constrict; this constriction compensates for the failure of the nasal port to close.

The child with a facial cleft faces a variety of problems. One of the first likely to be encountered is difficulty in feeding, with some possible consequences of poor nutrition. As the child grows older, there are frequently dental conditions that require orthodontia. Teeth may fail to erupt, or they may grow in an irregular alignment. The child tends to suffer from the effects of colds, with chronic infection of the nasal areas and of the Eustachian tube. These may produce conductive hearing loss. Pannbacker (1969) found that about two thirds of a population of 103 cases of cleft lip and cleft palate (60 males and 43 females) had hearing losses of 15 decibels or more on audiometric assessment. However, cases with cleft lip alone, and those with congenital palatal insufficiency, did not have "socially significant audiological defects." Based on their review of the literature, Westlake and Rutherford (1966, p. 18) state: "All researchers agree that there is a high incidence of hearing loss in the cleft-palate population." Essentially the same observations are made by Prather and Kos (1968).

LINGUISTIC COMPETENCE

Although we are inclined to think of the cleft-palate child as one whose primary difficulties are with voice and articulation, recent evidence suggests that language competence as a whole may be delayed or improficient in many such children. In a population of 107 cleft-palate children between the ages of two and 15, Morris (1962) found an overall below-age-level expectation of language skills based on standardized test measurements. These included the Ammons Picture Vocabu-

---

[3] For a detailed discussion of the speech and voice characteristics, see K. L. Moll, "Speech Characteristics of Individuals with Cleft Lip and Cleft Palate," in D. C. Spriestersbach, and D. Sherman, eds., *Cleft Palate and Communication* (New York: Academic Press, 1968).

lary Test and the vocabulary subtest of the Wechsler Intelligence Scale for Children. In addition, mean length of sentence used and structural complexity of sentences were also below age-level expectation.

Smith and McWilliams (1968) assessed the linguistic abilities of 136 cleft-palate children ranging in age from 3.0 to 8.11. The population included 86 males and 50 females. Of these, 71 had both cleft lip and cleft palate, 46 had cleft palates without cleft lip, and 19 had cleft lip alone. Smith and McWilliams used the Illinois Test of Psycholinguistic Abilties (ITPA) as their investigative instrument. They compared the standard age scores for the nine subtests of the ITPA with the scores for their experimental population. "The data revealed that cleft-palate subjects manifest a general language depression with particular weakness in vocal expression, gestural output, and visual memory. Moreover, in the samples studied, there was a tendency for language weaknesses to become more marked as age increased." Both male and female subjects with cleft lip alone showed relative weaknesses in motor expression and visual memory, and generally similar linguistic profiles to the children with cleft palate.

Moll (1968, p. 110) after reviewing the literature concludes:

> it appears that individuals with cleft lips and cleft palates are retarded in some degree in language development. This retardation seems to exist on almost every dimension measured in the various studies: these children exhibit less verbal output and a more simple language structure than children without clefts.
>
> . . . it must be emphasized that the conclusions about retarded language development refer to cleft palate subjects on the average; obviously not all children exhibit retardation in language skills.

Intelligence

Another factor deserving study and consideration in determining the therapeutic needs of the cleft-palate child is his intellectual development. A carefully conducted control study by Goodstein (1961), in which the Wechsler Intelligence Scale for Children was used to assess the intellectual status of cleft-palate children and a matched group of children without cleft palate, indicates that there are significant differences in intelligence levels between the two groups. An appreciably larger percentage of the cleft-palate children fell in the categories of dull normal, borderline, and mentally defective intellectual classifications than did the control children. The latter group of children tended to distribute very much according to the expected intellectual classification levels. This study points to the need for the individual assessment of the intelligence of the cleft-palate child as well as the related need to adjust the therapeutic program so that the objective, materials, and rate of progress are realistically geared to the child's intellectual capacity.

Westlake and Rutherford (1966), after reviewing some of the literature on the intelligence of cleft-palate children, suggest that one of the reasons for the somewhat lower intelligence test scores may be in involvements, such as hearing loss, that are associated with, or etiologically related to, the clefts. They conclude (Westlake and Rutherford, 1966, p. 17) that "present information gives little reason for assuming that a person with a cleft is more likely to have a lower I.Q. than any other person." This observation is consistent with the general position taken by Westlake and Rutherford that cleft-palate persons vary individually as much as persons without cleft, and that generalizations are to be avoided in favor of intensive study of the individual who may have a facial cleft.

Based on his own study and a review of the literature, Goodstein (1968, pp. 209–212) concludes: "The findings . . . suggest a generally mild to moderate degree of intellectual impairment, with the distribution of I.Q. for the group of children with cleft palate displaced to the lower end of the distribution." The differences are generally more pronounced in the verbal than in the performance areas. Though the mean I.Q. of cleft-palate children ranged from 94 to 99, it needs to be reemphasized that a given child with cleft palate can be found anywhere on the intelligence range, including genius.

Therapy: Surgical

The first step, if possible, is the repair of the oral mechanism to the fullest extent that can be achieved for life processes and speech. The first step may in fact be a series of steps taken over a period of years, through infancy and childhood. The primary goal of surgery is to provide the cleft-palate child with the best possible functioning of the palate and the vocal mechanism as a whole. A secondary but exceedingly important goal is cosmetic; to do whatever can be done to make the child as good-looking and as normal in appearance as possible.

A variety of procedures is used to close the palate, to lengthen it if possible, and to provide an oral cavity that will serve both the functions of articulation and reinforcement (resonance). Often, as we have indicated, the teeth need to be arranged or rearranged, or dentures provided when this is not possible.

Usually the repair of extensive facial clefts requires a series of operations. Since surgical repair of facial clefts is a highly specialized area in medicine, most of the work is done in fairly large medical centers. Surgeons must not only make the oral cavity adequate for the present but must also predict how future growth will be affected by the surgery.

Descriptions of some of the surgical procedures are presented in Westlake and Rutherford (1966, pp. 79–82), and Perkins (1971, pp. 188–190 and 197–200).

Prosthetic Appliances

In some cases, the surgeon may advise against or postpone an operation. It may be desirable for the child to be older or to be in better health before surgery. The surgeon may decide that the available tissue is insufficient for the purpose of "covering" the area of the cleft. In such instances the physician may recommend that the child be fitted with an obturator, a prosthetic device that substitutes or "supplements" the cleft palate according to need. Some prosthetic appliances are inserted into the hard palate, others are inserted into the soft palate area, and still others "cover" both the hard and soft palates. Soft palate appliances usually include a bulb for the area of the nasopharynx, which, if carefully fitted, may help considerably in reducing nasality. If the bulb is too large, denasality may result.

In some instances, prosthetic appliances are used temporarily, while the child is growing. These devices may need changing as the child grows. With maturity, if surgery is not indicated ,"permanent" prosthetic appliances may be designed and fitted.

Descriptions of prosthetic appliances and their use may be found in Van Riper (1972, pp. 362–365).

COOPERATION OF ALL SPECIALISTS

The treatment of the child with a facial cleft may require long and continuous cooperation and coordination of services. The speech clinician, surgeon, orthodontist, psychologist, and prosthodontist must work together carefully and well. They must have a fairly intimate knowledge of each other's goals and their methods of achieving them.

The classroom teacher must work with the specialists and understand their work.

SPEECH CORRECTION

MUSCLE STRENGTHENING

The speech clinician must help the child to make maximum use of the oral cavity musculature as modified either by the surgeon or by the prosthodontist. Objectives should include making the oral musculatures stronger and more flexible so that they may be used more adequately for speech. Control of breath and the prevention or reduction of leakage of breath into the nasal cavities are the primary goals. This may be accomplished through nonenergetic "blowing exercises."[4] The gentle, sustained blowing of a feather, a Ping-Pong ball, a candle flame, or a paper butterfly helps to improve the child's ability to direct the breath stream outward toward the front of his mouth, and so to increase oral resonance when application is made to speech production. Swallowing, sucking through a straw, and yawning are also of some help in strengthening the soft palate and throat muscles. Young children may enjoy the interesting noise effects of blowing through the teeth of a comb against which a piece of tissue paper is fixed. A more musical result may be obtained from playing a harmonica.

It must be emphasized, however, that all of these exercises are merely token indicators of what a child may be able to do in nonspeech activities. A child may be able to achieve complete success in blowing exercises and yet not be able to control his velum in a manner and at a rate necessary to avoid nasality while speaking. In the final analysis, what matters is how a child with a repaired cleft, or one with an oral prosthesis, uses his mechanism for intelligible and, if possible, appropriate nasal reinforcement. Of the two, *intelligibility should be the primary objective.*

Realism should dictate the remedial speech efforts and objectives for the cleft-palate child. Along this line we accept the basic philosophy for speech therapy of Van Riper (1972, pp. 369–370):

"We make the person's speech better and we make him a happier person. . . . Within the limits of our time and energy and knowledge, and with an awareness of the limitations which the case also possesses, let

---

[4] Note that we use the term *nonenergetic blowing*. Energetic blowing that requires great tension is contraindicated. Further, at no time should the child be permitted or directed to constrict the nostrils to achieve blowing. Such constricted blowing efforts may produce a backing up of the nsasal fluids and may result in middle-ear infection.

us do our utmost and be content with that." So, with the clinician's direct help and the teacher's support, cleft-palate children should be taught to speak as well as they can. This means with as little abnormality as possible, and with major emphasis on intelligible communication.

VISUALIZING PALATAL MOVEMENT

Actual movement of the palate and the oral mechanism as a whole can now be visualized by means of X-ray photography, taken while the patient is talking. Perhaps the best technique is that of X-ray motion pictures (cinefluorography), which is now available in many medical centers. Information derived from such films enables the clinician to know what needs to be done to improve palatal action and to counteract the tendencies of a person with repaired cleft to use inappropriate articulatory movements. It may be possible to see as well as hear the differences when the child speaks slowly and when the child speaks at what may be a normal rate of utterance, but not an optimum rate for this child. However, X-ray photography is not always available, so that other less sophisticated methods may need to be used. Simple devices include the use of long bits of light feather glued to the end of a tongue depressor or, perhaps better, an ice cream stick. Placed under the nostrils, the feather should respond to the emitted air. If the air is inappropriately emitted, the clinician and child have a visual cue for this misfunction. Westlake and Rutherford (1966, p. 91) also suggest the use of a small plastic rectangular box, fashioned so that an open space on one of the shorter ends fits against the upper lip so that the nose may extend into the area of the box. Air escaping from the nostrils will cause the feather or paper to move about in the box. Westlake and Rutherford (1966, p. 91) realistically observe that "all these methods are difficult to use with young children, many of whom seem diabolically driven to make the papers fly instead of trying to speak without moving them." We would suggest a counterdiabolic procedure by directing the child alternately to make things move and to talk without producing such movement. This is an application of the principle of negative practice in learning!

In some instances, a child may have a short palate, insufficient in length to close the nasal part. Excessive nasality is then almost inevitable. A physician can advise whether this is the situation and whether a prosthetic device is considered advisable as an adjunct to the soft palate. Occasionally we find a child who sounds like one with a cleft palate but who, upon cursory examination, appears to have a complete palate. In some instances, the palate does indeed have a cleft, but is covered by a thin layer of tissue (submucous cleft), which results in hypernasality as well as deviant articulation.

IMPROVING THE VOCAL QUALITY

Careful ear training and voice training often reduce the excessive nasality. We are not sure how excessive nasal resonance is produced, although we do know that it occurs when the opening of the nasal cavity is too large as compared with the opening of the mouth cavity. The clinician will strive for a satisfactory acoustic balance of nasal and oral resonance. Thus, if the child speaks with a "tight" (hypertensive) oral musculature and a small oral opening, effort should be directed to help the child change to the use of a more relaxed and larger mouth opening. It is often not possible to get rid of all hypernasality. Continued effort to achieve the not realistically achievable may frustrate both the clinician and the child.

For extended discussions and specific details for vocal therapy for cleft-palate children see Shelton *et al.* (1968) and Van Riper (1972, pp. 370–379).

CORRECTING ARTICULATORY DEFECTS

Although excessive and inappropriate nasality is a major problem of most cleft-palate children, constant attention should be paid to improving articulation. Investigations indicate that cleft-palate speakers with intelligible articulation are likely to be judged as having less nasality then do cleft speakers with poorer articulation (Moll 1968, 96–97).

The speech clinician must help the cleft-palate child to improve his overall articulatory efforts. Exercises should be directed at increasing the child's mobility and control of jaw, lip, and tongue movements.

In some instances, a hearing loss may increase the difficulties of the cleft-palate child. Impaired hearing may account for the misarticulation of some of the sounds. If the hearing loss is moderate or severe, the use of a hearing aid may be indicated.

The clinician first teaches the sounds that are easiest for the child. For example, *h* is usually fairly easy to teach. Some of the later sounds to be established are *k*, *g*, *s*, and *z*. Since *k* and *g* involve the soft palate and since the stream of air for *s* and *z* needs very careful control, these four sounds are difficult for the child with a cleft palate. In many instances, there is a persistent tendency for sibilant sounds to be emitted nasally. Considerable effort and time are needed to overcome this tendency.

Voice and speech therapy for the cleft-palate child require patience, sustained effort, and continued motivation. Because the results often seem small for the time and energy involved, both child and clinician may become discouraged. But most children can be helped a great deal if the objectives of intelligible communication are kept realistically in mind.

The Role of the Classroom Teacher

Classroom teachers must augment the efforts of the clinician. Teachers appreciate that the degree of normalcy of the child's speech will depend on the condition of the speech mechanism after its repair, as well as on speech training, motivation, intelligence, and hearing. At times a teacher is the liaison between the clinician and the home. The teacher and the clinician advise the parents that the training period for correcting the child's speech may be long and that the work will be hard. They explain to the parents how the parents can help the child. Such advice includes providing good speech models, recognizing and rewarding small increments of improvement, and not rejecting or punishing the child for deficiencies that are not the fault of the child.

The teacher helps the child to carry over the work from the correction class into everyday speech. The teacher promotes such activities as creative dramatics, in which the child may sell newspapers on the corner or popcorn at the ball park. This activity gives the child practice in the use of the acceptable speech.

Children with cleft palates must be helped to "accept" and adjust to their difficulties. Adjustment includes efforts to improve the child's voice and overall speech intelligibility. Beyond this, cleft-palate children must be helped to feel that they are worthwhile, adequate, and loved. In the classroom the teacher must help the cleft-palate child to such attitudes. It may also be necessary to modify the reactions of the classmates so that the child is neither ridiculed nor pitied. The teacher's attitude of acceptance will go a long way to influence the behavior of the classmates.

Parents often unconsciously and sometimes even consciously may reject their child with a facial cleft. The rejection may be accompanied by feelings of shame and guilt. If these feelings become apparent to the teacher or to the clinician, recommendation for counseling is in order. In some instances, the teacher's attitude of acceptance may help the parents to modify their own attitudes.

Another result of rejection by parents may be overprotection. So some parents who, because of their concern about their cleft-palate child, overindulge the youngster and do more than they should if social, psychological, and intellectual development are to have a chance for normal potential. Oversolicitude may also be shown by the teacher. The child with a facial cleft must be encouraged to perform according to his/her potential. In the interests of the child, it should be made clear that classroom obligations are to be carried out, and the child's best performance effort is regularly to be expected. Allowances when they are made, are based on knowledge of a given child's limit-tions, but these should not be flaunted. Allowance must, of course, be made on the basis of hazards to health. Here a physician's guidance is important.

Problems and Projects

1. What are the types of facial clefts? What are the chief causes of clefts?
2. What is meant by the term *cosmetic problem*? What can be done to avoid or minimize such a problem in cleft-palate children?
3. Contrast the positions of Westlake and Rutherford and Van Riper (see References) on the psychological and social implications of a facial cleft for a child or an adult. Compare those with Goodstein's findings.
4. What problems, other than speech, are often associated with cleft palate?
5. The voice of the cleft-palate child, even after repair, is often excessively nasal. Why? When may the voice become denasal?
6. Why is it especially important to ameliorate any hearing loss that may be associated with cleft palate? Why are the hearing losses usually conduc-tive?
7. One of the new surgical procedures for reducing nasality is called the "surgical flap." Check the literature for a description of this operation and the circumstances that indicate when it is the procedure of choice.
8. Why is the strengthening of the oral musculature important in the therapeutic program for a child with cleft palate?
9. What should be the primary objective in speech training for a cleft-palate child?
10. What are the most frequent articulatory errors made by young cleft-palate children? How are these errors different from those made by most young children?
11. Describe some techniques that may be used by clinicians to help them, and their cleft-palate children, to visualize excessive nasal emission?
12. What is a prosthetic appliance? When is its use indicated for a person with a cleft palate?
13. What are the findings relative to the intelligence of cleft-palate children?
14. Can you explain the bases for the findings that as a total "special" population, cleft-palate children are behind their age peers in early language development?

References and Suggested Readings

ASHA Report No. 1, *Proceedings of the Conference: Communicative Problems in Cleft Palate*, Washington, D.C.: American Speech and Hearing Association, 1965.

Goodstein, L. D., "Psychosocial Aspects of Cleft Palate," in D. C. Spriestersbach, and D. Sherman, eds., *Cleft Palate and Communication*, New York: Academic Press, 1968.

Moll, K. L., "Speech Characteristics of Individuals with Cleft Lip and Cleft Palate," in D. C. Spriestersbach, and D. Sherman, eds., *Cleft Palate and Communication*, New York: Academic Press, 1968.

Moller, K. T., C. D. Starr, and R. R. Martin, "The Application of Operant Conditioning Procedures to the Facial Grimace Problem," *Cleft Palate Journal*, **6** (July 1969), 193–201.

Morris, H. L., "Communication Skills of Children with Cleft Lips and Palates," *Journal of Speech and Hearing Research*, **5** (March 1962), 79–90.

Pannbacker, M., "Hearing Loss and Cleft Palate," *Cleft Palate Journal*, **6** (October 1969), 50–56.

Perkins, W. H., *Speech Pathology*, St. Louis: C. V. Mosby Co., 1971.

Powers, G. L., and C. D. Starr, "The Effects of Muscle Exercises on Velopharyngeal Gap and Nasality," *Cleft Palate Journal*, **11** (1974), 28–35.

Prather, W. F., and C. M. Kos, "Audiological and Otological Considerations," in D. C. Spriestersbach, and D. Sherman, eds., *Cleft Palate and Communication*, New York: Academic Press, 1968.

Smith, R. M., and B. J. McWilliams, "Psycholinguistic Abilities of Children with Clefts," *Cleft Palate Journal*, **5** (April 1968), 238–249.

Shelton, R. L., E. Hahn, and H. L. Morris, "Diagnosis and Therapy," (chap. 7), in D. C. Spriestersbach, and D. Sherman, eds., *Cleft Palate and Communication*, New York: Academic Press, 1968.

Shprintzen, R. J., G. N. McCall, and M. L. Skolnick, "A New Therapeutic Technique for the Treatment of Velopharyngeal Incompetence," *Journal of Speech and Hearing Disorders*, **40**, 1 (1975), 69–83.

Spriestersbach, D. C., and D. Sherman, eds., *Cleft Palate and Communication*, New York: Academic Press, 1968. (A high level scientific approach by ten contributors to the multiple aspects of cleft palate.)

Van Riper, C., *Speech Correction*, 5th ed., Englewood Cliffs, N.J.: Prentice-Hall, Inc., 1972, pp. 357–379. (Has excellent illustrations for types of cleft palate. Discusses the psychological and social problems of persons with cleft palate that Van Riper believes are often as severe as for many stutterers.)

Westlake, H., and D. Rutherford, *Cleft Palate*, Englewood Cliffs, N.J.: Prentice-Hall, Inc., 1966. (A study guide for the understanding of the problems of persons with cleft palate. Emphasis is on the individual with cleft palate and the need to determine therapy based on his special problems.)

Yules, R. B., and R. A. Chase, "Pharyngeal Flap Surgery: A Review of the Literature," *Cleft Palate Journal*, **6** (1969), 303–308. (Indicates that there is a lack of available criteria for determining when the pharyngeal flap procedure should be used.)

16. Brain Damage, Brain Difference, and Brain Dysfunction

In this chapter we consider the implications of brain damage and brain difference for the acquisition and development of speech. Three groups, whose syndromes are by no means always clearly defined, are discussed. These groups are the "minimally" brain-damaged (minimal brain dysfunction), the congenitally aphasic (dyslogic), and the cerebral palsied.

The Concept of Minimal Brain Dysfunction

During recent years, and increasingly since the 1960s, teachers and clinicians have been confronted with the terms *minimal brain damage* and *minimal brain dysfunction*. The second term assumes the presence of the first, but not on the basis of the "hard signs"—the physiological, and structural alterations that many neurologists require as evidence of brain damage. In brief, the child with minimal brain dysfunction is not frankly (obviously) cerebral-palsied. He does not have clear and unquestioned indications of sensory and motor impairments, or of aberrant reflexes, that are the "hard-sign" indications of brain damage. Neurologists, psychologists, and teachers who do accept the concept of minimal brain dysfunction do so on the assumption that there are relationships between brain functioning and dysfunctioning, and behavior. So, they agree:

we must accept certain categories of deviant behavior, developmental dyscrasias, learning disabilities, and visual motor perceptual irregularities as valid indices of brain dysfunctioning. They represent neurologic signs of a most meaningful kind, and reflect disorganized central nervous system functioning at the highest level. To consider learning and behavior as distinct and separate from other neurologic functions echoes a limited concept of the nervous system and of its various levels of influence and integration (Clements 1966, pp. 6–7).

THE SYNDROME OF MINIMAL BRAIN DYSFUNCTION (MBD)[1]

The term *minimal brain dysfunction* (MBD) refers to a combination of manifestations (syndrome) present in children who are of near-average, average, or above-average intelligence. These manifestations, all of which are not necessarily present for any given child, include problems of attention and memory, impulsivity, mild motor disabilities (awkwardness, delayed laterality), perception, conceptualization, and speech and language development. These children are *perceptually* and *intellectually inefficient*, so that they do not meet the expectations for educational achievement based on their intelligence test scores, especially for those scores derived from "nonlanguage" or performance inventories. Often, in fact, they present problems in learning during the school years, and so become identified. They are often among the "underachievers," especially in the language subjects—reading, spelling, and often arithmetic as well. Their thinking tends to be concrete and ego-oriented and they may have difficulty with abstract conceptualization and abstract language. Occasionally, however, some children show surprising flashes of insight as well as an ability to appreciate the abstract. Thus, they may be inconsistent and puzzling performers who show wide day-to-day variations in their accomplishments. For a detailed testing of the symptomatology of the child with minimal brain dysfunction, see Clements (1966, pp. 11–12) and Kenny and Clemmens (1975, pp. 48–57).

Kenny and Clemmens (1975, p. 48) point out that we have no clearly defined clinical prototype of minimal brain dysfunction. Usually the child is identified between the ages of six and nine because of behavior and learning problems. Other behavioral "symptoms" include awkwardness, difficulty in fine motor coordination, hyper-

---

[1] We prefer the use of the term *minimally brain different* to the term *minimally brain damaged.* The notion of a "different" brain, even one that may be "minimally" different, has implications for deviant functioning. The term *damage*, even though it is presumed to be minimal, is difficult to establish. Moreover, the term *damage* has semantic implications that may be excessive and discouraging.

activity, distractability and associated tendencies, tendency to act impulsively (acting out), low frustration tolerance, and perseveration.

In general, the term *minimal brain dysfunction* is employed to describe a group of children who have determined deficiencies in learning and/or motor functioning. However, the children's intellectual level is usually well above the range for the mentally retarded. The concept of minimal brain dysfunction implies that there are brain abnormalities that underlie and contribute directly to the aberrations observed (Kenny and Clemmens, p. 48).

The learning problems of these MBD children are especially apparent in their language. Often they are delayed in language acquisition and present a variety of speech problems that suggest articulation defects, but may in reality be problems of syntax (such as failure to understand plural and tense endings). Writing problems include both legibility and those that parallel difficulties in oral language development. Despite these characteristics, most MBD children come well within the normal range on nonverbal tests of intelligence. Their potential for learning must, therefore, be presumed to be adequate.

We agree with Kenny and Clemmens (p. 50) that "It is obvious that the current state of our knowledge about minimal brain dysfunction is far from complete and acceptance is far from universal." These children, insofar as they can be identified, constitute problems and challenge for classroom teachers and speech and language clinicians. Fortunately, their intellectual potential provides a basis for an optimistic outlook for most MBD children. We believe that many MBD children are probably congenitally aphasic (dyslogic). We discuss this problem in the succeeding pages.

Developmental Aphasia (Dyslogia) and Brain Difference

In a literal sense, *aphasia* means without language or without speech. However, the terms *aphasia* and *aphasic* are used by professional persons concerned with problems of language related to brain damage as designations for language impairments that were acquired at a stage after language was established. These include impairments in the comprehension and production of spoken as well as written language. The terms may also be used for a child who incurs damage and language impairment following accident or disease of the brain (encephalopathies). Fortunately, the young child, up to the age of early adolescence (12 to 14 or so) has such great plasticity of the brain and such great reorganizational and recuperative capacity that recovery and resumption of language functioning may ordinarily be expected. Exceptions are found, however, among children who incur bilateral or profuse damage of the cerebrum.

In our earlier discussion of minimal brain damage and minimal brain dysfunction, we anticipated our consideration of children whose impairments are so severe as to make them essentially nonverbal. We use the terms *developmental aphasia, congenital aphasia,* and *dyslogia* synonymously to designate such severely linguistically delayed and impaired children.

DEVELOPMENTAL APHASIA (DYSLOGIA) AND BRAIN DYSFUNCTION[2]

Children who are born with brain damage because of a prenatal condition, or who have incurred brain damage as a result of a birth injury or a cerebral pathology before the age at which speech usually begins, are frequently severely retarded in their speech onset and development. Often, even after these children begin to speak, their articulation, voice, and vocabulary development are impaired. In very severe cases, usually associated with damage to both hemispheres of the brain, even the comprehension of language may be severely and sometimes completely impaired. It is likely that most of these children who do learn to understand speech also suffer from an appreciable degree of mental impairment, and others suffer from hearing loss with or without mental deficiency. Our own experience with brain-damaged children leads us to believe that, where hearing loss and mental deficiency are not complicating factors, language learning may be delayed but is usually established by age four or five. In most cases where hearing and intelligence are relatively normal, language is acquired and speech, however defective, is usually established by the time the child has reached school age.

There are, however, a small group of children with slow maturation of the central nervous system, or who, because of minimal brain damage and considerably more than minimal brain dysfunction, do not "spontaneously" acquire speech. *These children must be taught directly what most children acquire naturally—by listening, identifying, and finally by imitating*

---

[2] F. R. Kleffner in *Language Disorders in Children* (New York: The Bobbs-Merrill Co., 1973), pp. 16–17 takes exception to the use of the term *aphasia* to designate failure to have language develop in children. He argues that *aphasia* should apply only to disorders in which there is a loss or impairment of previously established language competence. Kleffner prefers the use of the terms *congenital* or *developmental* disorders of language, which can result from input and/or output capacities including central nervous system defects.

and then creating on their own an infinite number of utterances they could not possibly have learned through imitation. These children who do not acquire language "naturally" are *developmentally* or *congenitally aphasic* or *dyslogic* (without language). Following are some critical differences that distinguish such children from their speaking as well as nonspeaking age peers.

1. The developmentally aphasic (dyslogic) child has perceptual difficulties related to one or more sensory modalities, but primarily for the perception of those auditory events that constitute the sounds of speech. [See Eisenson (1972, chap. 4) for an exposition of this point.]

2. The dyslogic child is often slow in developing laterality. At the age of five or even later he/she may not have established a preferred hand or foot or an eye or an ear. Often associated with this developmental lag is confusion in directional and spatial orientation.

3. Inconsistency of response is almost a universal characteristic of the dyslogic child. A response made to a situation on one occasion may not be made on a succeeding occasion. A response that may be completely appropriate when first made may simply fail to be made on successive occasions.

4. Morbidity of attention is associated with inconsistency of response. Occasionally the dyslogic child may become so completely absorbed with the situation to which he/she is attending that he/she cannot shift attention to new situations, despite the intensity of a new stimulus. Thus, loud noises may be ignored, or at least are not immediately able to compete for attention with what is already concerning the child. In contrast with this compulsive and persistent manner of attending to a situation, the dyslogic child may sometimes have such fleeting attention as to seem to be reacting to everything, and adequately to nothing.

5. Associated with inconsistency of response and morbidity of attention is lability (instability) of general behavior. The dyslogic child may behave excessively and exhibit uncontrolled emotionality because of seemingly trivial disturbances. If the child is disturbed at all, he/she is disturbed a great deal. Along with emotional lability there is accompanying hyperactivity. The child may suddenly change from being relatively docile to being active beyond easy control.

6. A characteristic feature of the language development of the dyslogic child, aside from the initial retardation, is unevenness of ability. Even after this child begins to use language, he/she does

not show the expected increments or the "ordered" pattern by which most children increase their linguistic abilities for day-to-day communication. Many dyslogic children learn to say a few words at intervals far apart, but during these periods may have a normal or better than normal increase in their comprehension vocabularies. They may show parallel disparities in learning to read and write. The result may be that even after the children are in the midprimary grades, their educational achievements are so uneven as to cause considerable concern to their teachers, their parents, and to themselves. They are often painfully slow in achieving an integrated pattern of development with those features that go together and that are ordinarily found together.[3]

The features we reviewed of the developmentally aphasic child may be understood in terms of the impaired efficiency of their neurological mechanisms. The overall effects of the cerebral differences in this brain different child are to aggravate any sensory impairments they may have—some have slight to moderate degrees of hearing loss—and to reduce their perceptual and intellectual potentials. Functionally, these children do not hear as well as audiometric results would suggest they should be able to hear. Otherwise stated, they do not hear (in reality, listen) as proficiently as nonbrain-damaged children do with the same amount of "objectively measured" hearing. Similarly, and more generally, they often function considerably below the upper limits of their mental potential. They disturb easily and have very good cause for such reactions.

CLINICAL ASSESSMENT

Severely linguistically retarded children who are suspected of being dyslogic should be evaluated by highly competent specialists. These children are often not easy to diagnose into clear-cut categories. They often respond, or fail to respond, in the manner of deaf children. Sometimes they seem to respond with the slowness and limited understanding of severely mentally retarded children. Often they behave as if they were emotionally disturbed. It is essential, therefore, that a team of clinicians, including a physician and, if possible, a neurologist, an audiologist, a psychologist, and a language clinician (speech pathologist), make the assessment. It may well be that a given child may have

---

[3] For example, most children begin to combine words into rudimentary two-word utterances when they have a base vocabulary of about 50–75 words. Dyslogic (aphasic) children usually do not begin to produce two-word utterances until they have a base vocabulary of from 250 to 500 words.

brain damage and hearing loss, and the general lability may be a reaction to his/her own impairments. Even when language learning is proceeding, the child as well as the teachers and parents, may be responding to the child's uneven abilities with repeated frustration.

The most severely developmentally aphasic children do not have enough language when they reach school age to enter and perform competently in regular classes. In some school districts they may be accepted in special classes for aphasic or neurologically handicapped children. Usually they need prior training to be prepared for such classes. Such training is now offered in clinics or in medical or educational centers here and abroad. Approaches that have been found useful emphasize speech-sound discrimination, visual stimulation in association with oral language, sequencing of visual materials and of oral language presented more slowly and in smaller units than in normal speech utterance, and the direct teaching of syntax. We have found that many preschool developmentally aphasic children do well by an almost exclusively visual approach that introduces arrangements of pictures to tell something (visual semantic sequencing), which later becomes associated with oral language. Essentially, the child learns that utterances, whether visual or audible, have "law and order," or rules out of which sense and meanings are derived. By approaching the child primarily through the visual and less impaired modality, which incidentally and importantly permits looking as long and as often as necessary to derive meaning from the input, the notion of representation and symbolization becomes established. Thus, some children begin to be able to read on a primer level before they are able to do much talking.

Programs for congenitally aphasic children are now being developed at the Institute for Childhood Aphasia at San Francisco State University (Eisenson, 1972). Programs with a different emphasis and orientation have been published by Barry (1961), McGinnis (1963), and Gray and Ryan (1973).

THERAPEUTIC APPROACHES

Such approaches to improve the speech and language impairments of the school-age dyslogic child should be shared by the language clinician and the classroom teacher. Many dyslogic children continue to need specialized help—either ancillary to regular class teaching or, as we have indicated, in special classes—throughout the primary grades, and some even beyond this level. If the child has made sufficient progress to be attending grade school, he/she still requires the additional therapy that is a product of understanding and patience. The classroom teacher may help the child to work to maximum level of ability by motivation that is timed to the child's periods of best effort. Dyslogic children more than most children, need encouragement because they are never quite certain what they may expect of themselves. In the absence of severe sensory or motor disability, many, if not most, dyslogic children may be helped to achieve at least a normal level of overall proficiency. Care must be exercised that they are not pushed too hard, or urged too soon, as they begin to acquire language and learn how to behave in a world of linguistic symbols. With good timing, and with an educational schedule geared to awareness of their labile inclinations and their intellectual limitations, the teacher and clinicians can balance their demands to the children's abilities so that proficiencies may develop despite early unevenness in developmental patterns.

The Cerebral-Palsied: Definition and Problems

In a narrow and literal sense the term *cerebral palsy* refers to motor involvement (palsy or paralysis) on the basis of brain damage. The motor involvement may vary in type or degree and may include obvious severe paralysis, motor weakness, and/or motor incoordination. It is usually possible to relate the nature of the motor disability with localized pathology in the brain. However, in some instances, pathology and manifest impairment are not easily associated.

In a broader sense, cerebral palsy refers to several conditions that are associated with the cerebral pathology, but not necessarily specific to the motor impairments. Perhaps it would be more accurate to say that many cerebral-palsied individuals have such impairments as hearing loss, visual difficulties, other sensory difficulties such as the integration of sensory stimuli, perceptual and intellectual decrement, and related behavioral problems. These involvements, which all too often occur multiply among the cerebral-palsied, underlie general learning disabilities and specific difficulties in the comprehending of speech and in acquiring and developing language proficiency, both oral and written. We should note and emphasize that many individuals who are known to have congenital brain damage, and who have manifest motor involvements are essentially free of any other associated impairments. Thus, we cannot stress the point too strongly that for any child, regardless of whether motor or sensory involvements are evident, a complete assessment of potential abilities as well as limitations is in order. High-level intelligence and high-level potential achievement are definitely represented among the population of the frankly cerebral-palsied.

INCIDENCE

Figures as to the incidence of cerebral palsy vary considerably according to criteria. The incidence would be high if the collector of the data assumes that the existence of any of the conditions mentioned previously is presumptive evidence of cerebral palsy, or if the condition cannot be attributed to some other specific cause. Behavioral disturbances, especially of the "acting out" variety, are perhaps all too frequently considered to be associated with brain damage. The incidence is likely to be considerably lower if the investigator demands clear-cut positive evidence of brain damage, such as would satisfy a pediatric neurologist who might be concerned with "hard-sign" indications of neuropathology. Psychologists, and neurologists as well, who view the assessment of perceptual and cognitive functioning as an extension of a neurological examination, would stress the significance of findings of perceptual impairment (the failure to derive meanings from sensory input) and impairment of intersensory integration as evidence of brain damage, even when motor disabilities are minimal. Investigations along this line are reviewed in monographs by Birch (1964) and Allen and Jefferson (1962). A conservative estimate of the incidence of cerebral palsy is about 1.7 per 1,000 of population (Wilson, 1973, p. 466). Interestingly, this incidence may have been somewhat higher in the 1960s than in previous decades because many children who survived the conditions that make them cerebral-palsied would have died in the first half of the century. We may hope, however, that immunization against measles and rubella may continue to reduce this incidence sharply in future years.

CAUSES OF CEREBRAL PALSY

The causes of cerebral palsy are, unfortunately, both numerous and varied. By definition, whatever the specific cause, it must be one that damages or retards the development of one of the centers of the brain that is involved in the production and control of motor activity. There is also a high incidence of sensory defects, predominantly hearing and vision, as well as mental retardation. These impairments are associated with pathologies of the cerebrum, cortical and subcortical, in the cerebral palsied.[5]

---

[5] See B. Crothers and R. S. Paine, *The Natural History of Cerebral Palsy* (Cambridge, Mass.: Harvard University Press, 1959) for medical considerations. A brief summary of the pathology of cerebral palsy may be found in S. F. Brown, in W. Johnson, et al., *Speech Handicapped School Children* (New York: Harper & Row Publishers, Inc., 1967), pp. 376–378.

The major causes of cerebral palsy include developmental maturational failure beginning in the embryonic stage. In many intances, such failure is associated with illness incurred by the mother during the early months of pregnancy. Rubella, or German measles, is high among such illnesses. Trauma affecting the brain, associated with the mother's prolonged labor or precipitous labor, is also one of the more frequent causes. Any condition that cuts off or sharply reduces the oxygen supply to the child's brain and that occurs immediately before, during, or after the child is born may cause cerebral palsy. Such conditions include maternal hemorrhaging, a tightened umbilical cord around the child's neck, an injury that occasionally, but fortunately rarely, may result from forceps delivery, or cerebral hemorrhaging of the child from unknown causes. Prematurity (babies born before full term and weighing less than five pounds) is high among the conditions associated with cerebral palsy. Even after the child has survived his first hazardous journey through the mother's birth canal, damage to the brain may be incurred from head trauma or from some infectious involvement that produces brain damage.

Although all causes of brain damage cannot be specifically related to the type of cerebral palsy a child may have, certain etiological correlates are recognized. External trauma to the brain (head injury that affects the brain) is likely to produce spastic cerebral palsy. Anoxia (a cutting off or sharp reduction in the supply of oxygen to the brain) tends to be associated with athetoid cerebral palsy. In the embryonic state, the stage of the development of the child's central nervous system may be affected by the illnesses of the mother.[6]

Disturbances Related to Cerebral Palsy

As we have indicated, many cerebral-palsied children have multiple handicaps usually associated with the basic brain damage. On the physical side these handicaps include epilepsy and impairments of hearing and vision. Many children also show considerable mental retardation even when allowances are made for the inadequacy of the test instruments. In addition, there are often subtle disturbances in perceptual

---

[6] E. T. McDonald and B. Chance, *Cerebral Palsy* (Englewood Cliffs, N.J.: Prentice-Hall, Inc., 1964), chap. 2 present an excellent brief review of the neurophysiology and etiology of cerebral palsy.

W. H. Perkins, *Speech Pathology* (St. Louis: The C. V. Mosby Co., 1971), pp. 135–141 discusses the types of cerebral palsy, their neuropathologies, and related disorders of speech (language, voice, and articulation).

ability, such as the ability to recognize and reproduce forms and appreciate spatial relationships. This impairment interferes with the children's learning potential and with their attempts at adjusting to their physical environment.[7] Another area of difficulty is emotional stability. Many cerebral-palsied children are disturbed children. Some of the disturbances arise out of a reaction to their multiple handicaps. Other disturbances arise out of the reactions of the parents and siblings to the cerebral-palsied children, and theirs in turn to their parents and siblings. Perhaps an even greater cause of emotional disturbance may be attributed to the frequent failures in attempts at communication, which may have the unfortunate result of allowing quick and chronic frustration to become an established mode of behavior.

INTELLIGENCE AND EDUCABILITY

INTELLIGENCE

Until very recently, testing instruments used for estimating the intelligence of cerebral-palsied children have had severe limitations. Most tests used were initially standardized on populations that did not include a significant number of children with motor handicaps or the other handicaps often associated with cerebral palsy. Tested by such instruments, the cerebral-palsied population showed a large incidence of mental retardation. Fortunately, several instruments are now available that require little or no verbalization and call instead for relatively gross motor actions in the test situations. Such tests enable us to make a more adequate estimate of the intelligence of the cerebral-palsied. These tests include the Ammons Full Range Picture Vocabulary Test, the Revised Peabody Vocabulary Test, the Revised Columbia Mental Maturity Scale, and Raven's Progressive Matrices. The results obtained from surveys employing these tests suggest that there is probably less mental retardation among the cerebral-palsied than was earlier reported. There is little question, however, that the incidence of mental retardation is considerably greater among the cerebral-palsied than among the population at large. Estimates as to the amount of mental retardation among the cerebral-palsied range from 25 per cent to more than 50 per cent.

---

[7] See W. M. Cruickshank's discussion of the multiple-handicapped child in *Psychology of Exceptional Children and Youth* (Englewood Cliffs, N.J.: Prentice-Hall, Inc., 1970), pp. 3–12 for an explanation of these factors; also the discussions by C. Kennedy and L. Eisenberg in H. S. Birch, ed., *Brain Damage in Children* (Baltimore: The Williams & Wilkins Co., 1964), pp. 13–26 and 61–76.

While becoming aware of the intellectual limitations of many of the cerebral-palsied, we should not overlook the important fact that intellectual genius is also present in this physically handicapped group. Taken as a whole, all levels of intellectual capacity are represented among the cerebral-palsied, as they are among the population at large.[8]

Perhaps the most realistic as well as the fairest way to deal with the results of psychological (intelligence) testing is to accept the scores as minimal indicators of a child's intellectual potential. They provide a baseline, a place from where to begin and to plan education and other treatment programs. The test results should not be regarded as the ceiling of a child's intellectual capacity.

EDUCABILITY

Because many cerebral-palsied children have multiple handicaps, including mental retardation, a large percentage of the children have been classified as uneducable. Many are "trained" in resident institutions rather than in schools. Of late, increasing numbers of cerebral-palsied children are being educated in special classes in regular public schools. Private schools specializing in the treatment of the handicapped are also accepting the cerebral-palsied and giving them the benefit of improved understanding and teaching techniques. A majority of cerebral-palsied children have sufficient intellectual capacity for education along with the nonhandicapped in the normal classroom situation. Many of these children, however, will require special attention from the speech clinician as well as understanding from the classroom teacher.

Therapy for the Cerebral Palsied

THE CEREBRAL PALSY TEAM

For children with more than minimum or residual cerebral palsy, a program of training calls for the cooperation of a team of professional specialists. Included in the team are the physician, the psychologist,

---

[8] R. M. Allen and T. W. Jefferson, in their manual on the *Psychological Evaluation of the Cerebral-Palsied Person* (Springfield, Ill.: Charles C Thomas, Publisher, 1962) describe tests and suggestions for the modification of procedures needed in the assessment of the cerebral-palsied. See also T. E. Newland, in Cruickshank, W. M., ed., *Psychology of Exceptional Children and Youth*, 3rd ed., (Englewood Cliffs, N.J.: Prentice-Hall, 1971), pp. 141–146.

the social worker, the physical therapist, the occupational therapist, the teacher, and the speech clinician.

The physician or physicians must estimate to what extent the child's neurological involvements may affect his/her learning. Frequently, an orthopedic surgeon is called upon for recommendations as to how class-room equipment or home furnishings are to be constructed or adapted to the child's needs. The orthopedic surgeon's advice is also needed in matters relating to the improvement of motor abilities and the prevention of physical disabilities.

The physical therapist, working with the physician, strives to improve the child's performance in coordination and motor activity. Specific therapeutic measures may be employed which may help the child to learn how to control speech musculature so that a proper degree of relaxation and synergy of movement is achieved. Such therapy prepares the cerebral-palsied child for the work of the speech clinician.

The occupational therapist functions as an observer of the child's motor activity and trains the child specifically in "occupational" skills. Essentially, the occupational therapist supplements the work of the physical therapist.

The psychologist, through testing and observation, makes an appraisal of the intellectual capacities and the present and potential abilities as well as the disabilities and limitations of the cerebral-palsied child. Recommendations as to the child's educability and type of education are made by the psychologist. Periodic reappraisals are made so that objectives and goals may be changed according to the manner and rate of the child's development.

The social worker investigates the home situation of the cerebral-palsied child. This specialist obtains information about the child's home and the attitudes of the parents and other key members in the household. In addition, the social worker helps to adjust the members of the family to their problem in relationship to the child and in the interest of the child.

The speech clinician evaluates the child's speech problems and trains him to improve communicative skills. Speech disabilities are found in 50 to 75 per cent of cerebral-palsied children. Some of the disabilities can be considerably improved; others can be modified only slightly. Realistic goals must be established that are consistent with the child's sensory and motor abilities and intellectual capacity. Progress, it must be recognized, is often slow and amounts of improvement are not likely to be discerned on a day-to-day basis.

We cannot overemphasize the point that the establishment of some functional language system should be the first and immediate objective for the communicatively impaired cerebral-palsied child. If the communicative system to be established is the aural-oral one, then reasonable intelligibility and not refined and precise articulation is the goal. We should also expect that many cerebral-palsied children are severely delayed in their acquisition of language. Procedures for delayed language children are, therefore, indicated. Such procedures include establishing a base vocabulary of at least 100 words (it may be as many as 300–500) before expecting the child to produce two-word utterances. Language teaching should include providing models of syntactic structures that incorporate features of grammar that approximate the order of a normal child's language acquisition. A program based on their principle is provided in *Aphasia in Children* (Eisenson 1972).[9]

The suggestions that follow pertain primarily to the motor aspects of speech. They include procedures for enhancing intelligibility and so communication. At all levels, realism should determine expectations.

Specific speech therapy for the cerebral-palsied child with speech disabilities must be adapted to the child in terms of specific involvements. If a child has a hearing loss, speech signals must be intensified. This can be accomplished through the use of a hearing aid or through the use of amplification and headset earphones. For many cerebral-palsied children, an overall program would include the following:

1. Relaxation and voluntary control of the speech musculature. Often much of this work has been accomplished through the training given by the physiotherapist.

2. The establishment of breath control for vocalization and articulation. Many cerebral-palsied children breathe too deeply or too shallowly for purposes of speech. Frequently children attempt to speak on inhaled breath. For most cerebral-palsied children, a normal length of phrase is not to be expected. Short, uninterrupted phrasing is a more modest and more possible achievement. Devices such as blowing through a straw, "bending" a candle flame, and moving ping-pong balls on flat surfaces and up inclined planes are helpful in establishing breath control. Application to speech must follow if the technique is to be more than a game.

3. Control of the organs of articulation. Considerable exercise is needed to establish directed and independent action of the tongue and to overcome the frequently present tendency of the cerebral-palsied child to move his jaw as he attempts to move his tongue. Children enjoy such exercises as licking honey from their lips, or reaching for a

---

[9] At the risk of being simplistic, we emphasize that no syntactic structure is taught by rote. The clinician or teacher must be certain that the child understands the content—the contextual meaning—of any given syntactic structure. It follows that both the meaning and the structure should be functionally useful to the child.

bit of honey or peanut butter placed on the upper gum ridge. A lollipop held outside the mouth for licking provides a sweet objective for the tip of the tongue. The child should be shown what he or she does by observing himself or herself and the speech clinician in a mirror.

4. Work on individual speech sounds. The sounds most frequently defective are those that require precise tip-of-the-tongue action. These include *t*, *d*, *l*, *n*, *r*, *s*, and *z*. Intense auditory stimulation, even if the child has no significant hearing loss, often helps to create awareness of what the child is expected to produce. Sound play, calling for repetition of sounds the child can produce, may give him or her a feeling of accomplishment in the early stages of speech training. For many children, normal proficiency of articulation may not be expected. The production of "reasonable facsimiles" of sounds so that speech, though defective, is intelligible is frequently all that we have a right to expect.

5. Incorporation of sounds in words and phrases. Many cerebral-palsied children have considerable difficulty in making the transition from the production of individual sounds to connected speech. Abrupt stops are frequent, especially when words include stop plosive sounds or others that call for rapid articulatory action. The child should be encouraged to keep the sounds moving, to keep the articulators in action, even if there is a resultant lack of precision in the effort as a whole. Articulation must, of course, be coordinated with breathing and vocalization.

Van Riper (1972, pp. 383–386) describes an approach to speech therapy that coordinates with the Bobath system of physical therapy for cerebral-palsied children. A more detailed explanation of this and other procedures is provided by McDonald and Chance (1964, pp. 63–75).

THE CLASSROOM TEACHER'S RESPONSIBILITY FOR CEREBRAL-PALSIED CHILDREN

Because the cerebral-palsied child may look different, because frequently the child is unable to participate in many of the activities of other children, because the family may have been oversolicitous or may have unconsciously rejected the child, the cerebral-palsied is likely to have difficulty in adjusting to a group. When the teacher accepts this situation, appears to be casual about it, but still demands performance that is within reach and is compatible with the child's capabilities, the teacher is doing the child a real service. If the teacher does not let his/her sympathy show but accepts the child in a friendly fashion with cheerful affection, the child's adjustment is made easier. The child should participate in such regular classroom activities as going on visits. As far as possible, the teacher should consider the cerebral-palsied child as just another member of the group who enjoys and likes living with the classmates, and should provide new experiences that give adequate scope for individual abilities and energies.

Cerebral-palsied children speak better when they are relaxed. They do better when they have confidence in themselves and in their abilities. When they are anxious or frustrated, cerebral-palsied children have more difficulty with their speech. When the teacher can help a child to feel that he or she is making a contribution to group living, and that he or she is accepting and carrying through responsibilities for successful group activity, a feeling of "belongingness" with the classmates and a feeling of security in this particular environment may be established. The teacher must provide the cerebral-palsied child with frequent opportunities to relax. At times, the teacher or children may make things easy for the cerebral-palsied child physically; for example, the child's seat may be moved to a particular spot that is more readily accessible for the current activity. Whatever is done should be done in as casual a manner as possible so that no attention is attracted to the activity and the cerebral-palsied child will be able to feel comfortable rather than self-conscious.

Problems and Projects

1. Children now referred to as being cerebral-palsied were once generally referred to as spastics. Why is the term *cerebral-palsied* more appropriate than spastic?
2. What are characteristics of the chief types of cerebral-palsy conditions?
3. Why are many cerebral-palsied children multiply handicapped? What are the most frequent types of handicaps?
4. Why is it difficult to be certain about the intellectual assessments of cerebral-palsied children?
5. Is it reasonable to believe that all cerebral-palsied children can achieve normal speech? Justify your answer.
6. Can a cerebral-palsy condition be acquired by an adult? Justify your answer.
7. What is meant by *minimal brain dysfunction?* What are the arguments for and against this concept? Why might *minimal brain difference* be a better term?
8. What does the term *perceptual dysfunction* imply?
9. Compare an obviously (frankly) cerebral-palsied person with one designated as having minimal brain dysfunction and so presumably minimally brain damaged. What are some similarities? What are some essential differences?

10. What does the term *emotional lability* signify when applied to the brain-damaged child?
11. What is developmental aphasia (dyslogia)? In what respects does the developmentally aphasic child resemble the one with minimal brain damage?
12. Why may it be said that a developmentally aphasic child often shows maximal brain dysfunction and minimal brain damage?
13. What is the rationale for approaching the developmentally aphasic child through the visual modality?
14. Why is the developmentally aphasic child described as one who is perceptually and intellectually inefficient?
15. What is the difference between hearing impairment and auditory perceptual dysfunction?
16. How would you go about establishing a differential diagnosis for the developmentally aphasic child and one who may be either mentally retarded or severly impaired in hearing?
17. Compare the approaches of Barry and McGinnis (see References) for the developmentally aphasic child. What are the chief similarities? The chief differences?
18. Compare the approaches of Gray and Ryan to those of Eisenson (see References). What is the basic rationale of each of the approaches?
19. Why do we emphasize the need for intelligibility rather than "standard" diction for cerebral-palsied children?
20. Check the literature for some writers who have reservations about the use of the term *aphasic* for children. What is the nature of the reservations or objections? What is your position?

References

Allen, R. M., and T. W. Jefferson, *Psychological Evaluation of the Cerebral-Palsied Person*, Springfield, Ill.: Charles C Thomas, Publisher, 1962.

Barry, H., *The Young Aphasic Child*, Washington, D.C.: Alexander Graham Bell Association for the Deaf, 1961.

Birch, H. G., ed., *Brain Damage in Children*, Baltimore: The Williams & Wilkins Company, 1964. (Includes a selective annotated bibliography on brain-damaged children.)

Brown, S. F., in W. Johnson et al., *Speech-Handicapped School Children*, New York: Harper & Row, Publishers, Inc., 1967.

Clements, S. D., *Minimal Brain Dysfunction in Children*, NINDB Monograph 3, Washington, D.C.: U.S. Department of Health, Education, and Welfare, 1966.

Crothers, B., and R. S. Paine, *The Natural History of Cerebral Palsy*, Cambridge, Mass.: Harvard University Press, 1959. (An authoritative medical presentation of cerebral palsy, based on a review of 1,800 cases.)

Cruickshank, W. M., ed., *Psychology of Exceptional Children and Youth*, 3rd ed., Englewood Cliffs, N.J.: Prentice-Hall, Inc., 1971.

Eisenson, J., "Perceptual Disturbances in Children with Central Nervous System Disfunctions and Implications for Language Development," *British Journal of Disorders of Communication,* **1,** 1 (1966), 21–32.

––––––, "Developmental Aphasia: A Speculative View with Therapeutic Implications," *Journal of Speech and Hearing Disorders,* **30,** 1 (February 1968), 3–13.

––––––, *Aphasia in Children,* New York: Harper & Row, Publishers, Inc., 1972. (Considers the nature, assessment, and treatment of children with congenital or developmental aphasia).

Gray, B., and B. Ryan, *A Language Program for the Non Language Child,* Champaign, Ill.: Research Press, 1973.

Kenny, T. J., and R. L. Clemmens, *Behavioral Pediatrics and Child Development,* Baltimore: The Williams & Wilkins Co., 1975.

Kleffner, F. R. *Language Disorders in Children,* New York: The Bobbs-Merrill Co., 1973

McDonald, E. T., and B. Chance, *Cerebral Palsy,* Englewood Cliffs, N.J.: Prentice-Hall, Inc., 1964.

McGinnis, M., *Aphasic Children,* Washington D.C.: Alexander Graham Bell Association for the Deaf, 1963.

Myklebust, H. R., "Childhood Aphasia: An Evolving Concept," and "Childhood Aphasia: Identification, Diagnosis, Remediation," in L. E. Travis, ed., *Handbook of Speech Pathology and Audiology,* New York: Appleton-Century-Crofts, 1971, pp. 1181–1217. (Traces the concept of childhood aphasia and differentiates it from other disorders that are associated with severe language delay. Emphasizes the underlying problems in auditory perception and verbal sequencing, and stresses the need for identifying the aphasic child early, and developing special education programs that should begin at the preschool level.)

Perkins, W. H., *Speech Pathology,* St. Louis: The C. V. Mosby Co., 1971.

Perlstein, M., *Cerebral Palsy,* National Society for Crippled Children and Adults, Chicago: December 1961. (A booklet in the *Parent Series,* in which a medical authority on cerebral palsy provides answers to questions parents might ask about their cerebral-palsied child.)

Trombly, T., "Linguistic Concepts and the Cerebral-Palsied Child," *Cerebral Palsy Journal,* **29** (1965), 7–8. (A realistic approach to the basic language needs for cerebral-palsied children.)

Van Riper, C., *Speech Correction,* 5th ed., Englewood Cliffs, N. J.: Prentice-Hall, Inc., 1972.

Wender, P., *Minimal Brain Dysfunction in Children,* New York: John Wiley & Sons, Inc., Interscience, 1971.

Westlake, H., and D. Rutherford, *Speech Therapy for the Cerebral Palsied,* Chicago: National Society for Crippled Children and Adults, 1961.

Wilson, M. I., "Children with Crippling and Health Disabilities," in L. Dunn, ed., *Exceptional Children in the Schools,* 2nd ed., New York: Holt, Rinehart and Winston, Inc., 1973.

Author Index

Subject Index